Prenatal Screening and Diagnosis

Guest Editors

ANTHONY O. ODIBO, MD, MSCE
DAVID A. KRANTZ, MA

CLINICS IN LABORATORY MEDICINE

www.labmed.theclinics.com

Consulting Editor
ALAN WELLS, MD, DMSc

September 2010 • Volume 30 • Number 3

SAUNDERS an imprint of ELSEVIER, Inc.

W.B. SAUNDERS COMPANY
A Division of Elsevier Inc.

1600 John F. Kennedy Boulevard • Suite 1800 • Philadelphia, Pennsylvania 19103-2899

http://www.theclinics.com

CLINICS IN LABORATORY MEDICINE Volume 30, Number 3
September 2010 ISSN 0272-2712, ISBN-13: 978-1-4377-2462-2

Editor: Katie Hartner

Reprints. For copies of 100 or more, of articles in this publication, please contact the Commercial Reprints Department, Elsevier Inc., 360 Park Avenue South, New York, New York 10010-1710. Tel. (212) 633-3813, Fax: (212) 462-1935, E-mail: reprints@elsevier.com.

Clinics in Laboratory Medicine (ISSN 0272-2712) is published quarterly by Elsevier Inc., 360 Park Avenue South, New York, NY 10010-1710. Months of issue are March, June, September, and December. Business and Editorial offices: 1600 John F. Kennedy Blvd., Suite 1800, Philadelphia, PA 19103-2899. Periodicals postage paid at New York, NY and additional mailing offices. Subscription prices are $220.00 per year (US individuals), $347.00 per year (US institutions), $114.00 (US students), $253.00 per year (Canadian individuals), $438.00 per year (foreign institutions), $157.00 (foreign students). Foreign air speed delivery is included in all *Clinics* subscription prices. All prices are subject to change without notice. POSTMASTER: Send address changes to *Clinics in Laboratory Medicine*, Elsevier Health Sciences Division, Subscription Customer Service, 3251 Riverport Lane, Maryland Heights, MO 63043. **Customer Service: 1-800-654-2452 (US). From outside of the US and Canada, call 1-314-447-8871. Fax: 1-314-447-8029. E-mail: journalscustomerservice-usa@elsevier.com (for print support) or journalsonlinesupport-usa@elsevier.com (for online support).**

Clinics in Laboratory Medicine is covered in *EMBASE/Exerpta Medica, MEDLINE/PubMed (Index Medicus), Cinahl, Current Contents/Clinical Medicine, BIOSIS* and *ISI/BIOMED.*

Printed and bound by CPI Group (UK) Ltd, Croydon, CR0 4YY

Transferred to Digital Print 2012

Contributors

GUEST EDITORS

ANTHONY O. ODIBO, MD, MSCE
Associate Professor, Director, Fetal Care Center, Division of Maternal Fetal Medicine and Ultrasound, Department of Obstetrics and Gynecology, Washington University Medical Center, St Louis, Missouri; Decision and Economic Analysis in Reproduction and Women's Health Group

DAVID A. KRANTZ, MA
Director of Biostatistics, Biostatistics Department, NTD Labs/PerkinElmer, Melville, New York

AUTHORS

STEPHANIE ANDRIOLE, MS, CGC
Comprehensive Genetics, New York, New York

PEDRO ARGOTI, MD
Department of Obstetrics and Gynecology, Wayne State University, Detroit, Michigan

RAY O. BAHADO-SINGH, MD, MBA
Department of Obstetrics and Gynecology, Wayne State University, Detroit, Michigan

PETER BENN, PhD, DSc
Professor, Department of Genetics and Developmental Biology, University of Connecticut Health Center, Farmington, Connecticut

ADAM F. BORGIDA, MD
Associate Professor, Prenatal Testing Center, Division of Maternal Fetal Medicine, Department of Obstetrics and Gynecology, University of Connecticut School of Medicine, Hartford Hospital, Hartford, Connecticut

ALISON G. CAHILL, MD, MSCI
Assistant Professor, Department of Obstetrics and Gynecology, Washington University School of Medicine, St Louis, Missouri

WINSTON A. CAMPBELL, MD
Professor, Obstetrics and Gynecology; PHS Professor, Maternal-Fetal Medicine; Division Director and Clinical Chief, Division of Maternal-Fetal Medicine, Department of Obstetrics and Gynecology, University of Connecticut Health Center-School of Medicine-John Dempsey Hospital, Farmington, Connecticut

JEANINE F. CARBONE, MD
Clinical fellow of Maternal-Fetal Medicine, Division of Maternal-Fetal Medicine, Department of Obstetrics and Gynecology, Washington University School of Medicine, St Louis, Missouri

ANGELINA CARTIN
Division of Maternal-Fetal Medicine, Department of Obstetrics and Gynecology, Maine Medical Center, Portland, Maine

AARON B. CAUGHEY, MD, MPP, MPH, PhD
Professor and Chair, Department of Obstetrics & Gynecology, Oregon Health & Science University, Portland, Oregon; Decision and Economic Analysis in Reproduction and Women's Health Group

STEPHEN T. CHASEN, MD
Associate Professor, Department of Obstetrics and Gynecology, Weill Medical College of Cornell University, New York, New York

AMBER R. COOPER, MD, MSCI
Assistant Professor, Division of Reproductive Endocrinology and Infertility, Barnes-Jewish Hospital, Washington University School of Medicine, St Louis, Missouri

HOWARD CUCKLE, MSc, DPhil
Professor, Department of Obstetrics and Gynecology, Columbia University Medical Center, New York, New York

JAMES F.X. EGAN, MD
Professor and Chairman of Department of Obstetrics and Gynecology, University of Connecticut Health Center, Farmington, Connecticut

MARK I. EVANS, MD
Fetal Medicine Foundation of America; Comprehensive Genetics; Professor of Obstetrics and Gynecology, Mount Sinai School of Medicine, New York, New York

DEBORAH M. FELDMAN, MD
Assistant Professor, Prenatal Testing Center, Division of Maternal Fetal Medicine, Department of Obstetrics and Gynecology, University of Connecticut School of Medicine, Hartford Hospital, Hartford, Connecticut

KATHERINE R. GOETZINGER, MD
Fellow in Maternal Fetal Medicine, Department of Obstetrics and Gynecology, Washington University School of Medicine, St Louis, Missouri

LAURA GOETZL, MD, MPH
Associate Professor, Division of Maternal Fetal Medicine, Department of Obstetrics and Gynecology, Medical University of South Carolina, Charleston, South Carolina

TERRENCE W. HALLAHAN, PhD
Laboratory Directory/Research Director, Biostatistics Department, NTD Labs/PerkinElmer, Melville, New York

EMILY S. JUNGHEIM, MD, MSCI
Assistant Professor, Division of Reproductive Endocrinology and Infertility, Barnes-Jewish Hospital, Washington University School of Medicine, St Louis, Missouri

ANJALI J. KAIMAL, MD, MAS
Department of Obstetrics and Gynecology, Massachusetts General Hospital, Harvard Medical School, Boston, Massachusetts; Decision and Economic Analysis in Reproduction and Women's Health Group

MICHAEL KILPATRICK, PhD
Vice President of Biology, Ikonisys Inc, New Haven, Connecticut

DAVID A. KRANTZ, MA
Director of Biostatistics, Biostatistics Department, NTD Labs/PerkinElmer, Melville, New York

K. NICOLAIDES, MD
Professor, King's College School of Medicine and Dentistry, Harris Birthright Centre; Fetal Medicine Foundation, London, United Kingdom

MARY E. NORTON, MD
Regional Director, Perinatal Genetic Services, The Permanente Medical Group, Kaiser Permanente, Northern California, Oakland; Clinical Professor of Obstetrics, Gynecology and Reproductive Sciences, University of California, San Francisco, California

ANTHONY O. ODIBO, MD, MSCE
Associate Professor, Director, Fetal Care Center, Division of Maternal Fetal Medicine and Ultrasound, Department of Obstetrics and Gynecology, Washington University, St Louis, Missouri; Decision and Economic Analysis in Reproduction and Women's Health Group

EUGENE PERGAMENT, MD, PhD, FACMG
Northwestern Reproductive Genetics, Inc, Chicago, Illinois

MICHAEL G. PINETTE, MD
Division of Maternal-Fetal Medicine, Department of Obstetrics and Gynecology, Maine Medical Center, Portland, Maine

ROXANE RAMPERSAD, MD
Assistant Professor of Obstetrics and Gynecology, Division of Maternal-Fetal Medicine, Department of Obstetrics and Gynecology, Washington University School of Medicine, St Louis, Missouri

ALIREZA A. SHAMSHIRSAZ, MD
Maternal-Fetal Medicine Fellow, Department of Obstetrics and Gynecology, Division of Maternal-Fetal Medicine, University of Connecticut Health Center, Farmington, Connecticut

JOHN E. SHERWIN, PhD
Director of Lab Operations, Biostatistics Department, PerkinElmer, Melville, New York

J. SONEK, MD, RDMS
Clinical Professor, Wright State University; Fetal Medicine Foundation/USA, Dayton, Ohio

DIANE TIMMS, DO
Instructor, Division of Maternal Fetal Medicine, Department of Obstetrics and Gynecology, University of Connecticut Health Center School of Medicine, John Dempsey Hospital, Farmington, Connecticut

METHODIUS G. TUULI, MD, MPH
Clinical Fellow, Division of Maternal-Fetal Medicine and Ultrasound, Department of Obstetrics and Gynecology, Washington University School of Medicine, St Louis, Missouri

JOSEPH R. WAX, MD
Division of Maternal-Fetal Medicine, Department of Obstetrics and Gynecology, Maine Medical Center, Portland, Maine

Contents

has also increased. There are several challenges related to first trimester screening; foremost among them is the need to distinguish between screening and diagnosis. Additional challenges include the need to discuss not only Down syndrome but cardiac defects, developmental/genetic syndromes, adverse pregnancy outcomes, and preeclampsia. In the future, counseling will involve specific risk assessment for a broad range of chromosome abnormalities. This article provides a framework for providing genetic counseling to prospective parents undergoing first trimester screening. However, the counseling session has to be individualized based on the counselor's approach and unique issues and concerns related to the pregnancy.

Protocols that include first trimester screening for fetal chromosome abnormalities have become standard of care throughout the United States. Earlier screening allows for first trimester diagnostic testing in cases found to be at increased risk. However, first trimester screening requires coordination of the nuchal translucency ultrasound screening (NT) and biochemical screening, during early, specific, narrow, but slightly different gestational age ranges. Instant results can often be provided at the time of the NT ultrasound if preceded by the programs that perform the biochemical analyses; this optimizes the benefits of the first trimester approach while improving efficiency and communication with the patient. This article discusses the benefits and logistics of such an approach.

The first trimester (11–13 +6 weeks) ultrasound examination is useful for several reasons: determination of an accurate date of confinement, diagnostic purposes, and screening for fetal defects. Nuchal translucency measurement combined with maternal serum markers (free b-human chorionic gonadotropin and pregnancy-associated plasma protein A) is the mainstay of first-trimester screening for chromosomal defects. However, over the past decade additional ultrasound markers have been developed that improve the performance of this type of screening. The novel markers include evaluation of the nasal bone, fronto-maxillary angle measurement, and Doppler evaluations of the blood flow across the tricuspid valve and in the ductus venosus.

Nuchal translucency is the single most discriminatory marker for screening Down syndrome. When this marker is combined with concurrent maternal serum markers, the model-predicted performance is greater than for all second-trimester serum-only combinations. However, quality results for the marker are more difficult to achieve than for serum markers. Monitoring of images and proper training are essential, but the ongoing use of epidemiologic indicators is the only way to assure quality. The positive rate in the screened population may indicate a problem, but the average multiple of the normal median values and the standard deviation of the logarithm (base 10) of these values are the key indicators for the markers. If there is a 10% shift in the median or a 0.02 change in the standard deviation, the results will be compromised.

quantified. Several studies have examined the cost-effectiveness of screening for Down syndrome (DS). Given the current test characteristics, screening for DS is cost-effective across a wide variety of clinical situations. In fact, contingent screening is potentially a dominant strategy (costs less and leads to better outcomes). Understanding the methodology and salient issues of cost-effectiveness analysis is critical for researchers, editors, and clinicians to accurately interpret results of the growing body of cost-effectiveness studies in prenatal diagnosis.

age of 35 years or older as a risk factor to offer patients the option for prenatal diagnosis. The actual diagnosis used an invasive procedure (amniocentesis) to obtain fetal cells for processing to determine fetal karyotype. This had a potential risk for miscarriage. The development of noninvasive prenatal screening to better identify pregnant patients at high risk for Down syndrome improved the ability to detect cases of aneuploidy and limit amniocentesis to only patients considered at high risk. This approach has a higher detection rate and a lower procedure-related rate of fetal loss than use of maternal age of 35 years or older alone. This article presents an overview of how prenatal diagnosis has evolved and then focuses on the current status of using ultrasound to evaluate patients considered to be screen-positive for Down syndrome based on first-trimester screening (10–14 weeks) or second-trimester (15–22 weeks) maternal serum analyte screening.

Preterm birth is the leading cause of perinatal morbidity and mortality in developed nations. The heterogeneous causes of spontaneous preterm birth make prediction and prevention difficult. Recently developed biochemical and biophysical tests add significantly to clinicians' ability to evaluate and treat women at risk for spontaneous preterm birth. The primary importance of transvaginal cervical sonography and cervicovaginal fetal fibronectin lies in the high negative predictive values of the tests for reducing preterm delivery risk. Cervical length may be useful in identifying women who are candidates for cervical cerclage or progesterone therapy for preterm birth prevention. Together, cervical length and fibronectin can be used in the triaging of women symptomatic for preterm labor.

Several infections in adults warrant special consideration in pregnant women given the potential fetal consequences. Among these are toxoplasmosis, parvovirus B19, and cytomegalovirus. These infections have an important effect on the developing fetus depending on the timing of infection. This article reviews the modes of transmission as well as maternal and neonatal effects of each of these infections. In addition, recommended testing, fetal surveillance, and treatment where indicated are outlined.

Maternal serum screening for congenital anomalies began over 30 years ago with the advent of alpha-fetoprotein (AFP) screening for open neural tube defects. It was from these screening programs that the more complex multiple marker Down syndrome screening programs developed. However, today open neural tube defect screening remains a relatively simple

THE CLINICS ARE NOW AVAILABLE ONLINE!

Access your subscription at:
www.theclinics.com

Preface
Prenatal Screening
and Diagnosis

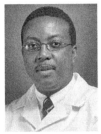 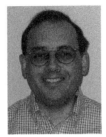

Anthony O. Odibo, MD, MSCE   David A. Krantz, MA
Guest Editors

It has been an honor to serve as guest editors for this special edition of *Clinics in Laboratory Medicine*, entitled Prenatal Screening and Diagnosis. The last issue devoted to prenatal testing was in June 2003. Since that time, a lot of development has occurred in the arena of prenatal testing, particularly with the development of new screening paradigms for Down syndrome. This edition may seem to have more articles dedicated to aneuploidy screening compared with prior editions. The reason for this is the proliferation of new screening strategies in the past 5 years and the struggle among clinicians to adopt what is best for their population.

As editors, we have made an attempt to avoid overlap in the articles submitted. Some degree of overlap is, however, inevitable in the articles devoted to aneuploidy screening. Dr Bahado-Singh begins by giving an overview of first-trimester screening. Others, such as Dr Egan and colleagues, review the impact of first-trimester screening on second-trimester screening for aneuploidy, whereas Campbell and colleagues provide an update on genetic sonogram. Drs Caughey and Odibo then review the economic considerations of the various aneuploidy screening paradigms. A review of aneuploidy screening would not be complete without an article on neural tube defects screening from which aneuploidy screening was derived. Such an article is provided by Krantz and colleagues.

Among the articles on aneuploidy, several relate to first-trimester screening with free β–human chorionic gonadotropin, pregnancy-associated plasma protein A, and nuchal translucency. Drs Sonek and Nicolaides focus on the addition of new ultrasound markers in the first trimester to improve screening performance. Although many studies have reported detection rates of 90% with first-trimester screening, Dr Cuckle focuses on the important issue of maintaining quality control of nuchal translucency measurements to maintain these high detection rates when nuchal translucency assessment is pushed into widespread clinical practice. Dr Chasen's article discusses the clinical implications of first-trimester screening, including the impact of early screening on the rate of invasive prenatal diagnosis, the gestational age of prenatal diagnosis and termination, as well as the side benefit of earlier prenatal

Clin Lab Med 30 (2010) xv–xvi
doi:10.1016/j.cll.2010.04.017
0272-2712/10/$ – see front matter © 2010 Elsevier Inc. All rights reserved.

diagnosis of certain major structural abnormalities. Dr Norton's article reviews the benefits of an instant results approach to first-trimester screening in which biochemistry is performed before ultrasound and, therefore, the final risk result is available at the conclusion of the ultrasound examination. Such an approach can improve screening performance in addition to the added clinical benefit of being able to communicate with patients at the conclusion of an ultrasound examination. Dr Pergament writes about the important role of genetic counseling in first-trimester screening given the general population's understanding of risk. Dr Goetzl's article discusses the adverse implications of extreme first-trimester aneuploidy markers when aneuploidy has been ruled out.

Drs Evans and Andiole discuss multiple pregnancy, which has a lower performance of serum screening protocols as compared with singleton pregnancies. The complexity of the invasive diagnostic procedures and the risk of loss of an unaffected twin due to the sequelae of the invasive procedures.

Although screening for cystic fibrosis is now a routine part of prenatal care, Drs Cahill and Goetzinger discuss the challenging aspects of offering such screening, especially as it relates to certain racial groups and populations. Another vexing area in prenatal testing is that of screening for thrombophilias, and Rampersad and Carbone provide a comprehensive review of the subject. Another medical disorder that has received a lot of screening attention is preeclampsia. Most of the focus is now on early detection and the first trimester provides a window for early screening. Tuuli and Odibo cover this area.

The use of ultrasound and biochemical methods to screen for preterm birth is now mainstream in prenatal care. Wax and colleagues performed a detailed review of the literature and provide an evidence-based summary of the subject. This is followed by a detailed review of the role of preimplantation genetic diagnosis by Jungheim and Cooper.

There has been a lot published in recent years about screening and treating infectious diseases, such as cytomegalovirus, during pregnancy. Borgida and colleagues performed a detailed review of this subject with particular emphasis on toxoplasmosis and cytomegalovirus.

Dr Evans provides an article on noninvasive prenatal diagnosis, a technology with huge potential. Unfortunately, the large number of technical approaches that have been used is testimony to the fact that none of them has been particularly successful.

Anthony O. Odibo, MD, MSCE
Division of Maternal Fetal Medicine and Ultrasound
Department of Obstetrics and Gynecology
Fetal Care Center
Washington University Medical Center
660 South Euclid
St Louis, MO 63110, USA

Decision and Economic Analysis in Reproduction
and Women's Health Group, USA

David A. Krantz, MA
Biostatistics Department
NTD Labs/PerkinElmer
80 Ruland Road
Melville, NY 11747, USA

E-mail addresses:
odiboa@wudosis.wustl.edu (A.O. Odibo)
david.krantz@perkinelmer.com (D.A. Krantz)

Preimplantation Genetic Testing: Indications and Controversies

Amber R. Cooper, MD, MSCI*, Emily S. Jungheim, MD, MSCI

KEYWORDS

- Preimplantation genetic testing
- Preimplantation genetic diagnosis
- Preimplantation genetic screening • Embryo research
- Embryo biopsy • In vitro fertilization

Clinically applicable preimplantation genetic testing was first brought to fruition in 1990, when it was announced that 2 women at risk for transmitting recessive X-linked diseases were pregnant with female fetuses as the result of in vitro fertilization (IVF) followed by embryo biopsy and sexing by polymerase chain reaction (PCR) for the Y chromosome.[1] Since then, use of preimplantation genetic diagnosis (PGD) has expanded to prevent the birth of children affected by several genetically lethal diseases.[2] There is no doubt that preimplantation genetic testing has helped to deliver remarkable gifts to many people; however, its use and application is not without risks or controversy. Preimplantation genetic testing techniques are also used clinically to prevent transmission of genes associated with late-onset diseases and increased, but not absolute, risk of disease. In addition, preimplantation genetic aneuploidy screening of embryos has been advocated as an adjunct to IVF for women of advanced reproductive age and women with recurrent pregnancy loss, although this application has failed to improve live birth rates among these women. Perhaps more contentious, preimplantation genetic testing is used to sex embryos for family balancing and to select for specific genetic traits.[2–5] With ever-increasing knowledge of the human genome and stem cell biology, the full potential of preimplantation genetic testing has yet to be realized. In this review the authors discuss the techniques and clinical application of PGD and the debate surrounding its associated uncertainty and expanded use.

Division of Reproductive Endocrinology and Infertility, Barnes-Jewish Hospital, Washington University School of Medicine, 4444 Forest Park Parkway, Suite 3100, St Louis, MO 63108, USA
* Corresponding author.
E-mail address: coopera@wustl.edu

Clin Lab Med 30 (2010) 519–531
doi:10.1016/j.cll.2010.04.008
0272-2712/10/$ – see front matter © 2010 Elsevier Inc. All rights reserved.

labmed.theclinics.com

HISTORY AND DEFINITION

In 1986, a group of experts met to discuss the feasibility of prenatal testing in the human preimplantation period to avoid the need for selective abortion associated with other antenatal screening techniques such as chorionic villus sampling (CVS) and amniocentesis.[6] These experts determined that 2 groups of people would be candidates for the screening: (1) among older mothers, those with low risk of having a child affected by sporadic genetic disorders like aneuploidy and (2) those at persistent high risk of having a child with a genetic disease. The experts concluded that the second group of patients was most likely to benefit from PGD, and they predicted that "pre-implantation genetic screening would not be widely applied to all IVF patients, but only in order to detect the specific disease or diseases for which a particular couple is at high risk".[6] Shortly after this meeting, in 1988, it was reported that the expression of the human genome occurs between the 4- and 8-cell stage of preimplantation development,[7] and in 1990, Handyside and colleagues[1] announced the pregnancies of 2 women who conceived female twins after transfer of IVF-created embryos that were biopsied and sexed by PCR for the Y chromosome. This breakthrough initiated the clinical application of preimplantation genetic testing.

In the first reported cases of preimplantation genetic testing, 5 women at risk for transmitting recessive X-linked diseases underwent ovarian stimulation with exogenous gonadotropins; oocyte retrieval was performed and the oocytes were fertilized in vitro. On day 3 of embryo culture, 1 to 2 cells were aspirated from the embryos after zona pellucida thinning and Y-chromosome–specific DNA from the biopsied cells was amplified by PCR, a technique that had only recently been developed. Day 3 embryos identified as female were transferred back, and 2 of the women became pregnant with twins. Sex of these fetuses was confirmed at 10 weeks by CVS. This application of preimplantation prenatal testing in which a specific genetic disease is being screened for is referred to officially as PGD. PGD is defined in the International Committee Monitoring Assisted Reproductive Technologies (ICMART) and the World Health Organization (WHO) revised glossary of Assisted Reproductive Technologies terminology as the "analysis of polar bodies, blastomeres, or trophectoderm from oocytes, zygotes, or embryos for the detection of specific genetic, structural, and/or chromosomal alterations."[8]

The application of preimplantation genetic testing in IVF for improving IVF success rates or decreasing the chance of offspring with sporadic genetic disorders is referred to as preimplantation genetic screening (PGS). PGS is defined in the ICMART/WHO glossary as the "analysis of polar bodies, blastomeres, or trophectoderm from oocytes, zygotes, or embryos for the detection of aneuploidy, mutation, and/or DNA rearrangement."[8] When experts convened in 1986, they predicted PGS as a means to increase live birth rates among women of advanced maternal age, and although used broadly, this application has yet to prove its ability to improve live birth rates in women undergoing IVF.[6] However, contrary to the experts' predictions in 1986, PGD and PGS are nowadays being offered to many patients in several settings.

INDICATIONS FOR PGD

The frequency of use and the indications for PGD in the United States and worldwide is increasing. In a 2006 survey, it was reported that 74% of IVF centers in the United States provided PGD to patients, and at least 5% of IVF cycles in 2005 included PGD for various reasons.[9] Although some researchers consider PGD to be an early type of prenatal diagnostic testing performed on the embryo in vitro before transfer to the uterus, prospective parents often choose PGD to avoid traditional prenatal testing (CVS or amniocentesis) and subsequent termination of an affected fetus. In its original applications PGD was primarily used for mendelian disorders. Mendelian disorders are single-gene defects often defined by describing their basic pedigree patterns: autosomal dominant, autosomal recessive, X-linked (recessive or dominant), and Y-linked (rare). These disorders require a particular genotype at a locus for expression of a character.[10] The widely used Online Mendelian Inheritance in Man (http://www.ncbi.nlm.nih.gov/omim/) is an online database created to describe the genes and phenotypes associated with all known mendelian disorders. Over the last 2 decades, the use of PGD in single-gene disorders has had tremendous expansion. Furthermore, more recently PGD has shown promise in polygenic disorders, sometimes referred to as nonmendelian, in which phenotypes or characters are dependent on multiple loci. In these conditions pedigrees do not follow traditional monogenetic heritability. More complicated is that often in nonmendelian disorders variability outside the nuclear genetic locus has an etiologic or influential role on the phenotype, such as epigenetic modifications, mitochondrial abnormalities (and abnormalities in mitochondrial DNA [mtDNA]), posttranslational modifications, and the recognized contributions from the environment.

Common mendelian disorders that require PGD in many centers include cystic fibrosis, β-thalassemia, sickle cell disease, myotonic dystrophy, Huntington disease, fragile X syndrome, and spinal muscular atrophy.[2,11–13] More recently, a portion of PGD cases include HLA typing in addition to monogenic testing for a particular condition, which aids treatment strategies for a living sibling or other relative. One example of this is with Fanconi anemia.[14,15] As discussed earlier, some of the first uses of PGD involved conditions with X-linked inheritance and amplification of a sequence on the Y chromosome to identify females who were presumably healthy for transfer.[1,13] Soon after, monogenic disorders such as cystic fibrosis were proposed as the most common indications for PGD as long as a probe containing the causative mutation could be created and used to amplify the DNA sequence in the genome of the embryonic cell. More than 200 single-gene disorders have been reportedly identified with PGD.[13] More ethically debated is the increasing use of PGD for single-gene disorders that either have late adult onset or undefined risk and penetrance profiles. Some examples of these disorders include Huntington disease, breast cancer caused by mutations (in the breast cancer gene [BRCA1] and BRCA2), and cancers caused by other mutations.

Nonmendelian disorders are much more complex scientifically and ethically. Many common multifactorial disorders such as congenital heart disease, cleft palate and lip, and some behavioral disorders are not conducive to PGD at present because the polygenic, epigenetic, and environmental contributions to such a phenotype are not completely understood. One of the few situations in which PGD may be helpful for nonmendelian or polygenic disorders is when there is unequal gender incidence.[16] For example, disorders such as breast cancer, rheumatoid arthritis, and multiple sclerosis have a significantly increased incidence in female offspring. On the other hand, a male sibling born to a family with an autistic child is much more likely to have autism than a female sibling.[17] In these cases, PGD may be utilized simply for sex selection of embryos to diminish the risk to offspring. Sex selection, even for medical indications, is ethically debatable and is likely to undergo continuous scrutiny.[18]

Another indication for PGD is in chromosomal disorders. Although numerical and structural chromosomal abnormalities are possible findings in spontaneous miscarriages and affected fetuses, overwhelmingly most are numerical.[19] Numerical chromosomal abnormalities include findings such as polyploidy, monosomy, and trisomies.

Although structural alterations cause a small number of miscarriages, they constitute the majority of PGD done for chromosomal abnormalities.[2] Structural alterations include translocations, inversions, deletions, and other rearrangements in the chromosomes. A parent may harbor an unrecognized balanced translocation that during segregation in gametogenesis and subsequent fertilization becomes an unbalanced abnormality in the offspring.

Finally, mitochondrial disorders are another growing indication for PGD, although more research in this area is needed. Several mitochondrial abnormalities are actually caused by mutations in the nuclear DNA, and thus a PGD process similar to that with a single-gene disorder can be carried out. When mitochondrial diseases are a result of a mutation in mtDNA, the phenotype or affected tissues do not become recognizable until the number of mutated mitochondria reaches an intolerable load within the cell. Many cells in identified mitochondrial diseases have heteroplasmy because a certain percentage of normal and mutated mitochondria exist within the same cell. Therefore, an individual would not be affected unless a critical threshold of mutated mitochondria is reached. Often, because of the primarily maternal inheritance of mtDNA from the ooplasm, the mother is a carrier of an unknown small percentage of mutated mtDNA that is propagated and expanded in her offspring. Such enhancement of the proportion of mutated mtDNA in the embryo or fetus is explained partially by the bottleneck theory, in which at some point in early oogenesis the number of mitochondria per cell is rapidly depleted to very few and subsequently is rapidly expanded in the fetus.[20–24] Once a woman is identified as having an increased risk of transmitting mutated mitochondria to her offspring, the only options to reduce this risk are to take a chance at spontaneous conception, use donor oocytes, try PGD if amenable to that condition, or try a nuclear transfer from the maternal oocyte into enucleated donor oocytes.[22,25] The potential to try to determine the ratio of mutated to normal mtDNA in an embryonic cell has led researchers to try to apply PGD to mitochondrial disorders caused by mutations in mtDNA. This application may not remove the risk of having an affected child but instead may dramatically lower it. One of the primary conditions that have shown promise in the techniques utilized is the more severe Leigh syndrome or neurogenic muscle weakness, ataxia, and retinitis pigmentosa, also called NARP, which results from a slightly lower mutation load.[5,26,27] Although certain mitochondrial disorders are showing increasing promise for PGD techniques, these are relatively new techniques that require continued research and follow-up.

TECHNIQUES

PGD requires multiple steps and manipulations of the gametes and embryos to select unaffected embryos for transfer and subsequent potential pregnancy. First, PGD requires use of IVF. An IVF procedure is necessary to have access to the oocytes and create multiple embryos for testing. An IVF cycle commences with controlled ovarian hyperstimulation using injectable gonadotropin and other medications in the mother. A transvaginal needle aspiration of multiple ovarian follicles is then performed to retrieve the oocytes when they are appropriately developed. The oocytes are then inseminated in vitro, and the resulting embryos are followed in culture for several days if viability continues. Fertilization of the oocytes can occur within hours of oocyte retrieval by 1 of 2 mechanisms: (1) conventional insemination, in which several hundred thousand sperm are placed around the oocyte and the 2 gametes are allowed to spontaneously fertilize, or (2) intracytoplasmic sperm injection (ICSI), in which 1 sperm is mechanically inserted into the oocyte. For most PGD cases, amplification of a very small amount of DNA (using PCR) is required to analyze and identify a particular genetic mutation.

Any contamination of DNA from either an abundance of additional sperm or cells embedded in the zona pellucida or maternal cells around the oocyte (cumulus or granulosa cells) can cause the PGD techniques to fail or produce erroneous results. Thus, stripping the oocyte of surrounding cells and ICSI is required for most PGD cases.

Once IVF has been performed, a biopsy is required to remove cells for preimplantation genetic testing. The DNA is obtained from either the first and/or second polar bodies given off from the oocyte or the embryonic blastomeres. In all cases the zona pellucida has to be breached and the cell or cells are extracted. The biopsy can actually be done at 1 of the 3 primary time points: (1) biopsy of the first and/or second polar body pre- or postfertilization depending on the indication for PGD (to examine the oocyte genotype), (2) biopsy of the cleavage-cell embryo (day 3 after fertilization, a 4–8-cell embryo) to remove 1 or 2 cells for testing, or (3) biopsy of the blastocyst embryo (formed on days 5–6 after fertilization, it is an embryo with an inner cell mass and a blastocele cavity) to remove trophectoderm cells. Polar body biopsy may be most useful for fluorescence in situ hybridization (FISH) technique utilized in aneuploidy testing, assuming that most cases result from abnormal divisions in the oocyte during meiosis.[28–30] Yet, most investigators still recommend sequential biopsy and testing of both polar bodies because of the significant chance for errors in meiosis I and II.[31,32] Polar body biopsy can be used for maternally inherited single-gene disorders but requires more complex techniques and often also the sequential biopsies of both polar bodies.[33,34] Most PGD cases use embryo biopsy techniques at either the cleavage or the blastocyst stage. Although occasionally debated, that removal of more than 1 cell in a cleavage (4–8 cells) embryo could have detrimental results on its development and viability, even though without a second cell to analyze, the proportion of absent, inconclusive, or incorrect results could increase.[35–38] Blastocyst-stage biopsy may be favored because of a significantly larger number of cells that can safely be removed, but this technique also limits the time available for genetic testing because of the need for transfer to the uterus that day or the next day (days 5–6 after fertilization). Furthermore, significantly fewer embryos survive in vitro to reach the blastocyst stage, producing fewer embryos that are available for biopsy at this time. On the other hand, one may argue that those that do survive to the blastocyst stage may be more likely to produce a live birth, the ultimate aim of the patients who desire PGD.[39] To allow for proper testing, the embryos may need to be frozen after biopsy and then transferred back in a separate frozen embryo transfer cycle weeks to months later.

GENOMIC TESTING

Most IVF centers in the United States that provide PGD continue to recommend subsequent prenatal testing (CVS or amniocentesis) to confirm the results because of the small frequency of errors that could occur during PGD.[9,40] Furthermore, genetic counseling of prospective parents before the start of a PGD cycle is essential because of the complexity of the multistep procedures, cost, alternatives, interpretation of testing, technical limitations, and outcomes.[40] Like much of technology, no single technique for PGD is perfect and they all carry a risk for misdiagnosis, an outcome that is often unacceptable for some couples.[41] Thus, technology is continually making strides for improved diagnostic accuracy while ensuring rapid and comprehensible results.

The 2 most utilized techniques for cellular analysis in PGD cycles at present are FISH and PCR.[15,42,43] FISH is a technique in which fluorescent-labeled DNA probes are used to bind to specific regions of a chromosome to identify a particular section or presence of a chromosome. FISH is primarily used to test for chromosomal abnormalities such as aneuploidy or translocations, and is also used for sex selection for X-linked disorders instead of PCR. The number of probes used in FISH in each round of hybridization is limited in PGD, which limits the expansion of testing of all 23 chromosome pairs; yet, FISH is technically easier than PCR with much less concern for contamination from other DNA material. The second widely used genetic testing mechanism, PCR, involves amplification of specific DNA fragments to produce enough material for subsequent analysis. Producing a large enough quantity of DNA from a single cell for mutation analyses is one of the main challenges with PCR. Improvements in PCR techniques have evolved over the last 2 decades to reduce the chances of erroneous results. The inclusion of additional processes such as nested PCR, fluorescent PCR, genetic haplotyping, whole-genome amplification, array comparative genomic hybridization (CGH), and multiplex PCR (additional polymorphic linked markers are also amplified with the region of interest to assure correct allele amplification) have improved accuracy.[15,28,42–52] Often a combination of these techniques is used.

DIAGNOSTIC ACCURACY

There are numerous decisions that must be made by a couple as they progress through an entire cycle of PGD. During the process, many complicated discussions ensue when an erroneous, inconsistent, or incomplete result is encountered. Precision in handling, manipulation, biopsy, and observation of the gametes and embryos is critical for reducing untoward outcomes. Numerous causes of misdiagnosis have been reported in the literature.[15,45] The most commonly discussed adverse outcomes are thought to be caused by human error, allele drop-out (ADO), contamination from other (usually maternal or paternal) DNA, and mosaicism. Human and/or laboratory error can occur at every step along the way, and laboratory personnel have an obligation to follow stringent quality-control mechanisms throughout the process. Furthermore, training not only in the laboratory techniques but also in the interpretation and delivery of reports and results is crucial. As the technology used in PGD becomes more complicated, interpretation of the results is more challenging and is often not as black and white as it may seem. Couples may be faced with the decision of whether or not to transfer an embryo based on a calculated estimate of risk, incomplete results, or limited to no information on the day of planned transfer rather than confirmation of a normal embryo. In addition, it is difficult to perform multiple testing mechanisms on a single embryonic cell. Just because an embryo may be negative for a particular single-gene mutation, an otherwise normal embryo void of other chromosomal or epigenetic abnormalities is not ensured. Thus, there is more recent movement toward more complex diagnostic procedures, such as microarray CGH, which would allow for broadened specific and generalized genomic screening in an embryonic blastomere, an application that shows technical promise yet remains quite complex and in its early stages.[13,51,53–57] It is vital that such information and potential outcomes be delivered to the patient pre- and postprocedurally.

ADO is a commonly cited cause of misdiagnosis, especially with PCR.[15,45] Any time one deals with a small amount of genetic material, especially from a single cell, there is a chance that 1 of the 2 alleles would fail to hybridize to the probe and not be amplified or detected. There is continuing debate about whether removing 2 cells at the cleavage stage could improve the diagnostic accuracy in such a situation. The improvements in PCR techniques, as discussed in the previous section, show more promise in their abilities to detect ADO and improve optimal results. Probe error can also occur with FISH procedures but is less common.

Contamination is another problem that must always be considered. The majority of PGD cycles use ICSI to remove the 2 most common DNA contaminant sources in conventional insemination: cumulus cells around the oocyte and remaining sperm surrounding the oocyte. This concept is particularly true with PCR because even a small amount of contaminant DNA can be dramatically amplified, making the results difficult to interpret or erroneously reported. On the other hand, contamination is still possible with FISH. For example, an additional X chromosome may be detected, due to the presence of maternal cumulus cell, in the process of gender selection for a particular monogenic disorder more prevalent in a certain gender, leading to the transfer of an embryo of a gender other than what was expected. Contamination can also occur as "carry-over" from either an operator or equipment used on a previous PGD case.[45]

Finally, mosaicism is likely always to be a factor that affects diagnostic accuracy in PGD cases. Germline and embryonic mosaicism can occur.[42] Inherent in any PGD case, removal of one or a few blastomeres from the embryo assumes that those cells represent the DNA make-up of the embryo and are identical to the cells that remain after biopsy. Yet, it is known that cells begin to differentiate into the inner cell mass and trophectoderm early in development. It is possible that the cells in the trophectoderm may not represent the cells in the inner cell mass, which is considered the developing fetus. Furthermore, the ratio of normal to abnormal cells within the embryo itself could vary and alter the ultimate phenotype. Also, there is the potential for an oocyte or an embryo to self-correct any chromosomal abnormality, a process called aneuploidy rescue in meiosis II or trisomy rescue in embryonic mitotic divisions.[31] Such suggestions only complicate testing protocols surrounding PGD and may ultimately lead to more biopsy requirements for confirmatory testing.

CONTROVERSIES
Controversies of Antenatal Testing

With advancing genetic technology, new social and ethical dilemmas constantly arise as applications of PGD and PGS and other prenatal genetic tests expand. Some questions include: (1) Should treatable diseases be considered for testing? (2) Should adult-onset diseases be considered for screening? (3) Is it all right to apply these techniques to screen for genetically linked traits associated with disease or even for nonmedical indications like fetal gender? And (4) if testing of embryos or fetuses is performed, should this information be shared with other family members who may share genetic risks? Also, as discussed earlier, misdiagnosis is possible with PGD and PGS, and diagnostic confirmation with CVS or amniocentesis is recommended, but these confirmatory procedures are not without their own associated risks.

Controversies Specific to Preimplantation Genetic Testing

For many people at risk for transmitting genetic disease, proceeding with PGD and PGS may be more palatable than prenatal diagnostic techniques like CVS or amniocentesis because PGD and PGS avoid the need for consideration of pregnancy termination. Because of this feature of PGD and PGS, along with the expanding knowledge of the human genome, some investigators have raised the concern that "potentially controversial genetic manipulations may be available" including selection for optimization of characteristics that may be considered desirable, such as intelligence or longevity.[58] Other investigators have argued that these possibilities are reasonable, allowing for procreative beneficence and setting a child up for the best possible life.[59] On the other hand, the definition of the best possible life is debatable because characteristics that are considered to be disease by some may be desirable to others. An example of this is genetically inherited deafness: some individuals have used PGD to prevent having a child with the disorder, whereas some individuals within deaf communities would consider options to increase their chances of having a deaf child.[3]

As discussed earlier, another issue that separates PGS and PGD from other antenatal diagnostic screening techniques is that PGS and PGD require the use of IVF. In standard IVF protocols, embryos in excess of what is needed for procreative needs are often created. With this excess, patients must decide on (1) which embryos to put back and (2) what to do with those embryos that they do not want to use for procreative purposes. When choosing the embryos to transfer after IVF with PGS and PGD, issues that clinicians need to address with patients include the potential inaccuracy of the PGS and PGD results, whether embryos carrying recessively inherited mutations or sex-linked disease are reasonable for transfer, and what other genetic information regarding the embryos should be revealed. It has been said that PGS/PGD should be used not as "a program of eugenics, to try and wipe out genetic disease," but rather to prevent a disease, meaning that embryos that are merely carriers of disease should be used for transfer.[60(p1544)] However, there are variations among clinicians as to how much patient autonomy they would allow in testing embryos.[61]

In addition to deciding which embryos to replace, patients must also decide what to do with embryos created in excess of what they need for their reproductive use. Some patients struggle with this decision.[62] Traditional options that have existed for patients with excess embryos after IVF/ICSI have included: (1) cryopreservation for future reproductive use, (2) discarding excess embryos, (3) donating excess embryos to research, or (4) donating embryos to other couples for reproductive uses. Some couples opt to fertilize only a few oocytes to reduce the chances of having excess embryos; however, with PGD and PGS, excess embryos are desirable to increase the chances that good-quality embryos with the desired genetic make-up are available for transfer. Alternatively, polar body biopsy of the oocyte could provide information regarding the potential maternal genetic contribution before fertilization. However, this technique is not well established and does not provide any paternal or postfertilization information.

Although there is legitimate concern that PGS/PGD could be used as a tool for eugenics, preimplantation aneuploidy screening is by and large the most widely practiced form of preimplantation genetic testing today,[2] and its use also raises concerns. Present techniques for preimplantation aneuploidy screening have not been shown to improve live birth rates after IVF,[63–65] and there is growing concern that newer genetic tests are being offered clinically without studies to support their utility.[66] Some researchers have argued that these newer techniques are more accurate, whereas other investigators have argued that clinicians are motivated by financial gain in offering these tests.[60] It may be that in time newer techniques may prove useful. However, neither PGS nor PGD guarantee disease-free children or even pregnancy, and this point needs to be made clear because some patients undergoing IVF may not fully grasp this concept.[3] It is also important to discuss with patients that the long-term health outcomes of children born after PGD and IVF/ICSI are unknown, because the first IVF child was only just born in 1978.[67]

Policy and Access

Many researchers have advocated increased monitoring of applications of preimplantation genetic testing[2] and of the long-term health outcomes of the children born from these technologies,[68] but there is no consensus on how this monitoring ought to be done. Some investigators have advocated government involvement and legislation.[69] In the United States there is little legislation, restriction, or monitoring of PGD use and application; however, the American Society for Reproductive Medicine (ASRM) provides reasonable practice guidelines for the use of preimplantation genetic testing.[40] The ASRM recommends thorough counseling of couples considering preimplantation genetic testing, including genetic counseling; discussion of the risks associated with IVF, embryo biopsy, and extended embryo culture, alongside discussion of the limitations of PGS and PGD including the risk for misdiagnosis. The ASRM also recommends a discussion of prenatal diagnostic testing options to confirm PGS and PGD results and the risks associated with the procedures, the possibility that all embryos may be affected, the disposition of embryos in which testing is inconclusive, the disposition of embryos not transferred, and a discussion of alternative options to avoid passing on genetic disease including the use of donor gametes.

In the United States and many other countries, reproductive decisions such as PGD, PGS, and IVF are left ultimately to individuals and their physicians.[40] On the other hand, there are some countries in which strict legislation and restrictions on PGD/PGS and IVF limit access to these treatments.[40,60,70] Some researchers have warned that these restrictions may contribute to the phenomenon of reproductive tourism in which patients travel to other countries for treatments that are not available in their own countries. This issue has raised further concern that a for-profit reproductive services market is being created, in which patients without sufficient financial resources will be "consigned to [genetic] fate."[71(p533)] In addition to legislation, reimbursement and financing for medical procedures may also influence the procedures that clinicians offer and can therefore limit the access patients have to different medical treatments.[40] Although health care reimbursement in the United States may change dramatically in the coming years, it is unlikely that clinicians in United States will stop offering techniques like PGD, PGS, and IVF, given that many of these procedures are by and large privately financed.[71,72]

Although controversy in techniques, application, and policy guiding PGS exists, innovations stemming from the present PGD technology may help alleviate some of these controversies. For example, regarding the use of PGD for sibling HLA matching, it was recently discovered that human embryonic stem cell lines could be derived from a single biopsied embryonic cell.[73] This discovery could allow for the development of stem cell lines without the destruction of embryos. Furthermore, it could potentially allow for study of specific diseases in affected embryos[74] and for matched tissue generation for children from biopsied PGD embryos; thus avoiding the controversy sparked by the birth of Adam Nash, the first child born after PGD for sibling HLA matching.[73,75]

SUMMARY

As predicted, preimplantation genetic testing has helped many individuals to prevent the birth of children with severe genetic diseases, and has also prevented the need for selective abortion associated with postgravid antenatal screening techniques.[6] Further work is needed to determine whether PGS for aneuploidy is an effective way to increase the chances of having a child after IVF. Also, increased knowledge of the human embryo and the genetic basis of human disease coupled with the development of new genetic tests will likely lead to increased application and use of preimplantation genetic testing.

Collaborative efforts among clinicians of different disciplines, scientists, and policy makers will be necessary to ensure that this increased application and use is done responsibly.

REFERENCES

1. Handyside AH, Kontogianni EH, Hardy K, et al. Pregnancies from biopsied human preimplantation embryos sexed by Y-specific DNA amplification. Nature 1990;344(6268):768–70.
2. Goossens V, Harton G, Moutou C, et al. ESHRE PGD Consortium data collection IX: cycles from January to December 2006 with pregnancy follow-up to October 2007. Humanit Rep 2009;24(8):1786–810.
3. Dennis C. Genetics: deaf by design. Nature 2004;431(7011):894–6.
4. Verlinsky Y, Rechitsky S, Schoolcraft W, et al. Designer babies—are they a reality yet? Case report: simultaneous preimplantation genetic diagnosis for Fanconi anaemia and HLA typing for cord blood transplantation. Reprod Biomed Online 2000;1(2):31.
5. Tajima H, Sueoka K, Moon SY, et al. The development of novel quantification assay for mitochondrial DNA heteroplasmy aimed at preimplantation genetic diagnosis of Leigh encephalopathy. J Assist Reprod Genet 2007;24(6):227–32.
6. Whittingham DG, Penketh R. Prenatal diagnosis in the human pre-implantation period. Meeting held at the Ciba Foundation on the 13th November 1986. Humanit Rep 1987;2(3):267–70.
7. Braude P, Bolton V, Moore S. Human gene expression first occurs between the four- and eight-cell stages of preimplantation development. Nature 1988; 332(6163):459–61.
8. Zegers-Hochschild F, Adamson GD, de Mouzon J, et al. International Committee for Monitoring Assisted Reproductive Technology (ICMART) and the World Health Organization (WHO) revised glossary of ART terminology, 2009. Fertil Steril 2009; 92(5):1520–4.
9. Baruch S, Kaufman D, Hudson KL. Genetic testing of embryos: practices and perspectives of US in vitro fertilization clinics. Fertil Steril 2008;89(5):1053–8.
10. Strachan T, Read A. Genes in pedigrees and populations. Human molecular genetics 3. 3rd edition. New York: Garland Science; 2004. 102–11.
11. Spits C, Sermon K. PGD for monogenic disorders: aspects of molecular biology. Prenat Diagn 2009;29(1):50–6.
12. Goossens V, Harton G, Moutou C, et al. ESHRE PGD Consortium data collection VIII: cycles from January to December 2005 with pregnancy follow-up to October 2006. Humanit Rep 2008;23(12):2629–45.
13. Fragouli E. Preimplantation genetic diagnosis: present and future. J Assist Reprod Genet 2007;24(6):201–7.
14. Verlinsky Y, Rechitsky S, Schoolcraft W, et al. Preimplantation diagnosis for Fanconi anemia combined with HLA matching. JAMA 2001;285(24):3130–3.
15. Yaron YGV, Gamzu R, Malcov M. Genetic analysis of the embryo. In: Gardner D, Weissman A, Howles C, et al, editors. Textbook of assisted reproductive technologies. 3rd edition. London: Informa; 2009. p. 403–16.
16. Amor DJ, Cameron C. PGD gender selection for non-Mendelian disorders with unequal sex incidence. Humanit Rep 2008;23(4):729–34.
17. Yeargin-Allsopp M, Rice C, Karapurkar T, et al. Prevalence of autism in a US metropolitan area. JAMA 2003;289(1):49–55.

18. Pennings G. Personal desires of patients and social obligations of geneticists: applying preimplantation genetic diagnosis for non-medical sex selection. Prenat Diagn 2002;22(12):1123–9.
19. ESHRE Capri Workshop Group. Genetic aspects of female reproduction. Hum Reprod Update 2008;14(4):293–307.
20. Instability of the human genome: mutation and DNA repair. In: Strachan T, Read A, editors. Human molecular genetics 3. 3rd edition. New York: Garland Science; 2004. p. 316–49.
21. Anderson S, Bankier AT, Barrell BG, et al. Sequence and organization of the human mitochondrial genome. Nature 1981;290(5806):457–65.
22. Poulton J, Kennedy S, Oakeshott P, et al. Preventing transmission of maternally inherited mitochondrial DNA diseases. BMJ 2009;338:b94.
23. Marchington DR, Macaulay V, Hartshorne GM, et al. Evidence from human oocytes for a genetic bottleneck in an mtDNA disease. Am J Hum Genet 1998;63(3):769–75.
24. Cree LM, Samuels DC, de Sousa Lopes SC, et al. A reduction of mitochondrial DNA molecules during embryogenesis explains the rapid segregation of genotypes. Nat Genet 2008;40(2):249–54.
25. Tachibana M, Sparman M, Sritanaudomchai H, et al. Mitochondrial gene replacement in primate offspring and embryonic stem cells. Nature 2009;461(7262):367–72.
26. Steffann J, Frydman N, Gigarel N, et al. Analysis of mtDNA variant segregation during early human embryonic development: a tool for successful NARP preimplantation diagnosis. J Med Genet 2006;43(3):244–7.
27. Bredenoord AL, Dondorp W, Pennings G, et al. PGD to reduce reproductive risk: the case of mitochondrial DNA disorders. Humanit Rep 2008;23(11):2392–401.
28. Moustafa H, Rizk B, Nagy Z. Preimplantation genetic diagnosis for single-gene disorders. In: Rizk B, Garcia-Velasco J, Sallam H, et al, editors. Infertility and assisted reproduction. New York: Cambridge University Press; 2008. p. 657–76.
29. Verlinsky Y, Ginsberg N, Lifchez A, et al. Analysis of the first polar body: preconception genetic diagnosis. Humanit Rep 1990;5(7):826–9.
30. Verlinsky Y, Cieslak J, Ivakhnenko V, et al. Preimplantation diagnosis of common aneuploidies by the first- and second-polar body FISH analysis. J Assist Reprod Genet 1998;15(5):285–9.
31. Kuliev A, Verlinsky Y. Meiotic and mitotic nondisjunction: lessons from preimplantation genetic diagnosis. Hum Reprod Update 2004;10(5):401–7.
32. Kuliev A, Cieslak J, Ilkevitch Y, et al. Chromosomal abnormalities in a series of 6,733 human oocytes in preimplantation diagnosis for age-related aneuploidies. Reprod Biomed Online 2003;6(1):54–9.
33. Strom CM, Verlinsky Y, Milayeva S, et al. Preconception genetic diagnosis of cystic fibrosis. Lancet 1990;336(8710):306–7.
34. Strom CM, Ginsberg N, Rechitsky S, et al. Three births after preimplantation genetic diagnosis for cystic fibrosis with sequential first and second polar body analysis. Am J Obstet Gynecol 1998;178(6):1298–306.
35. Goossens V, De Rycke M, De Vos A, et al. Diagnostic efficiency, embryonic development and clinical outcome after the biopsy of one or two blastomeres for preimplantation genetic diagnosis. Humanit Rep 2008;23(3):481–92.
36. Van de Velde H, De Vos A, Sermon K, et al. Embryo implantation after biopsy of one or two cells from cleavage-stage embryos with a view to preimplantation genetic diagnosis. Prenat Diagn 2000;20(13):1030–7.
37. Michiels A, Van Assche E, Liebaers I, et al. The analysis of one or two blastomeres for PGD using fluorescence in-situ hybridization. Humanit Rep 2006; 21(9):2396–402.

38. Tarin JJ, Conaghan J, Winston RM, et al. Human embryo biopsy on the 2nd day after insemination for preimplantation diagnosis: removal of a quarter of embryo retards cleavage. Fertil Steril 1992;58(5):970–6.

39. McArthur SJ, Leigh D, Marshall JT, et al. Blastocyst trophectoderm biopsy and preimplantation genetic diagnosis for familial monogenic disorders and chromosomal translocations. Prenat Diagn 2008;28(5):434–42.

40. Practice Committee of Society for Assisted Reproductive Technique, Practice Committee of American Society for Reproductive Medicine. Preimplantation genetic testing: a Practice Committee opinion. Fertil Steril 2008;90:S136.

41. Rechitsky S, Verlinsky O, Amet T, et al. Reliability of preimplantation diagnosis for single gene disorders. Mol Cell Endocrinol 2001;183(Suppl 1):S65–8.

42. Kearns WG, Pen R, Graham J, et al. Preimplantation genetic diagnosis and screening. Semin Reprod Med 2005;23(4):336–47.

43. Sermon K, Van Steirteghem A, Liebaers I. Preimplantation genetic diagnosis. Lancet 2004;363(9421):1633–41.

44. Hattori M, Yoshioka K, Sakaki Y. High-sensitive fluorescent DNA sequencing and its application for detection and mass-screening of point mutations. Electrophoresis 1992;13(8):560–5.

45. Wilton L, Thornhill A, Traeger-Synodinos J, et al. The causes of misdiagnosis and adverse outcomes in PGD. Humanit Rep 2009;24(5):1221–8.

46. Thornhill AR, deDie-Smulders CE, Geraedts JP, et al. ESHRE PGD Consortium 'Best practice guidelines for clinical preimplantation genetic diagnosis (PGD) and preimplantation genetic screening (PGS)'. Humanit Rep 2005;20(1):35–48.

47. Renwick PJ, Trussler J, Ostad-Saffari E, et al. Proof of principle and first cases using preimplantation genetic haplotyping—a paradigm shift for embryo diagnosis. Reprod Biomed Online 2006;13(1):110–9.

48. Sherlock J, Cirigliano V, Petrou M, et al. Assessment of diagnostic quantitative fluorescent multiplex polymerase chain reaction assays performed on single cells. Ann Hum Genet 1998;62(Pt 1):9–23.

49. Fiorentino F, Magli MC, Podini D, et al. The minisequencing method: an alternative strategy for preimplantation genetic diagnosis of single gene disorders. Mol Hum Reprod 2003;9(7):399–410.

50. Zhang L, Cui X, Schmitt K, et al. Whole genome amplification from a single cell: implications for genetic analysis. Proc Natl Acad Sci U S A 1992;89(13):5847–51.

51. Wilton L. Preimplantation genetic diagnosis and chromosome analysis of blastomeres using comparative genomic hybridization. Hum Reprod Update 2005; 11(1):33–41.

52. Bejjani BA, Shaffer LG. Application of array-based comparative genomic hybridization to clinical diagnostics. J Mol Diagn 2006;8(5):528–33.

53. Wells D, Sherlock JK, Handyside AH, et al. Detailed chromosomal and molecular genetic analysis of single cells by whole genome amplification and comparative genomic hybridisation. Nucleic Acids Res 1999;27(4):1214–8.

54. Hu DG, Webb G, Hussey N. Aneuploidy detection in single cells using DNA array-based comparative genomic hybridization. Mol Hum Reprod 2004;10(4):283–9.

55. Le Caignec C, Spits C, Sermon K, et al. Single-cell chromosomal imbalances detection by array CGH. Nucleic Acids Res 2006;34(9):e68.

56. Spits C, Le Caignec C, De Rycke M, et al. Whole-genome multiple displacement amplification from single cells. Nat Protoc 2006;1(4):1965–70.

57. Spits C, Le Caignec C, De Rycke M, et al. Optimization and evaluation of single-cell whole-genome multiple displacement amplification. Hum Mutat 2006;27(5): 496–503.

58. Ethical Issues in Genetic Testing. ACOG Committee Opinion No. 410. American College of Obstetricians and Gynecologists. Obstet Gynecol 2008;111: 1495–502.
59. Savulescu J, Kahane G. The moral obligation to create children with the best chance of the best life. Bioethics 2009;23(5):274–90.
60. Aarden E, Van Hoyweghen I, Vos R, et al. Providing preimplantation genetic diagnosis in the United Kingdom, The Netherlands and Germany: a comparative in-depth analysis of health-care access. Humanit Rep 2009;24(7):1542–7.
61. Wertz DC, Fletcher JC, Nippert I, et al. In focus. Has patient autonomy gone too far? Geneticists' views in 36 nations. Am J Bioeth 2002;2(4):W21.
62. Lyerly AD, Steinhauser K, Voils C, et al. Fertility patients' views about frozen embryo disposition: results of a multi-institutional U.S. survey. Fertil Steril 2010; 93(2):499–509.
63. Mastenbroek S, Twisk M, van Echten-Arends J, et al. In vitro fertilization with preimplantation genetic screening. N Engl J Med 2007;357(1):9–17.
64. Hardarson T, Hanson C, Lundin K, et al. Preimplantation genetic screening in women of advanced maternal age caused a decrease in clinical pregnancy rate: a randomized controlled trial. Humanit Rep 2008;23(12):2806–12.
65. Meyer LR, Klipstein S, Hazlett WD, et al. A prospective randomized controlled trial of preimplantation genetic screening in the "good prognosis" patient. Fertil Steril 2009;91(5):1731–8.
66. Kuehn BM. Prenatal genome testing sparks debate. JAMA 2008;300(14):1637–9.
67. Steptoe PC, Edwards RG. Birth after the reimplantation of a human embryo. Lancet 1978;2(8085):366.
68. Reddy UM, Wapner RJ, Rebar RW, et al. Infertility, assisted reproductive technology, and adverse pregnancy outcomes: executive summary of a National Institute of Child Health and Human Development workshop. Obstet Gynecol 2007; 109(4):967–77.
69. Simpson JL, Rebar RW, Carson SA. Professional self-regulation for preimplantation genetic diagnosis: experience of the American Society for Reproductive Medicine and other professional societies. Fertil Steril 2006;85(6):1653–60.
70. Jones HW Jr, Cohen J. IFFS surveillance 07. Fertil Steril 2007;87(4 Suppl 1): S1–67.
71. Spar D. Reproductive tourism and the regulatory map. N Engl J Med 2005; 352(6):531–3.
72. Jain T, Harlow BL, Hornstein MD. Insurance coverage and outcomes of in vitro fertilization. N Engl J Med 2002;347(9):661–6.
73. Klimanskaya I, Chung Y, Becker S, et al. Human embryonic stem cell lines derived from single blastomeres. Nature 2006;444(7118):481–5.
74. Mateizel I, De Temmerman N, Ullmann U, et al. Derivation of human embryonic stem cell lines from embryos obtained after IVF and after PGD for monogenic disorders. Humanit Rep 2006;21(2):503–11.
75. Crockin S. Adam Nash: legally speaking, a happy ending or slippery slope? Reprod Biomed Online 2001;2(1):6–7.

An Update on Cystic Fibrosis Screening

Katherine R. Goetzinger, MD*, Alison G. Cahill, MD, MSCI

- Cystic fibrosis • Prenatal diagnosis • Carrier screening
- CFTR • Pregnancy

Cystic fibrosis (CF) is a multisystem disease that is characterized by chronic airway infection, pancreatic insufficiency, gastrointestinal dysfunction, and male infertility. It is one of the most common single-gene disorders in the Caucasian population, with an incidence between 1 in 3000 to 1 in 3300 individuals.[1,2] Symptoms typically present in early childhood, but in a minority of cases, the diagnosis may not be evident until adulthood. Although there have been major advances in the medical care and treatment of CF, the median age of survival remains approximately 37 years. Because of the morbidity and mortality of this disease and the growing number of CF patients who are advancing into child-bearing years, prenatal screening for CF has become a topic of increasing interest over the past 2 decades. Currently, the American College of Obstetricians and Gynecologists[3] (ACOG) recommends that "it is reasonable to offer cystic fibrosis carrier screening to all couples regardless of race or ethnicity before conception or early in pregnancy." This article aims to review the genetics of CF, including its genotypic-phenotypic variations, current prenatal carrier screening and diagnostic recommendations, ultrasonographic markers of CF, and reproductive options for carrier couples.

THE GENETICS OF CF

The gene for CF was first cloned in 1989 and has paved the way for current screening protocols.[4–6] The responsible gene is located on chromosome 7 and encodes the protein called CF transmembrane conductance regulator (CFTR), a 170kDa cAMP-regulated chloride channel located on the apical membrane of epithelial cells. Absence of, or mutation in, CFTR leads to abnormal fluid and electrolyte membrane transport, resulting in dehydrated secretions, decreased mucus clearance in the lung, deficient secretion of pancreatic enzymes, gut dysmotility, and increased sodium chloride levels in sweat.[1,7]

Department of Obstetrics and Gynecology, Washington University School of Medicine, 660 South Euclid, Campus Box 8064, St Louis, MO 63110, USA
* Corresponding author.
E-mail address: goetzingerk@wudosis.wustl.edu

Clin Lab Med 30 (2010) 533–543
doi:10.1016/j.cll.2010.04.005
0272-2712/10/$ – see front matter © 2010 Elsevier Inc. All rights reserved.
labmed.theclinics.com

CF is inherited in an autosomal recessive manner, and more than 1000 different CFTR mutations have been described with differing prevalences depending on race and ethnicity (**Fig. 1**). The most common mutation is ΔF508, which is a frameshift mutation caused by a 3–base-pair deletion at codon 508 in exon 10 of CFTR, that results in the absence of a phenylalanine residue (**Fig. 2**). This particular mutation accounts for 70% of CF mutations in the Caucasian population. The ΔF508 mutation causes a protein misfold that inhibits migration of the CFTR protein from the endoplasmic reticulum to the cell membrane.[1,7] Other common mutations include G542X, R553X, W1282X, N1303K, 621+1 G-to-T, 1717-1 G-to-A, and R117H.[8] These result in a spectrum of protein dysfunction ranging from the production of unstable RNA to CFTR cell surface instability.[7]

PHENOTYPIC VARIATION IN CFTR MUTATIONS

Although 70% of CF patients are either homozygotes or compound heterozygotes for these 8 common mutations, there is tremendous variation in their phenotype. Multiple studies on CFTR genotype-phenotype relationships have been reviewed and conclude that although the CFTR genotype may be a good predictor of pancreatic function, it is an overall poor predictor of pulmonary disease severity.[9–11] For example, ΔF508 homozygotes generally have pancreatic insufficiency but exhibit mild-to-moderate pulmonary symptoms. Alternatively, R117H/ΔF508 compound heterozygotes tend to exhibit pancreatic sufficiency with varying pulmonary manifestations.[9] N1303K has been associated with yet another phenotype: the early onset of pancreatic insufficiency and a wide spectrum of pulmonary disease.[10] Experts have hypothesized that there are gene-environment interactions that may explain the variable pulmonary phenotype observed across the spectrum of CFTR genotypes.[12,13] For example, in 2008, Collaco and colleagues[12] demonstrated that any secondhand tobacco exposure had a negative long-term effect on lung function in CF patients. These adverse effects were amplified in the presence of variants in a CF modifier gene, transforming growth factor β1 (TGFβ1), thus providing support for gene-environment interactions.[14]

Another well-studied phenotypic variant is the R117H mutation and its association with the 5T/7T/9T polymorphism in intron 8 of the same allele. R117H paired with the 7T variant (in cis) and R117H paired with the 5T variant (in trans) have been observed in infertile but otherwise healthy men with congenital bilateral absence of the vas deferens (CBAVD).[15,16] When this same mutation is paired with the 5T variant (in cis), signs and symptoms of classical CF are observed.[17] This has led to extensive debate as to whether the R117H mutation should even be included in the prenatal screening panel

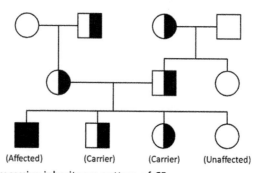

(Affected)   (Carrier)   (Carrier)   (Unaffected)

Fig. 1. Autosomal recessive inheritance pattern of CF.

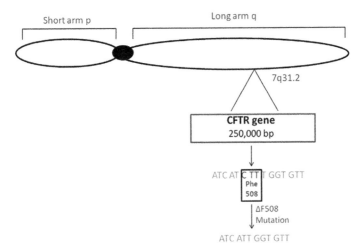

Fig. 2. Locus of the CFTR gene.

because of its complex genetic interactions and its potential to screen for both male infertility and classical CF. Despite this fact, the R117H mutation remains a part of the standard prenatal carrier screening panel, with a reflex test for the 5T/7T/9T variant performed if positive for this mutation.

CARRIER SCREENING FOR CF

Carrier screening for CF accomplishes 2 goals: (1) identification of carrier couples who have a 1 in 4 risk of having affected offspring in order to provide genetic counseling and offer prenatal diagnosis and (2) identification of individual carrier status that may have future reproductive and genetic implications. This has proven to be challenging for CF because of the sizeable number of detectable mutations and extensive ethnic and geographic variation. **Table 1** illustrates this variation and the rate of mutation detection by standard DNA mutation analysis. The Caucasian and Ashkenazi Jewish population have the highest incidence of disease and also the highest carrier detection rate. As previously noted, the most common mutation in the Caucasian population is ΔF508, and the most common mutation in the Ashkenazi Jewish population is W1282X followed by ΔF508.[18] Although Hispanics exhibit a relatively high incidence of disease, the sensitivity of carrier testing remains only 57% to 72% because detectable alleles account for only slightly more than half of the CF mutations observed in this population. African Americans, in contrast, have a relatively lower incidence of disease, and current screening only detects approximately 65% to 69% of carriers.[2] Sugarman and colleagues[19] reviewed results from CFTR mutation analyses in Hispanic and African American individuals with a CF diagnosis and those undergoing carrier screening using an 87-mutation panel. Five mutations currently not included in the current carrier screening panel accounted for 7.55% detection in CF patients and 5.58% detection in CF carriers in Hispanic patients. In the African American population, 10 mutations currently not included in the current carrier screening panel accounted for a 7.41% detection rate in CF patients. Twelve mutations identified in the CF carriers were not identified in the actual CF patients, although these mutations

Table 1
Differences in carrier testing across individual ethnic/racial groups.

Ethnic Group	Incidence of CF	Carrier Frequency	Detection Rate	[a]Estimated Carrier Risk after Negative Screen
Caucasian	1/3300	1/25	80%–88%	1 in 166 (1/125–1/208)
African American	1/15,300	1/65	65%–69%	1 in 198 (1/186–1/210)
Ashkenazi Jewish	1/3970	1/24	94%–97%	1 in 600 (1/400–1/800)
Hispanic	1/8900	1/46	57%–72%	1 in 135 (1/107–1/164)
Asian	1/35,000	1/94	30%–49%	1 in 159 (1/134–1/184)

[a] Approximate numbers based on ranges in detection rate.

Data from Cutting GR. Genetic epidemiology and genotype/phenotype correlations. NIH Consensus Development Conference on Genetic Testing for Cystic Fibrosis, 1997; ACOG Committee Opinion 325. Update on Carrier Screening for Cystic Fibrosis, 2005.

are known to express a variable phenotype. Monaghan and colleagues[20] also reviewed carrier screening results from 2189 African Americans patients. Two additional mutations also not included in the current carrier screening panel, G622D and Q98R, were incidentally identified. The mutation 3120+1 G to A was not identified, although this mutation has previously been known to account for 12% of CF mutations in the African American population. These data illustrate the heterogeneity of the CFTR genotypes observed in ethnic populations, even when examined individually, and give support to the current panethnic carrier screening panel.

In 1997, the National Institutes of Health (NIH) held a consensus conference to address the complex issues associated with CF carrier screening in a panethnic population. This conference was followed, in 1998, by another NIH conference directed at the implementation of this committee's recommendations. Based on these recommendations, CF carrier screening was to be offered to (1) adults with a positive family history of CF, (2) partners of known CF carriers, (3) couples currently planning a pregnancy, and (4) couples seeking prenatal care.[21] In 2001, recommendations were issued from yet another steering committee comprised of representatives from the American College of Medical Genetics (ACMG), ACOG, and the National Human Genome Research Institute. This group recommended narrowing the screening population to non-Jewish Caucasians and Ashkenazi Jews, while still making testing available to other ethnic groups with informed consent and recognition of the limitations of screening.[22] Finally, in 2005, the ACOG issued an update to their committee opinion stating that "it is reasonable to offer cystic fibrosis carrier screening to all couples regardless of race or ethnicity as an alternative to selective screening." This recommendation is based on the fact that it is becoming increasingly difficult to assign an individual to any one particular ethnic group. Patients opting for testing who have a negative screening result must be reminded that carrier screening is not 100% sensitive. Patients should undergo pretest and posttest counseling, with particular attention paid to ethnic background, detection rate, and residual risk estimate (see **Table 1**).[3]

The current CF carrier screening panel was introduced by the ACMG/ACOG steering committee in 2001 and was initially comprised of 25 mutations. These mutations were chosen based on an allele frequency of 0.1% or greater in the general US population, regardless of their phenotypic expression of mild versus severe disease.[22] In 2004, the ACMG conducted a second review of the standard mutation panel, which specifically evaluated mutation distribution amongst various ethnic groups. Based on this review, 2 mutations (1078delT and I148T) were removed from the standard screening panel, narrowing it to include only 23 mutations. (Appendix A) These 2 mutations were selected for removal based on observed frequencies of less than 0.1%. Although this review also identified other mutations that were observed at a frequency of greater than 0.1%, no additions were made to the panel as the investigators did not think that these would substantially increase the sensitivity of the screening test. It was recognized that these mutations may be considered for use in future potential ethnic-specific panels.[23]

There are currently 4 reflex mutations also included as part of the standard screening panel. When a patient is positive for R117H, a reflex test for the 5T/7T/9T variant is sent. If positive for 5T, determination as to whether the polymorphism is in cis or in trans with the R117H allele is undertaken.[22] As discussed previously, R117H in combination with the 5T variant in trans manifests as CBAVD, but if in cis with the 5T variant, classical CF is expressed. Given that 5% of the general population will test positive for the 5T polymorphism alone, this test is recommended only as a reflex to a positive R117H result.[22,23] Non CF-causing variants, including I506V, I507V, and F508C, can mistakenly cause a false-positive result based on laboratory and testing methodologies. For example, in patients who screen positive for ΔF508 carrier status and for one of the aforementioned mutations, a false-positive test for ΔF508 homozygosity may be obtained, although the patient is an otherwise healthy individual.[22] Although F508C has been associated with CBAVD, neither I506V nor I507V have been associated with any phenotypic manifestations of classical CF or CBAVD.[24] Therefore, reflex testing for I506V, I507V, and F508C should be performed in any healthy individual who tests positive for ΔF508 or ΔI507 homozygosity, but these mutations should not be otherwise used for a priori testing.

In patients with a personal or family history of CF, identification of the disease-causing mutation should be pursued by reviewing medical records and, if unattainable, proceeding with DNA sequencing of the CFTR gene in the proband. If the proband is unavailable, DNA sequencing of the CFTR gene in the fetus can be performed, although time constraints in the setting of prenatal diagnosis must be considered. Extended CF mutation panels may also be available at select laboratories, but their use should be reserved for particular clinical circumstances, including patients with reproductive partners with CF or CBAVD and no identified mutation, family history of CF with no identified mutation, or a positive newborn screening test with none or only one identified CF mutation.[2] There has been considerable debate over whether to routinely offer extended panel screening to couples who test positive/negative for CF carrier status using the standard 23-mutation panel. The ACMG consensus is that this should not be offered as a standard of care, because it would probably yield very little additional information. For example, although mutation 3876delA occurs at a frequency of 0.48% in the Hispanic population, it occurs at an approximately 0% frequency in other ethnic populations, therefore leading to an overall frequency of 0.03% in a panethnic population. For couples who request supplementary material, the existence of extended panels should be made known.[22,23]

Although the aim of prenatal carrier testing is to identify couples at risk of having an affected child, it is possible that carrier testing may identify an individual with 2 mutations in the CFTR gene. Secondary to the variation observed in phenotypic expression, this individual may be asymptomatic, be affected with a very mild form of CF, or be destined for a late-onset presentation of the disease.[25] Although uncommon, this possibility should be incorporated into pretest counseling, and referral for genetic counseling should be made immediately in the event of this diagnosis.

Currently, there are 3 approaches to carrier screening in pregnant couples or couples planning a pregnancy. The first is a stepwise method, during which one partner, usually the woman, is tested. If this test yields a positive result, then the other partner is tested (**Fig. 3**). Alternatively, a couples-based screening method can be used, during which specimens are taken from both partners and results are reported accordingly. A third option is an alternative couples-based method that was first described by Wald[26] in 1991. In this approach, samples are collected from both partners, but positive results are reported only when both partners are carriers. Negative couple results are given to couples who test positive/negative or negative/not-tested. Advantages to this method are that both partners must enroll before testing and, therefore, are making a joint decision regarding prenatal screening. Also, partner-specific genetic information is not divulged unless it has the potential to affect the pregnancy. A randomized controlled trial comparing this alternative couples-based method to standard stepwise screening revealed that although both methods were practically feasible, stepwise screening was the preferred method, because it provided overall lower levels of couple anxiety and false reassurance about their pregnancy.[27] Because of ethical concerns of nondisclosure and its future ramifications for affected family members and future partners, the ACMG does not endorse this alternative couples-based approach to carrier screening. The ACOG and ACMG currently support the standard couples-based approach and the stepwise screening approach. Concurrent couple-based screening may be more practical for couples of Northern European or Ashkenazi Jewish descent, where the carrier frequency and test sensitivity is high. Generally, it is more practical and cost-effective to perform stepwise-screening unless time constraints are present for prenatal diagnosis and/or decisions for pregnancy termination. Ultimately, providers should be educated in both techniques and counsel couples accordingly.[3,22]

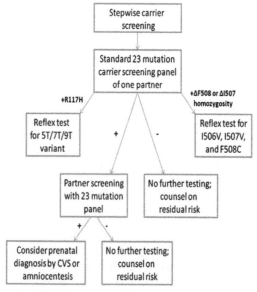

Fig. 3. Algorithm for prenatal stepwise carrier screening.

ANTENATAL ULTRASONOGRAPHIC FINDINGS ASSOCIATED WITH CF

In addition to genetic markers, ultrasonographic markers have also been linked to the prenatal diagnosis of CF. Echogenic bowel, defined as bowel with a sonographic density equal to or greater than that of surrounding bone, is observed in 0.1% to 1.8% of second-trimester ultrasound scans and is associated with CF (**Fig. 4**). Additional differential diagnoses include normal variant, fetal intestinal obstruction, aneuploidy, congenital viral infection, and intra-amniotic bleeding.[28–31] Meconium ileus is a syndrome observed in 10% to 20% of newborns affected with CF, and it presents with emesis, failure to pass stool, and abdominal distention.[1,7] Studies have suggested that meconium ileus may be detected on routine prenatal ultrasonography, manifested as echogenic bowel ± dilated intestinal loops. This appearance is thought to be due to dehydration of intestinal secretions, thereby leading to increased bowel viscosity and subsequent obstruction. Boue and colleagues[32] reviewed amniocentesis results for 200 pregnancies with a 25% risk of CF and found echogenic bowel in 50% to 60% of affected fetuses. Sepulveda and colleagues[33] prospectively studied 45 fetuses with echogenic bowel in a low-risk population, and none exhibited CF when evaluated by prenatal diagnosis or parental carrier screening. An additional study in 2002 revealed a 2.5% incidence of CF-affected fetuses with isolated echogenic bowel and a 2.9% incidence with isolated fetal bowel dilation. These 2 ultrasonographic findings in the same fetus increased the CF risk to 17%. Nonvisualization of the fetal gallbladder combined with either of the aforementioned signs further increased the risk to 25% in this particular study.[34]

Because the CF risk is variable among fetuses with echogenic bowel, counseling can become complex. Current recommendations for evaluation of fetal echogenic bowel include consideration of aneuploidy serum screening versus invasive testing, maternal studies for congenital infection, detailed anatomic survey to evaluate for other structural defects and growth restriction, and parental CF carrier screening.[28] Extreme ends of the prenatal diagnostic spectrum include identifying fetuses with 2 detected CF mutations (certain diagnosis) and fetuses with no detected mutation (extremely low risk). For fetuses found to have one detected CF mutation, the diagnosis cannot be certain and residual risk estimates vary based on carrier frequency, test sensitivity in the particular ethnic population, and risk association between echogenic bowel and CF (ranges reported from 0%–33%).[27,28]

PRENATAL DIAGNOSIS OF CF

Relative indications for prenatal diagnosis include "but are not limited to" 2 known parental mutations, family history of CF, and echogenic fetal bowel on

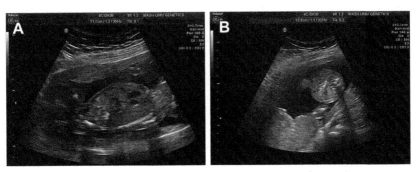

Fig. 4. Echogenic bowel identified on second-trimester ultrasound screening.

ultrasonography. The ACMG and ACOG recommend that each parent be tested for carrier status before pursuing invasive fetal diagnostic testing.[3,25] Testing can be performed using either chorionic villus samples or direct or cultured amniocytes. Although there does not appear to be a difference in test accuracy between chorionic villus sampling (CVS) and amniocentesis for diagnosing CF, gestational age, time constraints for decision-making, and risk of pregnancy loss must be considered. Recent studies from one academic center indicate a second-trimester amniocentesis loss rate of 0.13% and a CVS loss rate of 2.7%, neither of which were significantly different from loss rates in control groups.[35,36] For CVS, the fetal sample also must be examined in parallel with a maternal serum sample, and microsatellite markers should be analyzed to rule out maternal cell contamination. A positive diagnostic test is considered definitive, because the penetrance of the selected 23 mutations is quite high. However, variation in the expressivity of specific clinical manifestations must be considered when interpreting and counseling patients regarding their genotyping results. Clinical specificity approaches 100% because false-positive tests due to analytic error are exceedingly rare (1:1000–1:10,000).[25]

Many valid methods of DNA mutation analysis are available for carrier and diagnostic testing, and laboratories may elect to use original or commercially available reagents. Typically, carrier samples can be analyzed from serum, buccal washings, or mouthwash specimens. Common methods of mutation analysis include forward allele-specific oligonucleotide, reverse dot-blot hybridization, amplification refractory mutation system, and oligonucleotide ligation assay, each possessing strengths and weaknesses.[25] A review of each technique is beyond the scope of this article. In special situations with an unknown or only one known CF mutation in a patient with a personal or family history, linkage analyses and scanning technology can be used to detect sequence alteration in the CFTR gene.[25]

REPRODUCTIVE OPTIONS FOR CARRIER COUPLES

When couples are identified as CF carriers before conception, reproductive options include natural conception with its associated risk of an affected child, natural conception followed by prenatal diagnosis and possible pregnancy termination, the use of donor oocytes or sperm, adoption, or preimplantation genetic diagnosis (PGD). Although PGD allows couples to use their own genetic material, it does require the use of in vitro fertilization regardless of the couple's baseline fertility. Typically, oocytes are retrieved, fertilized, and then biopsied at a cleavage stage. One or two cells are then removed and PGD for single gene disorders is performed by a complex technique of short tandem repeat polymorphism analysis and mutation detection using polymerase chain reaction.[37,38] PGD for CF was first described in 1992, and, although a relatively new technology, has been associated with reported success.[37–39] A recent cost-benefit analysis revealed net economic benefits of PGD for CF carrier couples compared with prenatal diagnosis and subsequent pregnancy termination in women younger than 40 years.[40] Counseling for couples identified as CF carriers can be complex, encompassing a range of emotional, ethical, religious, and financial concerns. The ACOG and ACMG recommend genetic counseling in an experienced center for such couples.[3,22]

SUMMARY

CF is a common, monogenic, autosomal recessive disorder characterized by altered fluid and electrolyte transport across epithelial cells. This leads to thickened secretions, recurrent infection, and eventually, multisystem organ dysfunction with a subsequent decrease in life expectancy. Because of the sizeable number of mutations, expansive ethnic and racial variation, and variable phenotypic expression, carrier screening has presented a challenge. Current recommendations include providing carrier screening information to all couples in either the preconception or early prenatal period and offering carrier screening to couples in high-risk ethnic or racial groups or even universally, as an alternative to selective screening. A mutation panel consisting of 23 mutations is the standard of care for routine carrier screening, although an expanded panel or even complete CFTR gene sequencing is available for patients with a personal or family history of CF or CBAVD. Because of the aforementioned limitations, carrier screening is not 100% sensitive and should be perceived as a risk-reducing rather than risk-eliminating test. For CF carrier couples, reproductive options, including definitive prenatal diagnostic tests and preimplantation genetic diagnosis, are available. With advances in molecular diagnosis and an increase in the number of identifiable CFTR mutations, the current screening panel will probably continue to evolve and possibly be used in a more ethnic/race-specific manner. Obstetricians and gynecologists should be familiar with the current guidelines and testing availability/limitations and routinely incorporate CF counseling into early prenatal visits, with referral for genetic counseling in appropriate situations.

APPENDIX A: STANDARD 23-MUTATION PANEL FOR CF CARRIER SCREENING

ΔF508
G542X
G551D
W1282X
3849+10kbC$\rightarrow$T
N1303K
621+1G$\rightarrow$T
1717-1G$\rightarrow$A
R553X
R117H
G85E
2789+5G$\rightarrow$A
3120+1G$\rightarrow$A
ΔI507
R1162X
1898+1G$\rightarrow$A
3659delC
711+1G$\rightarrow$T
R334W
2184delA
A455E
R347P
R560T

REFERENCES

1. Boucher RC. Cystic fibrosis. In: Harrison TR, Kasper DL, editors. Harrison's principles of internal medicine. 16th edition. New York: McGraw-Hill; 2005. p. 1543–6.
2. Wapner RJ, Jenkins TM, Khalek M. Prenatal diagnosis of congenital disorders. In: Creasy RK, Resnik R, Iams JD, editors. Maternal-fetal medicine. Principles and practice. 6th edition. Philadelphia: Saunders Elsevier; 2009. p. 221–74.

3. American College of Obstetricians and Gynecologists. Update on carrier screening for cystic fibrosis. ACOG committee opinion #325. Washington, DC: American College of Obstetricians and Gynecologists; 2005.

4. Rommens JM, Iannuzzi MC, Bat-Sheva K, et al. Identification of the cystic fibrosis gene: chromosome walking and jumping. Science 1989;245(4922):1059–65.

5. Riordan JR, Rommens JM, Bat-Sheva K, et al. Identification of the cystic fibrosis gene: cloning and characterization of complementary DNA. Science 1989; 245(4922):1066–72.

6. Kerem B, Rommens JM, Buchanan JA, et al. Identification of the cystic fibrosis gene: genetic analysis. Science 1989;245(4922):1073–80.

7. Nussbaum RL, McInnes RR, Willard HL. The molecular, biochemical, and cellular basis of genetic disease. In: Thompson & Thompson genetics in medicine. 7th edition. Philadelphia: Saunders Elsevier; 2007. p. 364–7.

8. Tsui L- C. Mutations and sequence variations detected in the cystic fibrosis transmembrane conductance regulator (CFTR) gene: a report from the Cystic Fibrosis Genetic Analysis Consortium. Hum Mutat 1992;1(3):197–203.

9. The Cystic Fibrosis Genotype-Phenotype Consortium. Correlation between genotype and phenotype in patients with cystic fibrosis. N Engl J Med 1993;329(18): 1308–13.

10. Osborne L, Santis G, Schwarz M, et al. Incidence and expression of the N1303K mutation of the cystic fibrosis (CFTR) gene. Hum Genet 1992;89(6):653–8.

11. Gasparini P, Borgo G, Mastella G, et al. Nine cystic fibrosis patients homozygous for the CFTR nonsense mutation R1162X have mild or moderate lung disease. J Med Genet 1992;29(8):558–62.

12. Collaco JM, Vanscoy L, Bremer L, et al. Interactions between secondhand smoke and genes that affect cystic fibrosis lung disease. JAMA 2009;299(4):417–24.

13. Campbell PW III, Parker RA, Roberts BT, et al. Association of poor clinical status and heavy exposure to tobacco smoke in patients with cystic fibrosis who are homozygous for the F508 deletion. J Pediatr 1992;120(2 Pt 1):261–4.

14. Drumm ML, Konstan MW, Schluchter MD, et al. Genetic modifiers of lung disease in cystic fibrosis. N Engl J Med 2005;353(14):1443–53.

15. Chillon M, Casals T, Mercier B, et al. Mutations in the cystic fibrosis gene in patients with congenital absence of the vas deferens. N Engl J Med 1995; 332(22):1475–80.

16. Gervais R, Dumur V, Rigot M-M, et al. High frequency of the R117H cystic fibrosis mutation in patients with congenital absence of the vas deferens. N Engl J Med 1993;328(6):446–7.

17. Kiesewetter S, Macek M, Davis C, et al. A mutation in CFTR produces different phenotypes depending on chromosomal background. Nat Genet 1993;5(3): 274–7.

18. Shoshani T, Augarten A, Gazit E, et al. Association of a nonsense mutation (W1282X), the most common mutation in the Ashkenazi Jewish cystic fibrosis patients in Israel, with presentation of severe disease. Am J Hum Genet 1992; 50(1):222–8.

19. Sugarman EA, Rohlfs EM, Silverman LM, et al. CFTR mutation distribution among U.S. Hispanic and African American individuals: evaluation in cystic fibrosis patient and carrier screening populations. Genet Med 2004;6(5):392–9.

20. Monaghan KG, Bluhm D, Phillips M, et al. Preconception and prenatal cystic fibrosis carrier screening of African Americans reveals unanticipated frequencies for specific mutations. Genet Med 2004;6(3):141–4.

21. NIH Consensus Development Conference Statement. Genetic testing for cystic fibrosis. April 14–16, 1997. Arch Intern Med 1999;159(14):1529–39.
22. Grody WW, Cutting GR, Klinger KW, et al. Laboratory standards and guidelines for population-based cystic fibrosis carrier screening. Genet Med 2001;3(2): 149–54.
23. Watson MS, Cutting GR, Desnick RJ, et al. Cystic fibrosis population carrier screening: 2004 revision of American College of Medical Genetics mutation panel. Genet Med 2004;6(5):387–91.
24. Dork T, Dworniczak B, Aulehis-Schotz C, et al. Distinct spectrum of CFTR gene mutations in congenital absence of vas deferens. Hum Genet 1997;100(3–4): 365–77.
25. Richards CS, Bradley LA, Amos J, et al. Standards and guidelines for CFTR mutation testing. Genet Med 2002;4(5):379–91.
26. Wald NJ. Couple screening for cystic fibrosis. Lancet 1991;338(8778):1318–9.
27. Miedzybrodzka ZH, Hall MH, Mollison J, et al. Antenatal screening for carriers of cystic fibrosis: randomized trial of stepwise v couple screening. BMJ 1995; 310(6976):353–7.
28. Norton MF. Genetics and prenatal diagnosis. In: Callen PW, editor. Ultrasonography in obstetrics and gynecology. 5th edition. Philadelphia: Saunders Elsevier; 2008. p. 26–59.
29. Nyberg DA, Dubinsky T, Resta RG, et al. Echogenic fetal bowel during the second trimester: clinical importance. Radiology 1993;188(2):527–31.
30. Dicke JM, Crane JP. Sonographically detected hyperechoic fetal bowel: significance and implications for pregnancy management. Obstet Gynecol 1992; 80(5):778–82.
31. Sepulveda W, Hollingsworth J, Bower S, et al. Fetal hyperechogenic bowel following intra-amniotic bleeding. Obstet Gynecol 1994;83(6):947–50.
32. Boue A, Muller F, Nezelof C, et al. Prenatal diagnosis in 200 pregnancies with a 1 in 4 risk of cystic fibrosis. Hum Genet 1986;74(3):288–97.
33. Sepulveda W, Leung KY, Robertson ME, et al. Prevalence of cystic fibrosis mutations in pregnancies with fetal echogenic bowel. Obstet Gynecol 1996;87(1): 103–6.
34. Muller F, Simon-Bouy B, Girodon E, et al. Predicting the risk of cystic fibrosis with abnormal ultrasound signs of fetal bowel: results of a French Molecular Collaborative study based on 641 prospective cases. Am J Med Genet 2002;110(2):109–15.
35. Odibo AO, Gray DL, Dicke JM, et al. Revisiting the fetal loss rate after second-trimester genetic amniocentesis. Obstet Gynecol 2008;111(3):589–95.
36. Odibo AO, Dicke JM, Gray DL, et al. Evaluating the rate and risk factors for fetal loss after chorionic villus sampling. Obstet Gynecol 2008;112(4):813–9.
37. Ao A, Ray P, Harper J, et al. Clinical experience with preimplantation genetic diagnosis of cystic fibrosis (ΔF508). Prenat Diagn 1996;16(2):137–42.
38. Gutierrez-Mateo C, Sanchez-Garcia JF, Fischer J, et al. Preimplantation genetic diagnosis of single gene disorders: experience with more than 200 cycles conducted by a reference laboratory in the United States. Fertil Steril 2009;92(5): 1544–56.
39. Handyside AH, Lesko JH, Tarin JJ, et al. Birth of a normal girl after in vitro fertilization and preimplantation diagnostic testing for cystic fibrosis. N Engl J Med 1992;327(13):905–9.
40. Davis LB, Champion SJ, Fair SO, et al. A cost-benefit analysis of preimplantation genetic diagnosis for carrier couples of cystic fibrosis. Fertil Steril 2010;93(6): 1793–804.

An Overview of First-Trimester Screening for Chromosomal Abnormalities

Ray O. Bahado-Singh, MD, MBA*, Pedro Argoti, MD

KEYWORDS

• First-trimester screening • Nuchal transparency
• Alpha fetoprotein • Human chorionic gonadotropin

Significant advances in Down syndrome screening have occurred in the last two decades. Before the 1980s, screening consisted exclusively of the use of maternal age threshold greater than or equal to 35 years for the identification of women at elevated risk, to whom mid-trimester amniocentesis was offered. Reports of an association between depressed mid-trimester serum alpha fetoprotein (AFP), used for neural tube defect screening, and aneuploidies[1] led to the development of a Down syndrome screening algorithm combining AFP with maternal age.[2,3] The combination achieved a detection rate of 25% to 33% for a 5% false-positive rate. This represented a significant landmark in prenatal screening and formed the basis of subsequent biochemistry-based aneuploidy screening algorithms. The current state of the art for screening incorporates first trimester–based biochemistry plus ultrasound measurements. The endorsement of the combined first-trimester algorithm by the American College of Obstetricians and Gynecolgists[4] has coincided with a marked increase in the use of first trimester for risk determination.

In this article emphasis is placed on first-trimester markers of established clinical use; however, mention is also made of other markers that are being evaluated. Finally, although mid-trimester markers per se remain outside the brief of this article, the combination of first and mid-trimester is a clinical reality and for the sake of completion providing a concise account of the performance and current clinical status of such combined algorithms seems reasonable.

Women's preference constitutes an important justification for first-trimester screening. Priorities expressed by women polled include early testing; safety (ie, having low false-positive rate and reduced invasive testing in normal women); and

Department of Obstetrics and Gynecology, Wayne State University, Detroit, MI, USA
* Corresponding author. Harper Hospital, OB/Ultrasound, 3980 John R, Box 160, Detroit, MI 48201.
E-mail address: rbahados@med.wayne.edu

Clin Lab Med 30 (2010) 545–555
doi:10.1016/j.cll.2010.05.001
0272-2712/10/$ – see front matter © 2010 Elsevier Inc. All rights reserved.

high detection rates.[5] Interestingly, studies report that health care professionals place a greater premium on earlier testing than their patients.[6,7] It should be noted, however, that consumers of prenatal screening services represent a significantly heterogeneous group, substantially affecting their screening preferences. Lo and colleagues[8] reported a study of 1967 primarily Chinese women greater than 35 years of age offered the option of first-trimester, fully integrated, partial integrated (first-trimester nuchal translucency [NT] and mid-trimester human chorionic gonadotropin [hCG] and AFP and second-trimester biochemistry) screening. Final choices were significantly affected by parity, history of fertility disorder, family history of chromosomal disorder, social class, and employment status. The authors found that the choice of screening test could be correctly predicted in 50% of the women based on these demographic and obstetric characteristics.

Having a menu of choices seems to be the best strategy for meeting the diverse expectations of pregnant women. Such a strategy is not without significant challenge. The nature of the required counseling becomes substantially more complex with the risk of confusing patients and possibly practitioners. Further complexities include the logistic and economic challenges of providing these choices. It can be safely concluded, however, that a screening algorithm that offers the highest possible diagnostic accuracy at the earliest gestational age meets the expectations of virtually all patients and practitioners. This is the ongoing challenge confronting clinicians and scientists interested in this discipline.

FIRST-TRIMESTER ULTRASOUND MARKERS

Contrary to what might have been anticipated given the difficulty of standardization, varying levels of expertise of practitioners and the differing make and capabilities of the equipment used, the ultrasound measurement NT has emerged as the single most sensitive marker for Down syndrome detection. The use of NT measurement has in turn created an opportunity for the evaluation of several other promising ultrasound markers in the first trimester.

NUCHAL TRANSLUCENCY

NT refers to the sonographic appearance of fluid collection localized to the space between the skin and deeper tissues at the back of the neck. The association between first-trimester nuchal fluid collection and major chromosome anomalies was reported more than a decade ago.[9,10]

The studies performed in the early and mid 1990s revealed a strong association between the depth of the first-trimester nuchal fluid pocket and the risk of mainly trisomy 21 and other chromosome defects. The etiology of this excessive fluid collection has been attributed to a number of plausible factors working individually or in concert. These include lymphatic dysplasia leading to accumulation of extracellular fluid, biochemical changes in the extracellular ground substance leading to increased water retention, transient cardiac failure often associated with cardiovascular abnormalities, and venous compression within the fetal chest or posterior cranial fossa.[11] Among first-trimester fetuses with increased NT approximately 28.7% have chromosome defects. Down syndrome accounts for 49.1% of these chromosomal disorders.[12] Among many of the earlier studies using NT for Down syndrome screening, marked variation in Down syndrome detection rates (33%–91%) were reported. This seemed initially to represent a significant challenge to the practical use and wide dissemination of the test.[13] The reasons for the extreme variability of results included lack of accepted technical standards for NT measurement at the time, varying definitions of "increased" NT, and gestational age differences between studies. Use of standardized techniques for measuring NT was subsequently shown to result in a high Down syndrome detection rate (72%), at a false-positive rate of 5%, in a large multi-center study of low-risk women.[12] In addition, between 60% and 87% of other major chromosome anomalies were detected. The detection of non–Down syndrome chromosome anomalies represented a significant accomplishment because Down syndrome cases constitute only 50% of major chromosomal abnormalities seen in the highest epidemiologic risk group (ie, women ≥ 35 years old).

Guidelines for the systematic measurement of NT have been published[14] and are now widely used. Specific training in obtaining standardized measurements is required for all individuals performing these assessments and ongoing audits of the quality of the measurements are critical components of effective NT-based screening programs.[15] Currently two organizations, the Society of Maternal Fetal Medicine and the Fetal Medicine Foundation of America, have established programs for training and quality assurance for NT measurement programs in the United States.

A commonly asked patient question is what NT threshold measurement value expressed in millimeters should be considered abnormal. It is important to bear in mind that in normal first-trimester fetuses the NT increases with crown-rump length and advancing gestational age.[16] Specific threshold definitions of abnormal NT in millimeters are less meaningful because the value changes with gestational age. To standardize for the variation of NT with crown-rump length, the measured value of the NT is divided by the expected average (median) NT value for that particular crown-rump length value. NT values are expressed as multiples of the normal median (MoM) average. It is this NT value, expressed as MoM rather than in millimeters, combined with maternal age and serum marker values, also expressed as MoM, which is used to derive a numerical Down syndrome risk estimate. Risk estimates of greater than 1 in 270 or 1 in 300 are commonly used to define the threshold for a high-risk group. It is also important to bear in mind that although these risk thresholds are somewhat arbitrary they are designed to achieve the optimal (maximum) sensitivity and specificity values for Down syndrome detection.

In 2004, Nicolaides and colleagues[11] systematically reviewed prospective Down syndrome screening studies using first-trimester NT in the preceding 10 years. There were greater than 200,000 first-trimester patients evaluated of which 871 had Down syndrome. First-trimester NT was found to have a detection rate of 76.8% with a false-positive rate of 4.2%.

The optimal time to schedule NT measurement seems to be 12 to 13 weeks,[17] although the measurement is valid from 10 4/7 to 13 6/7 weeks. Definitive confirmation of the validity of NT measurements obtained earlier in gestation is currently not available.

The first large American multicenter first-trimester study, the blood-urine-NT study, was performed in 2003. A total of 8514 singleton pregnancies of which 61 had Down syndrome were screened between 10 4/7 and 13 6/7 weeks in 12 centers.[18] NT combined with maternal age detected 68.8% of trisomy 21 at 5% false-positive rate. Corresponding values for trisomy 18 were 81.8% and 2.9%, respectively.

A subsequent prospective study, the FASTER trial, was also performed in the United States and evaluated NT performance between 10 3/7 and 13 6/7 weeks.[19] A total of 38,033 patients were enrolled with 92 Down syndrome cases. Unlike the prior study,[18] first-trimester cystic hygroma cases, increased NT measurements, and septations, a group known to have elevated risk of chromosome anomalies, were excluded from analysis. There were 134 of these cases of which 25 had Down syndrome. This affected the overall performance of the NT measurement. After excluding the cases designated as having first-trimester cystic hygromas, for a fixed 75% detection rate, NT measurement by itself had an 8.1%, 9%, and 12% false-positive rate at 11, 12, and 13 weeks gestation, respectively.

The SURUSS trial (serum, urine, and ultrasound screening study) was a large British multicenter study consisting of 25 participating centers.[20] A total of 47,053 singleton pregnancies were screened between 9 and 13 weeks and again between 14 and 20 weeks. Analysis was limited to 98 Down syndrome cases and a matched control group of 490 normals. At an 85% detection rate, the NT reportedly had 85% detection and 15% false-positive rate. The SURRUS trial included cases as low as 9 weeks gestational age. This was the case for 40% of the Down syndrome fetuses. Overall, in about 9% of normals and 16% of Down syndrome cases, NT measurements were not obtainable compared with less than 1% average for other large trials.[11] As noted previously, NT diagnostic accuracy is not proved to be optimal at such low gestational ages, and its validity remains to be demonstrated. Collectively, these large prospective studies performed both in the United States and overseas confirmed the diagnostic accuracy of the NT measurement by itself for the detection of Down syndrome fetuses.

FIRST-TRIMESTER SERUM ANALYTES

In contrast to the findings in the mid-trimester, most first-trimester studies suggest that maternal serum intact hCG is only moderately elevated in Down syndrome pregnancies compared with normal pregnancies. A meta-analysis of first-trimester Down syndrome cases revealed an average maternal serum intact hCG level of 1.33 MoM or 33% higher levels than normal controls.[21] This compares with an average elevation of 2.06 MoM for mid-trimester Down syndrome cases.[22] Currently, the dissociated free β subunit of hCG is more commonly used than intact hCG in first-trimester Down syndrome screening. The average level in the first-trimester Down syndrome pregnancies is 1.98 MoM.[22] Although a few studies had previously suggested no advantage to measuring free β-hCG over intact hCG,[23] extensive direct comparison of intact hCG and free β-hCG[24,25] show free β-hCG to be significantly elevated compared with total hCG in the serum of first-trimester women with Down syndrome fetuses.

PAPP-A is a glycoprotein that, like hCG, is produced by the trophoblast. Studies have consistently shown significantly reduced levels of this analyte in the serum of women carrying a first-trimester Down syndrome pregnancy. The average level of first-trimester serum PAPP-A in affected pregnancies is approximately 0.43 MoM, consistent with a greater than 50% reduction. This contrasts with free β-hCG, whose Down syndrome detection rate increases with gestational age during this period. By itself first-trimester PAPP-A has a Down syndrome detection rate of 38%. Combined with maternal age, the detection rate improves to 48%,[26] making it the more powerful of the widely used first-trimester biochemical markers.

GESTATIONAL AGE AND THE ACCURACY OF FIRST-TRIMESTER SCREEN

With widespread use of combined screen it has become apparent that the diagnostic value of individual markers changes with the gestational age at testing. The published literature was extensively reviewed by Palomaki and colleagues.[27] They reviewed 13 publications that measured median MoM PAPP-A levels in Down syndrome pregnancies from 9 to 14 weeks. Median MoM value increased progressively from 0.36 to 0.60 MoM and 0.59 MoM at 13 and 14 completed weeks, respectively. The discriminatory power of this marker decreased with advancing gestation within the first trimester and was highest at 9 weeks. Corresponding values for free β-hCG were 1.71 MoM at 9 weeks and increased to 2.17 MoM at 13 weeks and 2.52 MoM at 14 weeks. In contrast to PAPP-A, the discriminatory power of free β-hCG increases with advancing gestational age within the first trimester. A similar trend was noted with intact hCG levels in first-trimester pregnancies as seen for free β-hCG. Free β-hCG MoM values seemed consistently higher than intact hCG at each gestational age interval. These findings support the view that free β-hCG is advantageous to intact hCG for first-trimester screening.

Based on data from two studies reviewed by Palomaki and colleagues,[27] NT values in Down syndrome cases seemed to fall with advancing gestation, indicating a decline in the discriminatory power of this marker with advancing gestation. For the combined test, at a fixed detection rate of 75%, false-positive rates were modeled to be 1.9%, 2%, and 2.6%, respectively at 11, 12, and 13 weeks.

Based on the differential performance of serum and NT markers at varying gestational ages, the so-called "consecutive combined test" has been proposed wherein the serum markers are obtained between 8 and 13 weeks, whereas NT is measured between 11 and 13 weeks. The performance of first-trimester screening between 7 and 13 weeks was reported for 44,537 singleton pregnancies of which 120 had trisomy 21.[28] For cases in which serum samples were obtained between 7 and less than 10 weeks Down syndrome detection rate (combined screen) was 97% (confidence interval, 95%–99%), whereas cases in which blood was drawn greater than 10 to 13 weeks detection rate was 79% (confidence interval, 61%–91%). In addition, the screen positive rate was reportedly significantly lower in the less than 10 weeks group, although the actual value was not provided. It seems that significant further gains in diagnostic accuracy can be achieved with a strategy of early biochemistry combined with later NT measurement.

OTHER FIRST-TRIMESTER SERUM MARKERS

Other serologic markers of proved efficacy in the mid-trimester Down syndrome screening have also been evaluated in the first trimester. These include AFP, unconjugated estriol, and inhibin A. None of these have been shown to be of substantial clinical value in early pregnancy. Maternal serum AFP is reduced by approximately 13% in first-trimester Down syndrome cases compared with normal, for serum unconjugated estriol the reduction is approximately 30%, whereas inhibin A levels are modestly increased to between 25% and 40% in Down syndrome pregnancies.[29] This compares with an 85% increase in inhibin A in mid-trimester Down syndrome cases compared with normal.[30] Efforts continue toward the identification of additional first-trimester serum markers. In a small study by Koster and colleagues[31] additional first-trimester serum markers were evaluated with the traditional combined test. AFP, epidermal growth factor, extracellular rage binding protein, haptoglobin, insulin, and lipoprotein seemed to further improve detection rate over free β-hCG, PAPP-A, and NT. Using mathematical modeling, the combined test had a detection rate of 56.2% at a 5% false-positive rate. The six serum markers by themselves had detection and false-positive rates, respectively, of 38.7% and when combined with PAPP-A and free β-hCG this rose to 78.9%. When the new markers were added to the combined test detection rate was 82.5%. All sensitivity values were determined against a 5% false-positive rate.

COMBINED MATERNAL SERUM AND SONOGRAPHIC MARKERS

The combination of first-trimester biochemistry, free β-hCG, and PAPP-A with NT measurements constitutes the so-called "combined first-trimester screen." The results of the first large American-only multicenter first-trimester study, blood-urine-NT screening group in 2003, found that the combined screen had a 78.7% detection rate for trisomy 21 at 5% false-positive rate. In addition, 90.0% of trisomy 18 cases were detected for a 2% false-positive rate. The study first demonstrated the clinical feasibility of first-trimester screening in the general United States population. Among women greater than or equal to 35 years, the detection rate was 89.8% for trisomy 21 cases at a false-positive rate of 15.2%.

The FASTER trial[19] reported a 77% detection rate at 3.2% false-positive rate for the combined test after exclusion of cases designated as having first-trimester hygromas. When cystic hygroma cases were included the first-trimester detection rate increased to 82%.

The SURUSS trial[20] reported an 80% detection rate because the combined first-trimester test had a 2.3% false-positive rate. Other large trials have confirmed the diagnostic accuracy of the combined first-trimester test. A large prospective study of Avgidou and colleagues[32] evaluated first-trimester screening in 30,564 pregnancies between 11 and 13 + 6 weeks. There were 330 chromosome anomalies of which 196 had trisomy 21. The combined test detected 93.4% of Down syndrome, 92.3% of trisomy 18, 88.9% of trisomy 13, 84.2% of Turner syndrome, and 86.1% of other chromosome anomalies for a 7.5% false-positive rate. The accuracy of NT measurement in prenatal Down syndrome screening has been rigorously and extensively tested and it's central role has been confirmed.

COMBINING FIRST- AND SECOND-TRIMESTER SCREENING

Traditional Down syndrome screening was limited to the measurement of a group of markers all of which are obtained in the same trimester. Wald and colleagues[33] subsequently proposed an algorithm, the "integrated test," combining first-trimester (NT, PAPP-A) with second-trimester (AFP, hCG, unconjugated estriol, and inhibin A) markers along with maternal age. Using mathematical modeling, an improvement in Down syndrome detection rates over first-trimester combined test was projected. For example, at a fixed 5% false-positive rate, a detection rate of 94% versus 85% was projected for integrated versus combined first-trimester test, respectively. Based on these projections, women who screened positive on integrated test had a higher likelihood of actually having a Down syndrome fetus (ie, a higher positive predictive value). Other projected benefits of integrated screening include fewer invasive tests (chorionic villus sampling or amniocentesis) and fewer iatrogenic miscarriages caused by invasive procedures.[19,20] An important feature of the integrated test is that testing is not considered complete until both first- and second-trimester markers have been obtained. As a consequence no results are provided before the second trimester. Reportedly, only a small percentage of women screened would have a first-trimester Down syndrome risk level so high that the mid-trimester marker results could not possibly reduce the overall risk level to within the normal range. By this reasoning, a policy of releasing risk estimates at the end of the first-trimester component of the test would not be worthwhile because second-trimester blood test would only rarely be avoidable.[34] One of the largest prospective studies of integrated tests reported a detection rate of 85% at 0.9% false-positive rate compared with a false-positive rate of 4.3% at the same detection rate for the combined first-trimester test in the case control SURRUS trial.[20] The largest such American trial[19] found a 94% to 96% detection rate for integrated testing versus 82% to 87% for combined first-trimester test at a 5% false-positive rate. An outcomes analysis using medical cost assumptions relevant to the United States health care system found the integrated screening performed in the United States population would be more expensive than combined screening.[35] However, integrated screening would avert a moderately higher number of Down syndrome livebirths and significantly reduce the number of iatrogenic miscarriages caused by invasive procedures. Integrated screening cost slightly more for each trisomy 21 livebirth averted. Both strategies averted substantially more trisomy 21 livebirths than mid-trimester serum screening. Largely similar findings were reported in another analysis with more cases of Down syndrome liveborns averted with overall higher cost with the integrated test.[36]

Potential disadvantages and concerns raised with integrated screening include ethical issues occasioned by a delay in reporting significant first-trimester information, such as increased Down syndrome risk on first screen, patient anxiety generated by having to wait 3 to 4 weeks between initiation and completion of the test, and the loss of the benefits of early screening.[37] The possibility that significant numbers of patients in a clinical setting might fail to complete the test after performing the first-trimester component is a potential disadvantage. An argument in favor of integrated screening is that even with a positive first-trimester screen some patients may decline all invasive testing or elect to wait for mid-trimester amniocentesis and present an opportunity for mid-trimester serum analysis in any case. There is in addition some evidence that although patients generally value early testing, many are willing to delay the testing for a few weeks if it results in improved detection rate. Strategies by which the results of the first-trimester test can be disclosed to the patient with subsequent mid-trimester "stepwise sequential screening" have been proposed. This involves reporting positive first-trimester results to patients, with negative first-trimester screen cases going on to have additional mid-trimester serum testing. This algorithm doubled the false-positive rate compared with the integrated screening.[19] Finally, the development of other first-trimester sonographic markers, such as nasal bone measurement and ductus venosus Doppler velocimetry, has raised the possibility that screening performance similar to that reported for the integrated test may be achievable within the first trimester.[37,38]

Recently, a new algorithm of "contingent" screening has also been proposed. Patients are given their first-trimester results and offered invasive testing if positive and no further testing if negative, whereas cases with "intermediate" risk levels are offered additional mid-trimester testing. The purposed advantages are earlier screening and diagnosis overall with only a marginal increase in false-positive rates compared with the integrated test. It is hoped that extensive prospective testing in a patient population will be forthcoming.[39] The serum integrated test using first trimester PAPP-A and the mid-trimester QUAD screen has been proposed for circumstances in which NT measurement expertise is not available. This was found to have a Down syndrome detection rate of 85% to 88% detection rate at 5% false-positive rate.[19] Combining first- and second-trimester mid-trimester Down syndrome screening results as if they are independent, "sequential" screening, increases in the Down syndrome detection rate up to 94% to 98% but the false-positive rate is unacceptably high at 11% to 17%.[40,41] This particular approach is not generally recommended because of the high false-positive rate.

Overall, the currently available evidence suggests that at a false-positive rate of 5%, the integrated screen improves the Down syndrome detection rate by between 5% and 10% over combined first-trimester screen. Conversely, at a fixed detection rate of 85% the integrated test reduces the false-positive rate and the number of patients needing to undergo invasive testing (false-positive rate) by approximately 4 percentage points to a range of 0.9% to 2.8%, compared with the combined first-trimester screen. The implication is that integrated testing could lead to fewer invasive tests to detect the same number of Down syndrome cases compared with the current combined first-trimester test. Factoring in no-show rate for the second portion of the test decreases the effectiveness of this algorithm.

CURRENT STATUS OF FIRST TRIMESTER–BASED ANEUPLOIDY SCREENING IN THE UNITED STATES

A few national surveys have tracked the use of first-trimester and combined first- and mid-trimester Down syndrome screening among maternal-fetal medicine specialists in the United States. Fang and colleagues[42] and Egan and colleagues[43] documented survey responses from 543 maternal-fetal medicine specialists in 2001 and 448 in 2007. Over the survey period, a highly significant increase in the percentage of maternal-fetal medicine specialists performing first-trimester screen was documented (43.1% vs 97.3%; $P<.0001$). Similarly significant increase in the use of NT in first-trimester screening (48.5% vs 96.6%; $P<.0001$) was also observed. The relative rates of use indicated that the combined screen was the most frequently used of the first trimester–based screening strategies at 56%. Stepwise sequential (first-trimester results immediately reported and final risk based on combined first- and second-trimester results) was used by 29% of specialists, the integrated test (first-trimester results withheld with reporting of risk based on combined first- and second-trimester tests) by 13.6%, and contingency screening (offering invasive testing, no further testing, or second-trimester screen based on certain cut off values from first-trimester test) by 11.8%.

In a similar study, Driscoll and colleagues[44] surveyed 348 general obstetrician gynecologists. In their response, 42% frequently used the combined test, 28% used it on a case-by-case basis, and 30% rarely or never used the test. For the sequential test the frequencies were 15%, 21%, and 64%. For the serum integrated test (PAPP-A plus QUAD screen) the rates were 5%, 11%, and 64%. Of further interest were the physicians (obstetricians, gynecologists, and maternal-fetal medicine specialists) estimation of the acceptance rate for Down syndrome screening among their patients.[44] Estimated acceptance rates were consistently higher in women greater than or equal to 35 years. Acceptance rates also appeared highest in the Northeast and West and lowest in the Midwest, with the South occupying in intermediate position. In all regions, the estimated acceptance rates were greater than 58%, with the exception of women less than 34 years in the Midwest (estimated acceptance 48.01% $\pm$ 3.42%).

There has been dramatic progress in Down syndrome screening marker development. The nucleus of this advance has been the discovery and development of first-trimester ultrasound and biochemical markers. Recent surveys indicate that both physicians and patients in the United States have embraced first trimester–based screening where available. A collateral benefit of this progress has been high detection rates for all the other common aneuploidies and significant chromosomal structural anomalies.

The central role played by the ultrasound marker NT had been completely unanticipated more than two decades ago. The collateral benefits of this marker are only now being sufficiently acknowledged. There seems to be an association between NT measurement and nonchromosomal structural defects and the risk of miscarriage and stillbirths. One of the greatest practical benefits of routine first-trimester ultrasound is the opportunity to precisely date a pregnancy by measuring the crown-rump length. Implications for common pregnancy diagnoses and practice, such as fetal growth restriction, postdating pregnancy, and iatrogenic prematurity are profound and potentially supersede the value of ultrasound markers for fetal aneuploidy detection.

SUMMARY

NT measurement in the first trimester is the most sensitive individual marker for Down syndrome detection in the prenatal period. The diagnostic benefits extend to the detection of all common aneuploidies and an assortment of chromosomal aberrations including clinically significant deletions and inversions. The addition of biochemical markers further improves the detection of Down syndrome and other common aneuploidies. Current clinical guidelines now recognize the value of first-trimester screening making maternal age only a second-order risk predictor of use in patients who have declined or have not had the benefit of ultrasound or biochemical screening. Serial surveys indicate already significant and accelerating patient acceptance of this screening modality.

REFERENCES

1. Merkatz IR, Nitowsky HM, Macri JN, et al. An association between low serum alpha-fetoprotein and fetal chromosomal abnormalities. Am J Obstet Gynecol 1984;148(7):886–94.
2. Cuckle HS, Wald NJ, Lindenbaum RH. Maternal serum alpha-fetoprotein measurement: a screening test for Down syndrome. Lancet 1984;1:926–9.
3. DiMaio MS, Baumgarten A, Greenstein RM, et al. Screening for fetal Down's syndrome in pregnancy by measuring maternal serum alpha-fetoprotein levels. N Engl J Med 1987;317(6):342–6.
4. ACOG Committee on Practice Bulletins. ACOG Practice Bulletin No. 77: screening for fetal chromosomal abnormalities. Obstet Gynecol 2007;109(1): 217–27.
5. Grant SS. Options for Down syndrome screening: what will women choose? J Midwifery Womens Health 2005;50(3):211–8.
6. Bishop AJ, Marteau TM, Armstrong D, et al. Women and health care professionals' preferences for Down's syndrome screening tests: a conjoint analysis study. BJOG 2004;111(8):775–9.
7. Lewis SM, Cullinane FN, Carlin JB, et al. Women's and healthcare professionals' preferences in prenatal testing for Down syndrome in Australia. Aust N Z J Obstet Gynaecol 2006;46(3):205–11.
8. Lo TK, Lai FK, Leung WC, et al. Screening options for Down syndrome: how women choose in real clinical setting. Prenat Diagn 2009;29(9):852–6.
9. Bronstein M, Rottem S, Yoffe N, et al. First-trimester and early second-trimester diagnosis of nuchal cystic hygroma by transvaginal sonography: diverse prognosis of the septated from the nonseptated lesion. Am J Obstet Gynecol 1990; 163(1 Pt 1):267–9.
10. Cullen MT, Gabrielli S, Green JJ, et al. Diagnosis and significance of cystic hygroma in the first trimester. Prenat Diagn 1990;10(10):643–51.
11. Nicolaides KH, Heath V, Liao AW. Nuchal translucency and other first-trimester sonographic markers of chromosomal abnormalities. Am J Obstet Gynecol 2004;191(1):45–67.
12. Snijders RJ, Noble P, Sebire N, et al. UK multicenter project on detection rate for other chromosome defects trisomy 18 assessment of risk of trisomy 21 by maternal age and fetal nuchal-translucency thickness at 10–14 weeks of gestation. Lancet 1998;352(9125):343–6.

13. Malone FD, Berkowitz RZ, Canick JA, et al. First-trimester screening for aneuploidy: research or standard of care? Am J Obstet Gynecol 2000;182(3):490–6.
14. Nicolaides KH, Heath V, Liao AW. The 11–14 week scan. Baillieres Best Pract Res Clin Obstet Gynaecol 2000;14(4):581–94.
15. Snijders RJ, Thom EA, Zachary JM, et al. First-trimester trisomy screening: nuchal translucency measurement training and quality assurance to correct and unify technique. Ultrasound Obstet Gynecol 2002;19(4):353–9.
16. Pajkrt E, Bilardo CM, Van Lith JM, et al. Nuchal translucency measurement in normal fetuses. Obstet Gynecol 1995;86(6):994–7.
17. Mulney S, Baker L, Edwards A, et al. Optimising the timing for nuchal translucency measurement. Prenat Diagn 2002;22(9):775–7.
18. Wapner R, Thom E, Simpson JL, et al. First trimester screening for trisomy 21 and 18. N Engl J Med 2003;349(15):1405–13.
19. Malone FD, Canick JA, Ball RH, et al. First-trimester or second-trimester screening, or both, for Down's syndrome. N Engl J Med 2005;353(19):2001–11.
20. Wald NJ, Rodeck C, Hackshaw AK, et al. SURUSS in perspective. BJOG 2004; 111(6):521–31.
21. Spencer K. Aneuploidy screening in the first trimester. Am J Med Genet C Semin Med Genet 2007;145C(1):18–32.
22. Wald NJ, Kennard A, Hackenshaw A, et al. Antenatal screening for Down's syndrome. Health Technol Assess 1998;2(1):9–32.
23. Haddow JE, Palomki GE, Knight GJ, et al. Screening of maternal serum for fetal Down's syndrome in the first trimester. N Engl J Med 1998;338(14):955–61.
24. Spencer K, Coombes EJ, Mallard AS, et al. Free beta human chorionic gonadtropin in Down syndrome screenings: a multicenter study of its role compared with other biochemical markers. Ann Clin Biochem 1992;30(Pt 5):512–8.
25. Wald NJ, Rodeck E, Hakenshaw AK, et al. First and second trimester antenatal screening for Down's syndrome: the results of Serum Urine and Ultrasound Screening Study (SURUSS). J Med Screen 2003;10(2):56–104.
26. Spencer K, Souter V, Tul N, et al. A screening program for trisomy 21 at 10–14 weeks using total nuchal translucency, maternal serum free ß-human chorionic gonadotropin and pregnancy. Ultrasound Obstet Gynecol 1999;13(4):231–7.
27. Palomaki GE, Lambert-Messerlian GM, Canick JA. A summary analysis of Down syndrome markers in the late first trimester. Adv Clin Chem 2007;43:177–210.
28. Torring N. Performance of first trimester screening between gestational weeks 7 and 13. Clin Chem 2009;55(8):1564–7.
29. Spencer K, Liao AW, Ong CYT, et al. Maternal serum levels of dimeric inhibin A in pregnancies affected by trisomy 21 in the first trimester. Prenat Diagn 2001;21:441–4.
30. Wald NJ, Kennard A, Hackshaw AK. First trimester serum screening for Down's syndrome. Prenat Diagn 1995;15(13):1227–40 [erratum in: Prenat Diagn 1996;16(4):387].
31. Koster M, Pennings J, Imholz S, et al. Bead-based multiplexed immunoassays to identify new biomarker in maternal serum to improve first trimester Down syndrome screening. Prenat Diagn 2009;29(9):857–62.
32. Avgidou K, Papageorghiou A, Bindra R, et al. Prospective first-trimester screening for trisomy 21 in 30,564 pregnancies. Am J Obstet Gynecol 2005; 192(6):1761–7.
33. Wald NJ, Watt HC, Hackenshaw AK. Integrated screening for Down's syndrome on the basis of tests performed during the first and second trimesters. N Engl J Med 1999;341(7):461–7.

34. Hackshaw AK, Wald NJ. Assessment of the value of reporting partial screening results in prenatal screening for Down syndrome. Prenat Diagn 2001;21(9): 737–40.
35. Biggio JR Jr, Morris TC, Owen J, et al. An outcomes analysis of five prenatal screening strategies for trisomy 21 in women younger than 35 years. Am J Obstet Gynecol 2004;190(3):721–9.
36. Odibo A, Stamilio DM, Nelson DB, et al. A cost-effectiveness analysis of prenatal screening strategies for Down syndrome. Obstet Gynecol 2005;106(3):562–8 [erratum in: Obstet Gynecol 2006;107(1):209].
37. Copel JA, Bahado-Singh RO. Prenatal screening for Down's syndrome–a search for the family's values. N Engl J Med 1999;341(7):521–2 [comment in: N Engl J Med 1999;341(25):1935–6; author reply: 1937; comment on: N Engl J Med 1999;341(7):461–7].
38. Nicolaides KH, Spencer K, Avgidou K, et al. Multicenter study of first-trimester screening for trisomy 21 in 75 821 pregnancies: results and estimation of the potential impact of individual risk-orientated two-stage first-trimester screening. Ultrasound Obstet Gynecol 2005;25:221–6.
39. Wright D, Bradbury I, Benn P, et al. Contingent screening for Down syndrome is an efficient alternative to non-disclosure sequential screening. Prenat Diagn 2004;24(10):762–6.
40. Platt LD, Greene N, Johnson A, et al. Sequential pathways of testing after first trimester screening for trisomy 21. Obstet Gynecol 2004;104(4):661–6.
41. Malone FD. Sequential pathways of testing after first-trimester screening for trisomy 21. Obstet Gynecol 2005;105(2):438 [author reply: 438–9].
42. Fang YM, Benn P, Campbell W, et al. Down syndrome screening in the United States in 2001 and 2007: a survey of maternal-fetal medicine specialists. Am J Obstet Gynecol 2009;201(1):97.e1–5.
43. Egan JF, Kaminsky LM, DeRoche ME, et al. Antenatal Down syndrome screening in the United States in 2001: a survey of maternal-fetal medicine specialists. Am J Obstet Gynecol 2002;187(5):1230–4.
44. Driscoll DA, Morgan MA, Schulkin J. Screening for Down syndrome: changing practice of obstetricians. Am J Obstet Gynecol 2009;200(4):459.e1–9.

First-Trimester Genetic Counseling: Perspectives and Considerations

Eugene Pergament, MD, PhD

KEYWORDS

• First trimester screening • Genetic counseling
• Chromosome abnormalities • Obstetric care

Over the past decade, first trimester screening has assumed an increasingly dominant role in the obstetric care of prospective parents. Initially introduced for purposes of identifying pregnancies at risk for Down syndrome,[1] first trimester screening now encompasses risk assessments for other chromosome abnormalities,[2] cardiac malformations,[3] congenital malformation syndromes,[4] adverse pregnancy outcome,[5,6] and preeclampsia.[7–9] As a consequence, first trimester screening has generated an indisputable need for intense genetic counseling, if all of its clinical implications are to be fully understood by prospective parents. This task is a daunting challenge indeed, given the general population's understanding of risk, particularly its formulation and meaning, a challenge that can be effectively addressed only by medical geneticists and genetic counselors knowledgeable in all aspects of first trimester screening. Here then is one view of what the genetic counseling should comprise following first trimester measurements of nuchal translucency and related ultrasound findings[10–14] and the maternal serum proteins pregnancy associated plasma protein A (PAPP-A) and free beta human chorionic gonadotrophin (hCG).

BACKGROUND

In the 1960s, when formal genetic counseling became recognized as an essential medical specialty, the primary focus addressed 3 parental questions generated by the birth of a child with a developmental/congenital malformation syndrome: (1) what happened (ie, why was my child born with birth defects), (2) why me (ie, why am I the parent of a child born with birth defects), and (3) will this happen again (ie,

Northwestern Reproductive Genetics, Inc, 680 North Lake Shore Drive, Suite 1230, Chicago, IL 60611, USA
E-mail address: e-pergament@northwestern.edu

Clin Lab Med 30 (2010) 557–563
doi:10.1016/j.cll.2010.05.004
0272-2712/10/$ – see front matter © 2010 Elsevier Inc. All rights reserved.

labmed.theclinics.com

what is the risk for recurrence of a similarly affected birth)? The introduction of prenatal diagnostic testing in the 1970s, almost exclusively for women of advanced maternal age at increased risk for a conception with a chromosome abnormality, generated another set of informational responsibilities for genetic counselors: (1) why am I being offered genetic testing that carries a risk to the pregnancy, that is, what are the risks (ie, pregnancy loss, harm to fetus and mother) and the benefits (ie, detecting a conception with a genetic disorder, such as a chromosome abnormality) of such testing; (2) how is the procedure performed (ie, first trimester chorionic villus sampling (CVS) or second trimester amniocentesis); and (3) what are the options if a genetic abnormality is identified in the fetus?

When second trimester maternal serum screening for open neural tube defects was introduced in the 1980s, all pregnant women were subject to testing not just those at high reproductive risk. Counseling for this developmental anomaly was primarily provided by obstetricians, maternal fetal medicine physicians, and ultrasonographers, a practice that for the most part continues to the present. Second trimester maternal serum screening, initially for Down syndrome and then for trisomy 18, generated the need for increased interaction between medical geneticists/genetic counselors and obstetricians. Concepts such as false positive and false negative became common parlance of obstetricians and their patients. And, because of these concepts and their consequences, second trimester maternal serum screening, even as practiced today, is also couched with considerable reservations on the part of many obstetricians and their patients. It is not uncommon, for example, to learn of health professionals or their patients who for a variety of reasons think that second trimester maternal serum screening for Down syndrome makes mistakes or is not accurate. This negative characterization has to some degree carried over to first trimester screening for Down syndrome, despite its higher detection rate and lower false positive rate when compared with second trimester maternal serum screening. The first challenge, therefore, in providing genetic counseling to prospective parents in the case of first trimester screening is to distinguish between screening and diagnosis, their advantages, disadvantages, and ramifications.

CONSIDERATIONS

Genetic counseling, as provided to prospective parents undergoing first trimester screening, requires both art and science, to use an old proverbial saying. Here, more likely than in the routine obstetric visit, both prospective parents are likely to participate in the discussion before or following first trimester screening. One of the many challenges to the medical geneticist/genetic counselor is to engage the male partner, recognizing that all of the screenings focus on the female partner in terms of her age, the ultrasound findings of the fetus, and the maternal serum measurements. That engagement also allows the medical geneticist/genetic counselor to gauge the level of patients' understanding and to make initial judgments as to how to proceed. In addition to inquiring about their pregnancy history and their occupations, past and present, one speaks to (ie, counsels) a pregnant couple and not to a pregnant woman. Formalized tutorials in genetic counseling in the past emphasized that counselors present themselves as objective, impartial, and nondirective at all times during the counseling session. This approach, although appropriate with certain couples, lacks the degree of expression of understanding, sympathy, and compassion that recognizes the nervousness, worry, apprehension, and fear that most pregnant couples bring to a counseling session, discussing for the first time the wellbeing of their pregnancy. If empathy toward these concerns requires that the medical geneticist/genetic counselor compromise objectivity, impartiality, and detachment, contrary to past teachings, this can be deemed a categorical imperative.

A counselor must not only be able to maintain objectivity but at the right time and under the right circumstance, the counselor must consider exposing their own feelings about what course of action would best meet, in the counselor's judgment, the needs of the pregnant couple. For example, following first trimester screening in patients of advanced maternal age, previously considered a mandatory candidate for invasive testing under the now defunct standard of being 35 years of age or older, the question generally arises as to what course of additional testing, if any, should be considered: screening or diagnostic. This experience is all too frequent because women aged 35 years and older may comprise, as a group, the largest number undergoing first trimester screening. In such cases, the medical geneticist/genetic counselor must not only act as the pregnant couple's personal advocate but also present meaningful alternatives to their decisions concerning further testing, in essence play the devil's advocate to help sharpen their decision making.

PERSPECTIVES

The current focus of first trimester screening, based on publications and presentations at national and international meetings, is detection rate: the detection rates for aneuploidy, cardiac defects,[3] developmental/genetic syndromes,[4] adverse pregnancy outcomes,[6] and preeclampsia.[7,9] This predominantly undivided attention to detection rates and their corollary parameters (false positive and false positive rates) fails to take into account the overwhelming majority of women, 97% and greater, who will not only complete their pregnancy but will complete their pregnancy with a healthy outcome. A major contribution of first trimester screening is the ability to demonstrate visually and through chemistry that within the context of these technologies a pregnancy is developing normally. It is all too common that following first trimester ultrasound evaluation of nuchal translucency, pregnant couples, particularly those with their first pregnancy, enter a counseling session with considerable apprehension that something is wrong with their pregnancy. Recognizing that the medical geneticist/genetic counselor must address the issues of detection rates (false positive rates and false negative rates), the counseling must put into proper perspective that first trimester screening not only assesses the current developmental status of the fetus but also serves as the most meaningful predictor of pregnancy outcome with regard to aneuploidy, cardiac defects, and developmental/genetic syndromes.

The main challenge to providing meaningful genetic counseling following first trimester screening is to conduct a discussion that leads the pregnant couple to make decisions about their pregnancy that meet their needs and their lifestyle, and with which they can feel responsible for the consequences. To attain this goal, it is important that the pregnant couple understand as completely as possible the concept of risk and, in particular, how to use risk assessment in reaching a responsible decision. In the course of these discussions, however, all too often there is tension between a pregnant couple's own risk assessment and their tendency to interpret results in black and white terms. For example, following a counselor's description of how measurement of nuchal translucency in their pregnancy will be converted into a risk assessment for Down syndrome, it is not uncommon for a couple to ask if that measurement is normal or abnormal.

The difficulty in properly interpreting the meaning and implications of risk is obviously not unique to first trimester screening. Rather, it reflects much of the general population's difficulty in thinking in terms of probability. In the case of first trimester screening, overcoming that inability, if present, is essential to successful genetic counseling. If pregnant couples are to be faulted, this failing must be shared not only by our educational system but also by the medical community. All too frequently an obstetrician or nurse assistant, instead of taking the time to define the relative risk for Down syndrome, simply inform prospective parents by telephone that their second trimester maternal serum screening is "normal" or "abnormal."

CONSIDERATIONS

First trimester screening does require face-to-face consultation by health care professionals with expertise in the interpretation of nuchal translucency and biochemical marker measurements and of the clinical implications and ramifications of the results. Such consultations should be limited to medical geneticists, genetic counselors, and obstetric geneticists certified by agencies specifically established for evaluating not just the quality of nuchal translucency and related ultrasound measurements (eg, presence or absence of nasal bone,[10] fetal heart rate,[2] ductus venosus flow,[11] tricuspid regurgitation,[12-14] and so forth) but of increasing importance, knowledge about the clinical associations of the biochemical markers(eg, low PAPP-A levels and prematurity,[6] reduced fetal growth,[5] and so forth).

Listed subsequently is an outline of the minimal components and content of a genetic counseling session devoted to informing prospective parents about the results of their first trimester screening for Down syndrome and trisomies 13 and 18. This outline also pertains to any discussion of pregnancies deemed at increased risk either for possible cardiac malformations or developmental/genetic syndromes because of increased nuchal translucency or adverse pregnancy outcome because of significantly reduced levels of the serum markers PAPP-A and free beta hCG.

1. The genetic counseling session should begin with an overview of the first trimester screening process, with emphasis on 2 major considerations presented to the prospective parents:

    All pregnancies are at risk for a conception with a chromosome abnormality, such as Down syndrome.

    Chromosome abnormalities are the cause of significant developmental disabilities, including mental and physical retardation and congenital malformations.

2. The main components of first trimester screening are identified and consist of assessing risk for a conception with a chromosome abnormality based on (1) maternal age, (2) nuchal translucency (and nasal bone presence, if possible), and (3) two maternal serum proteins, PAPP-A and free beta hCG. The concept of independent variables is introduced and how that allows the individual risk assessment of each screening component to be combined. The introduction to the description of the results of the first trimester screening concludes by stating the underlying philosophy of first trimester screening: the more independent variables that can be combined the more accurate the risk assessment.

3. Each component of the first trimester screening approach is subsequently detailed:

    The relationship between advancing maternal age and increased risk for a conception with a chromosome abnormality is well known by almost all prospective parents. A simple graph illustrating this relationship is useful. Attention is then given to the process by which the age-related risk for a chromosome abnormality is obtained specific to the individual pregnant couple.

The pregnant couple is then informed that the next risk assessment will be based on the ultrasound measurement of fluid in the neck of the fetus; that all fetuses have fluid in the neck and that fluid separates the skin on the surface of the body from the underlying muscle mass and, based upon the pregnancy outcome of nearly 200,000 women[15] undergoing the same ultrasound evaluation as the pregnant couple, it was found that the greater the distance between the skin and the underlying muscle mass the greater the risk for a conception with a chromosome abnormality (and an increased risk for cardiac malformations and developmental/genetic syndromes). The actual ultrasound prints comprising the fetus' crown-rump measurement to date the pregnancy, nuchal translucency measurements (at least 3), and nasal bone (present or absent) should then be shown to the prospective parents; the relationship between crown-rump length and size of the nuchal translucency should be elucidated at this time. Here, the risk assessment is actually given in 2 stages. First, a general statement is made that at 11 to 14 weeks' gestation, nuchal translucency measurements of most fetuses range between 1 and 2.5 mm and that measurements greater than 3 mm are expected to result in a *markedly increased risk* for a fetal chromosome abnormality, regardless of maternal age and levels of maternal serum markers; second, the approach by which the actual risk estimate will be derived for the specific pregnant couple is explained, namely, the pregnant couple's risk for a fetal chromosome abnormality is to be based on the pregnancy outcomes and experiences of the 200,000 women in the previously mentioned database. If the nuchal translucency is 3 mm or greater, the pregnant couple is informed that additional studies are to be anticipated. Four stages of evaluation will be proposed: (1) chromosome analysis either of chorionic villi or amniocytes to determine if a karyotypic abnormality is present, (2) an echocardiogram at 18 to 20 weeks' gestation to evaluate the cardiac status of the fetus,[3] (3) viral studies to rule out an infectious agent, and (4) ultrasound evaluation at 18 to 20 weeks' gestation to determine if any structural anomalies are present in the fetus.[16]

The final component of first trimester screening involves a discussion of the role of each of the 2 maternal serum proteins, PAPP-A and free beta hCG. The pregnant couple is first told that the 2 serum proteins were in fact not made by the prospective mother, rather they are both products of the placenta and therefore diet has no impact on their levels. In the case of PAPP-A, the inverse relationship between PAPP-A level and risk is described in general terms, that is, the lower the level of PAPP-A in maternal serum the higher the risk for an aneuploid conception and the higher the level of PAPP-A the lower the risk. In the case of free beta hCG, the pregnant couple is counseled that both high and low levels in maternal blood increase the risk for a fetal chromosome abnormality. High levels increase the risk for Down syndrome, in fact the higher the level of hCG the higher the risk for Down syndrome. Low levels increase the risk for trisomies 13 and 18, in fact the lower the level the higher the risk. Should there be a low level of PAPP-A (0.3 MoM or less) with or without low levels of free beta hCG, the possibility of an adverse pregnancy outcome[5–7] and how this issue will be addressed by their obstetrician as the pregnancy progresses is raised. This and related findings following first trimester screening may necessitate separate and additional counseling be made available for the prospective parents.

4. Recognizing that first trimester screening reassures the overriding majority of pregnant couples, if first trimester screening identifies the pregnancy to be at increased risk for trisomies 13, 18, and 21, the pregnant couple can be presented several courses of action:

   Diagnostic testing either by first trimester CVS or midtrimester amniocentesis

   Additional noninvasive screening by means of second trimester triple/quad screening and combining the risk assessments for both trimesters before making a decision of invasive testing

   Combination of 3 series of evaluations (first trimester screening, second trimester screening, and ultrasound evaluation) for any significant structural change associated with increased risk for a conception with a chromosome abnormality before making a decision on invasive testing.

Genetic counseling involving diagnostic testing requires that detailed information be provided concerning the procedure (CVS or amniocentesis), particularly a discussion of the cost and benefits; the cost being the risk of losing a pregnancy as a direct consequence of the procedure itself and benefits determined on the basis of what patients would do with the information derived from diagnostic testing.

The outline previously mentioned is meant only to serve as a possible framework for providing genetic counseling to prospective parents undergoing first trimester screening. The counseling session has to be individualized based on the individual counselor's approach and recognizing that each counseling session engenders its own unique set of questions, issues, and concerns (eg, multiple gestations,[17] IVF pregnancies[18]).

Future developments in first trimester screening will involve specific risk assessments for a broad spectrum of chromosome abnormalities, including Turner syndrome; triploidy; and the different sex chromosome abnormalities, such as 47,XXY, 47,XYY, and so forth. It should also be possible to combine these individual risk assessments into a single, overall risk assessment for a chromosome abnormality (numerical and structural) given the fact that the risk for any chromosome abnormality is well established based on maternal age.

REFERENCES

1. Spencer K, Souter V, Tul N, et al. A screening program for trisomy 21 at 10–14 weeks using fetal nuchal translucency, maternal serum free β-human chorionic gonadotropin and pregnancy-associated plasma protein-A. Ultrasound Obstet Gynecol 1999;13:231–7.

2. Kagan KO, Wright D, Valencia C, et al. Screening for trisomies 21, 18 and 13 by maternal age, fetal nuchal translucency, fetal heart rate, free beta-hCG and pregnancy-associated plasma protein-A. Humanit Rep 2008;23:1968–75.

3. Atzei A, Gajewska K, Huggon I, et al. Relationship between nuchal translucency thickness and prevalence of major cardiac defects in fetuses with normal karyotype. Ultrasound Obstet Gynecol 2005;26:154–7.

4. Souka AP, Von Kaisenberg CS, Hyett JA, et al. Increased nuchal translucency with normal karyotype. Am J Obstet Gynecol 2005;192:1005–21.

5. Spencer K, Cowans N, Avgidou K, et al. First-trimester biochemical markers of aneuploidy and the prediction of small-for-gestational age fetuses. Ultrasound Obstet Gynecol 2008;31(1):15–9.

6. Spencer K, Cowans N, Molina F, et al. First-trimester ultrasound and biochemical markers of aneuploidy and the prediction of preterm or early preterm delivery. Ultrasound Obstet Gynecol 2008;31(2):147–52.
7. Spencer K, Cowans N, Nicolaides KH. Low levels of maternal serum PAPP-A in the first trimester and the risk of pre-eclampsia. Prenat Diagn 2008;28(1):7–10.
8. Poon L, Maiz N, Valencia C, et al. First trimester maternal serum PAPP-A and pre-eclampsia. Ultrasound Obstet Gynecol 2009;33:23–33.
9. Khaw A, Kametas N, Turan O, et al. Maternal cardiac function and uterine artery Doppler at 11–14 weeks in the prediction of pre-eclampsia in nulliparous women. BJOG 2008;115:369–76.
10. Kagan KO, Cicero S, Staboulidou I, et al. Fetal nasal bone in screening for trisomies 21, 18 and 13 and Turner syndrome at 11–13 weeks of gestation. Ultrasound Obstet Gynecol 2009;33:259–64.
11. Maiz N, Valencia C, Kagan KO, et al. Ductus venosus Doppler in screening for trisomies 21, 18 and 13 and Turner syndrome at 11–13 weeks of gestation. Ultrasound Obstet Gynecol 2009;33(5):512–7.
12. Kagan KO, Valencia C, Livanos P, et al. Tricuspid regurgitation in screening for trisomies 21, 18 and 13 and Turner syndrome at 11+0 to 13+6 weeks of gestation. Ultrasound Obstet Gynecol 2009;33:18–22.
13. Falcon O, Faiola S, Huggon I, et al. Fetal tricuspid regurgitation at the 11 + 0 to 13 + 6-week scan: association with chromosomal defects and reproducibility of the method. Ultrasound Obstet Gynecol 2006;27:609–12.
14. Falcon O, Auer M, Gerovassili A, et al. Screening for trisomy 21 by fetal tricuspid regurgitation, nuchal translucency and maternal serum free beta-hCG and PAPP-A at 11 + 0 to 13 + 6 weeks. Ultrasound Obstet Gynecol 2006;27:151–5.
15. Spencer K, Spencer CE, Power M, et al. Screening for chromosomal abnormalities in the first trimester using ultrasound and maternal serum biochemistry in a one stop clinic: a review of three years prospective experience. BJOG 2003;110:281–6.
16. Dagklis T, Plasencia W, Maiz N, et al. Choroid plexus cyst, intracardiac echogenic focus, hyperechogenic bowel and hydronephrosis in screening for trisomy 21 at 11 + 0 to 13 + 6 weeks. Ultrasound Obstet Gynecol 2008;31:132–5.
17. Spencer K, Kagan K, Nicolaides KH. Screening for trisomy 21 in twin pregnancies in the first trimester: an update of the impact of chorionicity on maternal serum markers. Prenat Diagn 2008;28(1):49–52.
18. Liao A, Heath V, Kametas N, et al. First-trimester screening for trisomy 21 in singleton pregnancies achieved by assisted reproduction. Humanit Rep 2001;16(7):1501–4.

First-Trimester Screening for Chromosomal Abnormalities: Advantages of an Instant Results Approach

Mary E. Norton, MD[a,b,*]

KEYWORDS

- Prenatal screening • Down syndrome • Nuchal translucency
- First trimester screening

Protocols that include first trimester screening for fetal chromosome abnormalities have become standard of care throughout the United States. Most such protocols allow provision of at least preliminary risk assessment after the nuchal translucency ultrasound screening (NT) and first trimester biochemistry results are available. Earlier screening allows for first trimester diagnostic testing in cases found to be at increased risk. For those patients with an abnormal karyotype who decide to terminate their pregnancies, first trimester abortion is safer, more readily available, and more acceptable to women.[1] However, first trimester screening requires coordination of the NT with biochemical screening during early, specific, narrow, but slightly different gestational age ranges. If these tests are done in the latter part of the gestational age window, results may not be available until the second trimester. The NT can often provide instant results if preceded by programs that perform the biochemical analysis, thus optimizing the benefits of the first trimester approach while improving efficiency and communication with the patient. This article discusses the benefits and logistics of such an approach.

[a] Perinatal Genetic Services, The Permanente Medical Group, Kaiser Permanente, 3505 Broadway, Northern California, Oakland, CA 94611, USA
[b] University of California, 505 Parnassus Avenue, San Francisco, CA 94143, USA
* Kaiser Permanente San Francisco, 2238 Geary Boulevard, 7SE, San Francisco CA 94115.
E-mail address: mary.e.norton@kp.org

Clin Lab Med 30 (2010) 565–571
doi:10.1016/j.cll.2010.04.015
0272-2712/10/$ – see front matter © 2010 Elsevier Inc. All rights reserved.

labmed.theclinics.com

BIOCHEMICAL SCREENING FOR FETAL ANEUPLOIDY

Screening for Down syndrome has historically involved triple-marker screening with maternal serum alpha fetoprotein (MSAFP), unconjugated estriol (uE3), and human chorionic gonadotropin (hCG), or "quad" screening with the addition of inhibin A; these tests are performed in the second trimester, between 15 and 20 weeks' gestation. AFP and uE3 are 25% to 30% lower in Down syndrome pregnancies, whereas hCG and inhibin A are increased with a median value about twice that of normal controls.[2-6] Gestational age, maternal weight, race, insulin-dependent diabetes mellitus, smoking, and number of fetuses affect analyte levels to different degrees and laboratory protocols are variably adjusted for them.[7]

Because AFP, uE3, hCG, and inhibin A are all independent of maternal age and only weakly correlate with each other, they can be used in combination to estimate fetal Down syndrome risk. Results are typically expressed as multiples of the median (MoM); this provides less interlaboratory variation, which can be considerable, and a way to report results across a range of gestational ages. The MoM results are used to calculate a likelihood ratio, which is multiplied by the a priori risk for Down syndrome based on maternal age to generate a patient-specific risk. In the United States, although some laboratories continue to use the triple test, most have moved to quad screening as the standard for second trimester screening, which has an 11% greater detection rate (the detection rate of quad screening is 81%) at a 5% screen-positive rate.[8]

In addition to using different combinations of markers for screening, laboratories use different risk cutoff levels. As with many screening tests, a trade-off is made between detection of the disorder and the number of individuals with a screen-positive result. In many programs, a Down syndrome risk cutoff approximating the risk of a 35-year old is applied. In others, a screen-positive rate of 5% is the goal and the risk cutoff is set accordingly.

FIRST TRIMESTER SCREENING AND INTEGRATED ALGORITHMS

A desire to provide earlier diagnosis has led to identification of informative first trimester markers. Nuchal translucency is a sonographic measurement of the layer of fluid normally present in the posterior aspect of the fetal neck in the late first trimester (**Fig. 1**). Larger measurements are associated with increased risk of aneuploidy, and the nuchal translucency measurement is used in the algorithm to assess Down syndrome risk in a manner similar to serum analytes. Screening at 10 and 14 weeks of gestation using measurement of the nuchal translucency with maternal serum hCG and pregnancy-associated

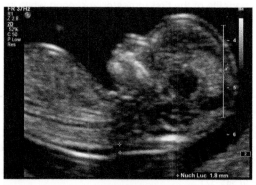

Fig. 1. Sonographic image of a 12-week fetus demonstrating a normal nuchal translucency measurement of 1.8 mm.

plasma protein A (PAPP-A) has been shown to detect 82% to 87% of Down syndrome fetuses at a 5% screen-positive rate.[8-10] The detection rate for other aneuploidies (T13, 18, 45X, triploidy) is about 78%.[11] The primary advantage of first trimester screening is earlier diagnosis of abnormalities (or early reassurance of the anxious patient), with the option of an earlier and safer pregnancy termination.

Various options to combine first and second trimester screening tests have been proposed or are currently in clinical use. With integrated screening, first and second trimester results are combined and given to the patient only after all testing is completed. This provides the optimal balance between detection and screen-positive rates (96% at a 5% false-positive rate) but patients do not receive a first trimester result, and most women prefer to receive results earlier.[12] Some investigators have expressed moral and ethical misgivings about this approach, which withholds results until all testing is completed, typically for several weeks.[13]

Other sequential strategies do provide first trimester risk information. In stepwise sequential screening, patients are provided a first trimester risk assessment and may elect to have invasive testing or decline further screening based on that information. For those who continue in the program, the second trimester quad test applies the first trimester screening results (as opposed to solely maternal age) as the a priori risk. This contrasts with independent sequential screening, in which the second trimester test uses maternal age as the a priori risk and ignores the first trimester screening results. However, as most aneuploid fetuses would have been identified and excluded by the first trimester screening, the maternal age-based background risk for aneuploidy is no longer accurate. Independent sequential screening will therefore result in high false-positive rates and should generally be avoided.

In contingent sequential screening, follow-up recommendations depend on the first trimester screening results. If the risk is high, invasive testing is offered, and if the risk is very low, no further testing is suggested. For patients in the middle range, second trimester screening is recommended to further clarify the risk. Although this allows the benefits of sequential testing, such protocols may be too complicated to be practical.

Cost-effectiveness analysis has been used to assess this complex array of testing strategies. Data from the First- and Second-Trimester Evaluation of Risk (FaSTER) trial compared 7 Down syndrome screening strategies: (1) triple screen, (2) quad screen, (3) combined first trimester screen, (4) integrated screen, (5) serum only integrated screen, (6) stepwise sequential screen, and (7) contingent sequential screen. The contingent sequential screen had the lowest costs, best outcomes, and highest quality-adjusted life years. The stepwise sequential strategy had the highest detection rate but at a higher cost per Down syndrome case diagnosed ($719,675 vs $690,427) as compared with contingent sequential.[14]

For the reasons outlined above, a stepwise sequential strategy seems the optimal approach, balancing early results, a high detection rate, a reasonable screen-positive rate, and the option of including screening for Down syndrome as well as open neural tube and ventral wall defects in a single testing strategy. The primary benefit of sequential over integrated screening is the provision of a first trimester result. The benefits of this include a shortened period of anxiety, the potential to have an earlier diagnostic procedure if indicated, and the improved safety of and access to first trimester termination instead of abortion later in pregnancy.

BENEFITS AND CONTROVERSIES IN FIRST TRIMESTER SCREENING

Although first trimester testing does provide these benefits, it has also been argued that some abnormal fetuses are miscarried between the first and second trimesters, thus early detection may actually result in some unnecessary pregnancy terminations of fetuses destined to abort spontaneously.[15] In addition, not all patients found to be at increased risk are able to avail themselves of early invasive diagnostic testing.

Chorionic villus sampling (CVS) is the standard first trimester diagnostic test and is typically performed between 10 and 13 weeks' gestation. Although it can be performed later, some CVS providers are unwilling to perform the test much after 13 weeks or will limit later procedures to a transabdominal approach, which is not feasible in all cases. Amniocentesis is most often performed between 15 and 20 weeks' gestation, and carries a higher risk of miscarriage and other complications when performed in the first trimester.[16] For patients seeking a diagnostic test after first trimester screening, then, a substantial number would either not have access to a CVS provider, or would receive results in the gestational age window between CVS and amniocentesis and be required to wait until amniocentesis is considered safe before they are a candidate for definitive testing.

Achieving the benefits of first trimester screening therefore requires that results be available as early as possible. If a patient undergoes her NT at the earliest possible gestational age (11 weeks 3 days of gestation) and has her blood drawn for first trimester biochemistry at the same time, her first trimester results would be available approximately one week later, at 12.5 weeks. If she is screen-positive, she will need to be contacted and an appointment scheduled for genetic counseling and, if desired, CVS. If circumstances are optimal and the appointment is scheduled within a day or two, the patient is now at 13 weeks' gestation. Turnaround time for karyotyping on CVS samples ranges from 7 to 14 days, so in ideal circumstances, the results might be available by 14 weeks' gestation. Again, the patient needs to be contacted and counseled, but clearly a pregnancy termination, even in ideal circumstances, is now no longer a true first trimester termination but is being performed at 14 to 15 weeks of gestation or even later.

LOGISTICS OF FIRST TRIMESTER AND SEQUENTIAL SCREENING PROGRAMS

The coordination of these 2 blood tests (in the first then second trimester) with the NT and obtaining a true first trimester result has therefore proven one of the most complex challenges of this evolving paradigm. Because the biochemical screening can be performed during an earlier period than the NT, it is possible to complete it and analyze its results before the NT, which has several advantages.

Numerous programs have been established that provide instant results at the time of the NT. Such protocols take advantage of the fact that first trimester biochemistry can be drawn and analyzed as early as 9 weeks' gestation (more than 2 weeks earlier than NT). If the biochemistry results are already available, the nuchal translucency measurement can be entered into a calculation package to immediately determine the risk, allowing instant results on the day of the NT. This approach has several advantages, including immediate genetic counseling when results are abnormal to explain the risks and options for follow-up. It eases the workload of busy genetic counselors or other providers, because difficulties in contacting patients to provide results are minimized. In some settings, a CVS can be offered at the same time if the patient so desires. This allows a decreased period of waiting, less anxiety and uncertainty, and a minimized delay in obtaining definitive information if that is the ultimate outcome. For patients who travel substantial distances to be seen at a referral center, receiving risk assessment and diagnostic testing, if needed, all during one visit, further increases the advantages of this approach.

OSCAR: The UK Approach

In the United Kingdom, instant results have been provided for many years through a program called OSCAR (One-stop clinic for assessment of risk). Biochemical testing of the mother, ultrasound examination of the fetus, and counseling are performed within a 1-hour visit. The maternal serum-free β-hCG and PAPP-A are drawn on arrival at the clinic and analyzed with an in-office Kryptor analyzer (Brahms AG, Berlin, Germany). An NT is performed and the NT and biochemistry results combined to determine the Down syndrome risk. The patients are counseled about their combined estimated risk and the available options for the subsequent management of the pregnancy explained. Those choosing to have an invasive test have the option of CVS during the same visit.[17]

A study published in 2004 to evaluate this program surveyed more than 1100 women attending antenatal clinics at 6 maternity units across the UK. A total of 75% of women selected a first trimester test as their first choice with 68.2% expressing a preference for the OSCAR approach. Twenty-four percent of women opted for integrated screening (with marginally higher detection rate that delivers results later in pregnancy) as their first choice with only 1% expressing a preference for second trimester screening. Timing and rapid reporting of results seemed to influence women's choice of test.[18]

The University of California, San Francisco Instant Results First Trimester Screening Program

The author and colleagues instituted an instant results protocol for provision of first trimester combined screening at the University of California, San Francisco in November 2003. This protocol involved blood collection by patients at home using a finger stick and filter paper mail-in card. Patients were instructed to complete their blood collection at least one week before the NT appointment so that biochemistry results would be available when the patient came to the clinic. On the day of the ultrasound appointment, biochemistry results were combined with the NT and risk assessment provided to the patient during the visit. In the first year of the program, this required a telephone call by the genetic counselor to the laboratory (NTD Laboratories, Melville, NY, USA) for result integration. Later, direct password-protected computer access was provided to streamline the process. Patients with abnormal results were offered genetic counseling, immediate CVS, or diagnostic testing with CVS or amniocentesis at a later date.

The outcomes of the first 2 years of the protocol were reviewed, including the effectiveness of providing instant results, predictors of success in performing the home blood test in a timely fashion allowing instant results, and patient decision-making regarding diagnostic testing. In the first 2 years of the program, 60.6% of patients received instant results. When biochemistry samples had been submitted before the visit, 80% received instant results. Women aged 35 years and older were more likely to complete the blood test in advance and receive instant results ($P = .001$), and patients' ethnicity and referring provider did not predict success with this part of the process. Reasons for not receiving instant results included collecting the blood sample at a time too close to the NT appointment, providing an insufficient sample that required repeat collection, or requiring assistance with obtaining the sample. Overall, diagnostic procedure volume was unchanged, although CVS increased by 12% ($P = .02$) and amniocentesis decreased by 6% ($P = .049$).[19]

The California Genetic Disease Screening Program

A state-sponsored prenatal genetic screening program has been in place since 1986 in the State of California. Initially, this involved MSAFP screening for neural tube defects and Down syndrome; in 1994, triple screening was introduced and in 2007, quad screening. In April 2009, the program introduced a first and second trimester serum integrated screening program, with the option of NT available to allow the provision of preliminary first trimester risk assessment. This program includes a Web-based tool that allows the NT to be combined with available biochemistry results for those patients who completed that screening in advance, and an instant result can be calculated and presented to the patient. Thus, in California, an instant results approach, at least for preliminary first trimester screening, has become the standard for all women seeking prenatal care.

SUMMARY

Integrated and sequential screening programs that provide first trimester risk assessment for Down syndrome and other chromosome abnormalities have improved performance characteristics when compared with second trimester triple or quad screening.[7–9] In 2007, the ACOG indicated that all pregnant women, regardless of age, should be offered screening for Down syndrome that included a first trimester option.[20] An increasing number of women are choosing to avail themselves of earlier testing with improved detection rates, and efficient and effective programs for provision of this service are increasingly important. Programs that provide instant results at the time of the NT benefit from several logistic as well as quality and service benefits for the patient, and such programs have been shown to be successful and preferred by women.

REFERENCES

1. Learman LA, Drey EA, Gates EA, et al. Abortion attitudes of pregnant women in prenatal care. Am J Obstet Gynecol 2005;192:1939–45.
2. Wald NJ, Cuckle HS, Densem JW, et al. Maternal serum screening for Down syndrome in early pregnancy. Br Med J 1988;297(6653):883–7.
3. Jorgensen PI, Trolle D. Low urinary oestriol excretion during pregnancy in women giving birth to infants with Down syndrome. Lancet 1972;2(7781):782–4.
4. Bogart MH, Pandian MR, Jones OW. Abnormal maternal serum chorionic gonadotropin levels in pregnancies with fetal chromosome abnormalities. Prenat Diagn 1987;7(9):623–30.
5. Lambert-Messerlian GM, Canick JA, Palomaki GE, et al. Second trimester levels of maternal serum inhibin A, total inhibin, alpha inhibin precursor, and activin in Down syndrome pregnancy. J Med Screen 1996;3(2):58–62.
6. Wallace EM, Swanston IA, McNeilly AS, et al. Second trimester screening for Down syndrome using maternal serum dimeric inhibin A. Clin Endocrinol (Oxf) 1996;44(1):17–21.
7. Palomaki GE, Lee JE, Canick JA, et al, ACMG Laboratory Quality Assurance Committee. Technical standards and guidelines: prenatal screening for Down syndrome that includes first-trimester biochemistry and/or ultrasound measurements. Genet Med 2009;11(9):669–81.
8. Malone FD, Canick JA, Ball RH, et al, First- and Second-Trimester Evaluation of Risk (FaSTER) Research Consortium. First-trimester or second-trimester screening, or both, for Down's syndrome. N Engl J Med 2005;353(19):2001–11.
9. Wapner R, Thom E, Simpson JL, et al. First trimester screening for trisomies 21 and 18. N Engl J Med 2003;349:1405–13.
10. Wald NJ, Rodeck C, Hackshaw AK, et al. First and second trimester antenatal screening for Down's syndrome: the results of the Serum, Urine and Ultrasound Screening Study (SURUSS). J Med Screen 2003;10(2):56–104.

11. Breathnach FM, Malone FD, Lambert-Messerlian G, et al, First and Second Trimester Evaluation of Risk (FASTER) Research Consortium. First- and second-trimester screening: detection of aneuploidies other than Down syndrome. Obstet Gynecol 2007;110(3):651–7.
12. Sharma G, Gold HT, Chervenak FA, et al. Patient preference regarding first-trimester aneuploidy risk assessment. Am J Obstet Gynecol 2005;193(4): 1429–36.
13. Sharma G, McCullough LB, Chervenak FA. Ethical considerations of early (first vs. second trimester) risk assessment disclosure for trisomy 21 and patient choice in screening versus diagnostic testing. Am J Med Genet C Semin Med Genet 2007;145(1):99–104.
14. Ball RH, Caughey AB, Malone FD, et al, First and Second Trimester Evaluation of Risk (FaSTER) Research Consortium. First- and second-trimester evaluation of risk for Down syndrome. Obstet Gynecol 2007;110(1):10–7.
15. Wenstrom KD. Evaluation of Down syndrome screening strategies. Semin Perinatol 2005;29(4):219–24.
16. The Canadian Early and Mid-trimester Amniocentesis Trial (CEMAT) Group. Randomised trial to assess safety and fetal outcome of early and midtrimester amniocentesis. Lancet 1998;351(9098):242–7.
17. Avgidou K, Papageorghiou A, Bindra R, et al. Prospective first-trimester screening for trisomy 21 in 30,564 pregnancies. Am J Obstet Gynecol 2005; 192(6):1761–7.
18. Spencer K, Aitken D. Factors affecting women's preference for type of prenatal screening test for chromosomal anomalies. Ultrasound Obstet Gynecol 2004; 24(7):735–9.
19. Norton ME, Hopkins LM, Pena S, et al. First-trimester combined screening: experience with an instant results approach. Am J Obstet Gynecol 2007;196(6):606, e1–5.
20. ACOG Committee on Practice Bulletins. ACOG Practice Bulletin No. 77: screening for fetal chromosomal abnormalities. Obstet Gynecol 2007;109(1): 217–27.

Additional First-Trimester Ultrasound Markers

J. Sonek, MD, RDMS[a,b,*], K. Nicolaides, MD[c,d]

KEYWORDS

- First-trimester screening • Nuchal translucency • Nasal bone
- Fronto-maxillary angle • Ductus venosus • Tricuspid valve

Over the past 15 years, the Fetal Medicine Foundation has developed and standardized the use of several first-trimester ultrasound markers for screening for fetal chromosomal abnormalities in the first trimester: nuchal translucency (NT), nasal bone (NB), fronto-maxillary facial (FMF) angle, ductus venosus (DV), and tricuspid valve (TCV) Doppler evaluation. For the sake of brevity, this discussion is primarily confined to their use in screening for trisomy 21. However, these markers have also been shown to be useful in screening for other types of aneuploidy (trisomies 18 and 13, monosomy X, other sex chromosome aneuploidies, and triploidy).

The goal of this review is primarily to describe the additional first-trimester ultrasound markers, that is, markers other than NT. However, the manner in which the new markers are used is inextricably connected with NT evaluation. NT thickness is arguably the most powerful marker in screening for fetal aneuploidy.[1] All first-trimester (11–13 +6 weeks) screening protocols that make use of ultrasonography should include an NT measurement, whether or not additional ultrasound markers are used. Therefore, a brief discussion regarding the acquisition and use of this marker is also included in this article.

In order for all of the ultrasound markers described in this review to be used effectively, in-depth knowledge of how the markers are used, training, experience, and ongoing quality assurance are crucial.

FIRST-TRIMESTER ULTRASOUND (11–13 +6 WEEKS' GESTATION)

There are several advantages that first-trimester ultrasound offers that extend beyond simply looking for markers of aneuploidy. First, the measurement of the crown rump

[a] Wright State University, Dayton, OH, USA
[b] Fetal Medicine Foundation/USA, Dayton, OH, USA
[c] King's College School of Medicine and Dentistry, Harris Birthright Centre, London, UK
[d] Fetal Medicine Foundation, London, UK
* Corresponding author. Wright State University, Dayton, OH.
E-mail address: jdsonek@mvh.org

Clin Lab Med 30 (2010) 573–592
doi:10.1016/j.cll.2010.04.004
0272-2712/10/$ – see front matter © 2010 Elsevier Inc. All rights reserved.

labmed.theclinics.com

length (CRL) in the first trimester is the most accurate way to establish gestational age.[2] In addition, with the advent of high-resolution ultrasound, a fairly complete evaluation of the fetal anatomy may be performed even at this early gestational age.[3–13] The majority of significant structural fetal defects are already detectable at this point in pregnancy.[14] Even if a specific fetal structural defect is not seen and the karyotype is normal, a significantly increased NT thickness (≥ 3.5 mm) has been shown to be associated with an increased risk of fetal abnormalities (cardiac anomalies and abnormalities of the great vessels,[15–29] several other fetal structural defects,[30–36] a multitude of genetic and nongenetic defects,[36–59] certain fetal infections,[60–62] and an increased fetal and neonatal morbidity and mortality in general).[63–72]

In the special case of multiple gestations, the first-trimester scan is even more beneficial. The first trimester is the best time to establish the chorionicity and amniocity. In a dichorionic gestation, the dividing membrane demonstrates a typical thickening ("lambda" or "twin peak" sign) as it approaches the placental surface.[73–75] However, in the case of a monochorionic/diamniotic gestation, the membrane is thin throughout its length, even at the point where it meets the placenta ("T" sign). Knowledge of chorionicity is not only useful in the overall management of the pregnancy but also helps to select the appropriate algorithm to establish the fetal risk of aneuploidy.[76–78] In addition, first-trimester evaluation of the DV helps to estimate the risk of twin-to-twin transfusion syndrome in monochorionic/diamniotic gestations.[79]

To gain the maximum benefit of the first-trimester ultrasound examination, it is crucial to perform it between 11 and 13 +6 weeks' gestation. There are several reasons for using the lower limit of 11 weeks' gestation. The success of a credible fetal anatomic survey is very low prior to 11 weeks' gestation and increases rapidly thereafter.[3–13] In addition, many of the organs that are usually not detectable before 11 weeks' gestation become much more readily visible starting after that point.[80] Physiologic exomphalos, which is consistently present prior to 11 weeks' gestation, makes the diagnosis of an omphalocele difficult.[81,82] The fetal skull is not yet ossified, which complicates the diagnosis of the exencephaly/anencephaly sequence.[83]

The additional ultrasound markers cannot be used prior to 11 weeks' gestation, as their effectiveness has not been described before this point.

The reason for placing the upper gestational age limit at 13 + 6 is threefold. First, the NT thickness as a marker for aneuploidy becomes less reliable as the gestational age progresses.[84] Second, the position of the fetus within the uterus tends to be such that the NT measurement is more difficult to acquire.[85,86] Finally, the first-trimester approach provides the patient a significant amount of information at a very early stage of pregnancy, thus preserving maximum privacy and safety regarding her reproductive choices. This advantage is lost beyond 14 weeks' gestation.

ULTRASOUND MARKERS

The following ultrasound markers are included in the currently used Fetal Medicine Foundation algorithm: NT,[87] NB,[88] FMF angle,[89] TCV evaluation,[90] DV evaluation,[91] fetal heart rate (FHR),[92] and presence or absence of certain fetal anomalies.[93–97] The FHR is useful mainly in screening for trisomy 13.[92] FHR does not contribute to the efficiency of screening for trisomy 21 and is not addressed in this article. There are several fetal anomalies that are recognized as markers for aneuploidy.[93–97] However, discussion regarding such anomalies is beyond the scope of this article.

The first-trimester ultrasound markers may be divided into those that are best evaluated using 2-dimensional (2-D) gray scale ultrasound (NT, NB, FHR, fetal anomalies), those that may be evaluated using 2-D ultrasound but where 3-D ultrasound is beneficial (FMF angle), and those that are evaluated using Doppler ultrasound (TCV and DV blood flow evaluations). The markers may also be divided based on whether they represent quantitative measurement (NT, FMF angle, FHR) or a qualitative determination (NB, TCV, DV, fetal anomalies).

MARKERS LOCATED ON THE FETAL HEAD AND NECK

These markers are based on the dysmorphic features observed in persons with Down syndrome.[98] Such markers may also be used in the second trimester but their efficacy decreases with advancing gestational age.

Nuchal Translucency Measurement

The NT is formed by a layer of fluid beneath the nuchal skin extending for a variable distance over the head and neck.[99] To standardize the measurement and to make the measurement accurate to one-tenth of a millimeter,[100] the Fetal Medicine Foundation has developed several requirements that the image of the fetus needs to meet, which are listed and demonstrated in **Fig. 1**. It is acceptable for the fetus to be either facing toward or away from the transducer. Ideally, at least 3 NT measurements should be taken and the largest measurement that meets the FMF criteria should be used for risk assessment. The amnion has to be clearly differentiated from the skin line of the NT, as both are seen as a thin line. Failure to do so may result in obtaining the incorrect measurement. The fetus should be in a neutral position, as neck extension artificially increases the NT measurement and hyperflexion decreases it.[101]

In approximately 5% to 10% of the cases, a nuchal cord is present.[102] This cord is usually first noted when a small section of the NT cannot be clearly delineated. Often, there are additional short echogenic lines seen in this area representing a cross section of the tortuous umbilical cord vessels. The best way to confirm the presence

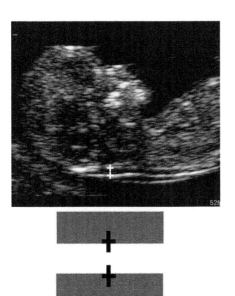

- **CRL : 45-84 mm** (Gestation ~ 11^{+0} to 13^{+6} wks)
- **Mid-sagittal view** (fetus can be either facing towards or away from the transducer)
- **Image size**: head and upper thorax occupies most of the screen (measurement accuracy **.1 mm**)
- Fetus **away from amnion**
- Fetus in **neutral position**
- Adjust for **nuchal cord** (5% of the cases)
- Caliper placement **"on-to-on"**
- Use **maximum lucency**
- Motivated **sonographer**

Caliper placement

Fig. 1. Nuchal translucency measurement protocol (Fetal Medicine Foundation).

of a nuchal cord is by using color Doppler. The nuchal cord may compress the NT and displace the nuchal fluid. To compensate for this redistribution of the fluid, NT measurements should be taken above and below the nuchal cord. The risk assessment is based on the average of the 2 measurements.

The appearance of the NT does not change the likelihood ratios based on the thickness of the NT. The risk assessment should be based on the NT measurement alone; the artificial differentiation between simple NT and a "cystic hygroma" has not been shown to be useful.[103]

The likelihood of fetal abnormalities being present increases as the NT thickness increases.[87,104] Several mechanisms have been proposed for the nuchal thickening: structural cardiovascular abnormalities and/or abnormalities of myocardial performance,[105–109] abnormalities of connective tissue composition,[110–114] abnormalities or delay in lymphatic system formation,[49,50,115,116] increase in intrathoracic pressure,[31,37–44] decrease in fetal movement,[33,53–55] fetal hypoproteinemia,[52,117] fetal anemia,[56–59] and fetal infection.[60–62,118] It is likely that in many cases, especially in fetuses with chromosomal defects, more than one mechanism is in effect.

The NT measurement must be adjusted for gestational age, as the normal ranges change with gestation.[84,87,99,104,119] NT measurement is independent of maternal serum biochemistry levels.[120] For a false-positive rate of 5%, the detection of trisomy 21 using the combination of maternal age and NT is 75%.[87] The detection rate increases to 90% with the addition of free β-human chorionic gonadotropin (free β-hCG) and pregnancy-associated plasma protein A (PAPP-A).[120–125] The detection rates for trisomies 18 and 13, monosomy X, and triploidy are at or in excess of 90% for the same false-positive rate.[126–128]

Nasal Bone Evaluation

In the first trimester, the purpose of an ultrasound evaluation of the nasal bone is to recognize whether the nasal bone is present or absent.[88,129–134] Unlike in the second trimester, it does not appear that measuring its length adds to the screening performance of this marker.[134,135] The use of 3-D ultrasound does not improve the success of NB evaluation.[136]

The requirements for the correct image acquisition are similar to those of NT measurement: a magnified mid-sagittal section of the fetal head (**Fig. 2**). However, the standard view used to evaluate the NB differs from the one used for NT measurement in 2 main aspects: the NB evaluation can be done only with the fetus facing the transducer, and the accuracy of the NB evaluation is highly dependent on the angle of insonation.

The angle of insonation needs to be 90° with respect to the longitudinal axis of the NB and the nasal bridge. In other words, the face of the transducer should be parallel to these structures. In this view, the NB is seen along its largest diameter and, if present, is relatively easy to see. However, the NB is extremely thin. Therefore, if the angle of insonation is closer to 0° (face of the transducer is perpendicular to the long axis of the NB), the NB may become sonographically undetectable.

It needs to be kept in mind that the skin over the nasal bridge is quite echogenic in the first trimester. Therefore if the NB is present, the correct view will demonstrate 2 echogenic lines: the skin on the surface of the nasal bridge and the NB located beneath the skin forming the "equal sign." Because faint echogenic lines are often seen within the nose even in the absence of the NB, in order to be able to say with certainty that the NB is present, the echogenicity of the NB must be equal to or exceed the echogenicity of the nasal skin.

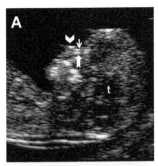

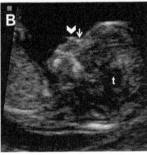

- **CRL : 45-84 mm** (Gestation ~ 11^{+0} to 13^{+6} wks)
- **Mid-sagittal view** (fetus must be facing towards the transducer)
- **Image size**: head and upper thorax occupies most of the screen
- The **face of the transducer** is parallel to the long axis of the nasal bone and the skin over the nasal bridge
- The **image includes**: 1. Echogenic line representing the skin over the nasal bridge (solid arrow) 2. echogenic line in front representing the nasal tip (chevron) 3. hypoechoic area within the brain representing the region of the thalamus (t) 4. if the nasal bone is present, a line within the nasal bridge is seen (notched arrow) – the echogenicity is higher than that of the skin
- The "equal sign" is formed by the skin and the nasal bone underneath (euploid fetus: Image A). It is not seen when the nasal bone is absent (trisomy 21: Image B)

Fig. 2. Nasal bone evaluation protocol (Fetal Medicine Foundation). (*A*) Present nasal bone in a euploid fetus. (*B*) Absent nasal bone in a fetus with trisomy 21.

A third echogenic line is seen anteriorly and slightly superiorly to the "equal sign." This line represents the skin over the nasal tip. If the fetal face is insonated in the mid-sagittal plane, this echogenic line and the "equal sign" are seen in the same view.

The prevalence of NB absence decreases with gestational age in both euploid and trisomy 21 fetuses. Therefore, the likelihood ratios change with gestational age. To reduce the false-positive rate, if the NB is noted to be absent between 11 and 11 +6 weeks' gestation it is reasonable to repeat the examination 1 week later and use the results of the latter examination for the risk assessment. The result of NB evaluation also needs to be adjusted for ethnicity. Specifically, NB absence is most common in fetuses of African origin, followed by those from Asia. The prevalence of NB absence is the lowest in Caucasians. The prevalence of NB absence increases as the NT measurement increases, but this does not appear to be significant until the NT thickness becomes very large (≥3.5 mm).[137] The presence and absence of nasal bone are independent of maternal serum biochemistries.[88,138–140]

A combined number of approximately 49,000 fetuses from several studies yields a prevalence of nasal bone absence of 65% in trisomy 21 and 1% to 3% in euploid fetuses.[134] The prevalence of nasal bone absence has also been shown to be increased in trisomy 18 (55%), trisomy 13 (34%), and Turner syndrome (11%), but not in triploidy.[137] In a study involving 19,614 fetuses, the combination of maternal age, NT measurement, NB evaluation, and maternal serum biochemistries (free β-hCG and PAPP-A) resulted in a 92% detection for trisomy 21 and 100% detection for trisomies 13 and 18, and monosomy X with a 3% false-positive rate.[140]

Fronto-Maxillary Angle Measurement

The image requirements to measure the FMF angle are similar to those for the nasal bone evaluation. The fetus also always needs to be facing the transducer. However, the attainment of a strictly mid-sagittal view is absolutely critical for the accuracy of the measurement; even small deviations from the midline may change this measurement significantly. 3-D ultrasound appears to aid in performing this evaluation.[141]

There are several ultrasonographic landmarks that help to establish that the fetal profile is being viewed in the precise midline section and that the image is suitable for FMF angle measurement (**Fig. 3**).[141] In the correct view, the hard palate is seen as a roughly trapezoidal structure that is somewhat wider at the posterior end than anteriorly. The skin over the forehead should be seen separately from another thin echogenic line, which is located a short distance beneath the skin. The latter represents the metopic suture, which is not yet calcified at this point in gestation.

In the precise midline view the space between the upper edge of the hard palate and the nose should be relatively echo-free. If the ultrasound plane is slightly off midline, an echogenic structure that runs upwards from the hard palate will come into view. This structure represents the zygomatic process of the maxilla and should be absent from the correct view for FMF angle measurement. The intracranial landmarks that are seen in the precise midline view consist of the hypoechoic regions of the thalamus, pons, and medulla oblongata.

The measurement of the FMF angle is demonstrated in **Fig. 3**. The first ray of the angle is drawn along the upper edge of the hard palate. This edge is composed of the maxillary and the vomer bones. The apex of the angle is located at the anterior edge of the maxilla. The second ray of the angle runs from the apex upwards; it is positioned so the inner edge of the line rests on the echogenic line beneath the skin, that is, the noncalcified metopic suture.

In the first trimester, the division between the vomer bones and the maxilla is usually difficult to see. However, toward the end of the first trimester, this division may become evident as an oblique hypoechoic line running from the upper edge of the

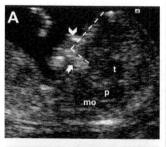
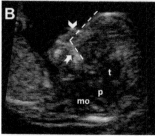

- **CRL : 45-84 mm** (Gestation ~ 11^{+0} to 13^{+6} wks)
- **Mid-sagittal view** (fetus must be facing towards the transducer)
- **Image size**: head and upper thorax occupies most of the screen
- The position of the **face of the transducer** is approximately parallel to the long axis of the nasal bone and the skin over the nasal bridge
- The **image includes**: 1. echogenic line in front representing the nasal tip (chevron), 2. hypoechoic areas within the brain representing the regions of the thalamus (t), pons (p), and medulla oblongata (mo) 3. trapezoid or rectangular echogenic structure of the hard palate (notched arrow)
- **Angle measurement**: 1. first ray is drawn along the upper edge of the hard palate 2. apex of the angle is at the anterior edge of the maxilla. 3. second ray of the angle runs from the apex upwards resting on the echogenic line beneath the skin (the non-calcified metopic suture)
- The angle is increased in trisomy 21 (Image B) as compared to a euploid fetus (Image A)

Fig. 3. Fronto-maxillary angle measurement protocol (Fetal Medicine Foundation). (*A*) Normal fronto-maxillary angle in a euploid fetus. (*B*) Shallow fronto-maxillary angle in a fetus with trisomy 21.

hard palate anteriorly to the lower edge of the hard palate posteriorly.[142] This line should not be used to form the lower ray of the FMF angle.

The increase in the FMF angle measurements in fetuses with trisomy 21 appears to be due to the deeper location of the front edge of the maxilla, which may be the result of maxillary hypoplasia, dorsal displacement of the maxilla, or a combination of the two.

The normal ranges for the FMF angle measurements change with gestational age; the angle measurements become smaller.[143] Therefore, the risk assessment based on these measurements has to be adjusted for gestational age. The FMF angle measurement is independent of the presence or absence of the nasal bone, the NT measurement, and the maternal serum biochemistries.[89,144]

Increased FMF angle measurements have been found not only in trisomy 21 but also in trisomies 18 and 13. The FMF angle measurements are above the 95th percentile in 45%, 58%, and 48% of trisomy 21, trisomy 18, and trisomy 13, respectively.[144–146] In a study involving 782 euploid fetuses and 108 fetuses with trisomy 21, the combination of maternal age, NT measurement, FMF angle measurement, and maternal serum biochemistries (free β-hCG and PAPP-A) resulted in a 92% detection for trisomy 21 with a 3% false-positive rate.[144]

MARKERS WITHIN THE FETAL CARDIOVASCULAR SYSTEM

The fetal heart has several qualities that make it respond to stress differently than hearts later on in life. This situation is especially true in early pregnancy. The main features are well known: less organized muscle arrangement in the myocardium, fewer sarcomeres per unit mass, lower compliance, and an increased pressure at any cardiac volume. Furthermore, the placental vasculature has a relatively high resistance in the first trimester, placing additional strain on the heart. As a result the fetal heart, especially early in pregnancy, functions at the upper limits of the Frank-Starling curve. Therefore, even relatively minor deviations from the normal that involve the structure and/or function of the myocardium may lead to detectable changes in the cardiovascular performance.

Ductus Venosus Doppler Evaluation

Approximately 50% of the oxygenated blood brought back from the placenta by the umbilical vein courses through the DV. The DV empties into the inferior vena cava at a point very close to the right atrium. Its proximity to the fetal heart makes it susceptible to changes in the cardiac performance.[147–149]

The DV waveform as seen on pulsed Doppler normally demonstrates forward flow throughout the cardiac cycle. However, it contains episodic changes that correspond to the various phases of the cardiac cycle. Normally, the blood flow significantly decreases during an atrial contraction (a-wave). The a-wave appears not only to be sensitive to changes in the fetal cardiovascular status but also lends itself to an objective evaluation.[147–149]

The exact reason for trisomy 21 being associated with a-wave abnormalities is unknown.[150–155] However, it is postulated that these findings are related to the abnormalities known to be present in the myocardium of individuals with Down syndrome (decreased number of myocytes, abnormal orientation of myocytes and myofibrils,[109] abnormal connective tissue).[113,114] If these changes result in an increased stiffness of the myocardial walls, the right ventricular filling pressure may be increased along with an increase in the right atrial systolic pressure. The increased pressure generated during an atrial contraction may also cause an increase in the central venous pressure, leading to an absence (absent a-wave) or even a reversal (reversed a-wave) of blood flow through the DV.

The protocol developed by the Fetal Medicine Foundation for Doppler evaluation of the DV blood flow is shown in **Fig. 4.** In the current protocol, the a-wave needs to be reversed to be considered abnormal. The image magnification and angulation of the interrogating Doppler beam are important. The Doppler gate needs to be small (0.5–1.0 mm) in order to minimize contamination of the signal by venous structures that are in close proximity, such as the hepatic veins and the inferior vena cava.

A reversed a-wave is seen in approximately 66% of fetuses with trisomy 21 but only in 3% of euploid fetuses. For fetuses with trisomies 18 and 13 and monosomy X, the prevalence of a-wave reversal is 58%, 55%, and 75%, respectively.[154] The prevalence of a-wave abnormalities varies with gestational age and increases with increasing NT measurements. Therefore, the algorithms that incorporate a-wave evaluation in the risk assessment must be able to adjust the likelihood ratios for these 2 variables.

In a study involving 19,614 fetuses, the combination of maternal age, NT measurement, DV Doppler evaluation, and maternal serum biochemistries (free β-hCG and PAPP-A) resulted in a 96% detection for trisomy 21, 92% for trisomy 18, and 100% for both trisomy 13 and monosomy X, with a 3% false-positive rate.[154]

It should be noted that a-wave abnormalities are also associated with an increased risk of cardiac anomalies.[155,156]

Tricuspid Valve Doppler Evaluation

The exact reason for the increase in the prevalence of tricuspid valve regurgitation (TR) seen in fetuses with trisomy 21 is also unclear.[90,157–159] However, the changes in the

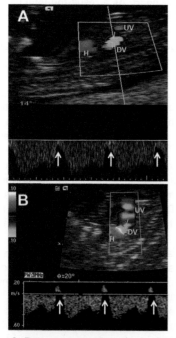

- **CRL : 45-84 mm** (Gestation ~ 11^{+0} to 13^{+6} wks)
- **Right ventral mid-sagittal view**
- **Image size:** thorax and abdomen occupy most of the screen
- **Color flow Doppler** is used to identify the umbilical vein (UV), fetal heart (H), and the ductus venosus (DV) located between them
- **Pulsed-wave Doppler:** 1. small gate (.5-1mm in width) is positioned in the ductus venosus (an area of increased velocity with respect to other venous structures) 2. the angle formed by the longitudinal axis of the ductus venosus and the Doppler beam must be <30°
- The filter should be set at a low frequency (50-70-Hz) so the a-wave is not obscured
- The sweep speed should be high (2-3cm/sec) – the spreading of the waveforms allows better assessment of the a-wave (solid arrows)
- Image B demonstrates a-wave reversal in a fetus with trisomy 21. The a-wave is normal in a euploid fetus (image A)

Fig. 4. Ductus venosus Doppler evaluation protocol (Fetal Medicine Foundation). (*A*) Normal a-wave in a euploid fetus. (*B*) Reversed a-wave in a fetus with trisomy 21.

myocardium and connective tissue known to exist in individuals with Down syndrome and which are described in the section on the DV almost certainly play a role. These changes may result in a relative dilatation of the right ventricle with a concomitant dilatation of the tricuspid valve annulus. In addition, it is known that the atrioventricular valves themselves are affected by the connective tissue abnormalities.[114] Both of these factors may lead to valvular incompetence and regurgitation.

The protocol for TCV evaluation is shown in **Fig. 5**. The magnification and angle of insonation are important. Unlike in the DV evaluation, the Doppler gate needs to be relatively large (2–3 mm) to make sure that both sides of the TCV are included in the Doppler evaluation. It must be kept in mind that the great vessels (aorta and pulmonary artery) are in close proximity to the tricuspid valve and may contaminate the Doppler waveform. There are 2 ways to distinguish between the regurgitant jet and the Doppler footprint of a great vessel. The most important way is to measure the velocity of the blood flow detected on Doppler during the time of ventricular systole. The velocity of the regurgitant jet is generally much higher (>60 mm/s) than the flow in the great vessels (<60 mm/s). In addition, the regurgitant jet on Doppler produces a typical "hissing" sound that is generally absent from sound of the Doppler waveform in the great arteries. The duration of regurgitation should last at least 50% of the ventricular systole to be considered significant.

The prevalence of TR changes with gestational age. There is also an association between an increase in the prevalence of TR and an increase in NT thickness. Therefore, just like the DV evaluation, the likelihood ratio based on the result of TCV evaluation must be adjusted for these 2 variables.[159]

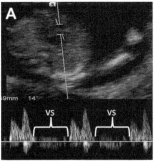
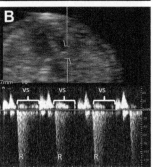

- **CRL : 45-84 mm** (Gestation ~ 11^{+0} to 13^{+6} wks)
- **Apical four-chamber heart view** (fetus may be facing towards or away from the transducer)
- **Image size:** thorax occupies most of the screen
- **Pulsed-wave Doppler:** large gate (2-3mm in width) is positioned across the tricuspid valve, angle formed by the ventricular septum and Doppler beam must be <30°
- **True tricuspid regurgitation (R):** 1. velocity > 60 cm/sec (in order to differentiate from a great vessel waveform). 2. duration ≥ 50% of the ventricular systole (VS)
- At least three sample volumes need to be obtained as the insufficiency may not be present in all three cusps
- Image B (trisomy 21)demonstrates tricuspid regurgitation (R). No evidence of blood flow is seen across the tricuspid valve during the ventricular systole in Image A (euploid fetus)

Fig. 5. Tricuspid valve Doppler evaluation protocol (Fetal Medicine Foundation). (*A*) Absent tricuspid regurgitation in a euploid fetus. (*B*) Tricuspid regurgitation in a fetus with trisomy 21.

The prevalence of TR in fetuses with trisomy 21 is 56% and is only 1% in euploid fetuses. For fetuses with trisomies 18 and 13 and monosomy X, the prevalence of TR is 33%, 30%, and 38%, respectively. In a study involving 19,614 fetuses, the combination of maternal age, NT measurement, TCV Doppler evaluation, and maternal serum biochemistries (free β-hCG and PAPP-A) resulted in a 96% detection for trisomy 21, 92% for trisomy 18, and 100% detection for trisomies 13 and monosomy X, with a 3% false-positive rate.[159]

It should be noted that the presence of TR is also associated with structural cardiac anomalies.[158]

ACQUIRING PROFICIENCY IN ULTRASOUND MARKER EVALUATION

To achieve proficiency in using the ultrasound markers currently available, there is a need for training, experience, and ongoing quality assurance. To be able to perform each of the evaluations correctly on a consistent basis, it is estimated that a sonographer needs to perform around 80 to 120 ultrasound examinations.[160–162] However, there is a steady improvement in performance starting after the first few examinations.

USE OF ADDITIONAL ULTRASOUND MARKERS IN SCREENING FOR TRISOMY 21

All of the ultrasound markers described in this review have been shown to be useful in screening for trisomy 21. However, the manner in which they are used depends on the availability of trained and experienced operators.

If a screening protocol that includes ultrasound markers is employed, NT measurement should be an integral part of it, not only because NT is the most robust marker in screening for aneuploidy but also because of its utility in estimating the risk of other fetal problems. The combined first-trimester screen includes both the NT measurement and maternal serum biochemistries (free β-hCG and PAPP-A) and, as discussed earlier, is very effective in screening for trisomy 21 (approximately 90% detection rate for a 5% screen-positive rate). It should be pointed out that free β-hCG has been rigorously tested in screening,[1,76–97,120–128,138–140,144,154,159] but the effectiveness of total hCG in screening is largely unknown.

It has been shown on a prospective basis that the addition of the new ultrasound markers significantly improves the detection rate of first-trimester screening while decreasing the false-positive rate. Such is the case regardless of whether this is done in every examination or on a first-trimester contingent basis.[140,144,154,159]

The use of first-trimester contingent screening protocols was first proposed by Nicolaides and colleagues.[124] Unlike the contingent screening protocols that have both first- and second-trimester components, a contingent screening protocol that is confined to the first trimester has the advantage of being completed early in pregnancy. The first step is a combined first-trimester screen. Patients are divided into 3 categories based on the results of the combined screen: high risk, intermediate risk, and low risk (see later discussion). In this type of schema, the high-risk group is offered invasive diagnostic testing without any additional screening and the low-risk group is reassured, with invasive diagnostic testing done only on maternal request. The intermediate-risk group is for the additional first-trimester ultrasound markers. If the additional markers are reassuring, the patient is treated in the same way as the low-risk group. If additional markers are abnormal, the patient is offered invasive diagnostic testing. Regardless of the results of the first-trimester screen, a second-trimester targeted scan at around 20 weeks' gestation is recommended to complete the fetal structural evaluation.

Mathematical modeling suggests that screening may be progressively improved by incorporating an increasing number of additional markers. Given the training and expertise required to master the new markers, it is likely that the evaluation of these markers will be done on a contingent basis. A contingent screening protocol that incorporates all of the additional markers in this review (singly or in combination) has been developed by the Fetal Medicine Foundation and is based on the most current data.[123,140,144,154,159] Each of the variables is appropriately adjusted based on the maternal history and ultrasound findings. Likelihood ratios are then generated and mathematically combined. The first step is a combined first-trimester screen and placement of the patients into 1 of the 3 categories described earlier. Based on this model, the high-risk group ($\geq$1:50) constitutes 1.3% of the population, the intermediate-risk group (1:51–1:1000) constitutes 12% of the population, and the low-risk group (<1:1000) constitutes 86.7% of the population. The high-risk, intermediate-risk, and low-risk groups contain 82%, 14%, and 4% of the trisomy 21 fetuses, respectively. Using a false-positive rate of 2%, the projected detection rates by using 1 additional marker is 90%, 2 markers 94%, 3 markers 95%, and all 4 markers 96%.

The use of additional ultrasound markers may be even more important in multiple gestations. Maternal serum markers in higher order multiple gestations (triplets and greater) are unreliable, and first-trimester ultrasound screening is the best option.[76–78] The use of ultrasound markers in multiple gestations also allows assignment of risk to each individual fetus, which cannot be done using maternal serum biochemistries.

SUMMARY

The addition of the newer markers for aneuploidy serves 2 purposes: it increases the detection rate for Down syndrome while decreasing the false-positive rate. The benefit of increased detection rate is self evident, as detection of fetal chromosomal defects is the very purpose of a screening program. The decrease in screen-positive rates leads to fewer prenatal diagnostic procedures; this in turn decreases the number of unaffected fetuses that are lost as a result of performing invasive procedures and is bound to decrease the cost of screening. Furthermore, with a decreased screen-positive rate, fewer women need to go through the anxiety of dealing with a positive screening result.

On the other hand, the addition of new ultrasound markers requires more training and expertise for the sonographer. It is clear that screening tests are useful only if the persons who administer them have the appropriate training, expertise, and equipment, and are monitored by an ongoing quality assurance program.

For further information and updated protocols, go to: http://www.fetalmedicine. com/fmf and click on "Certificates of competence" under "Training and certification".

REFERENCES

1. Cuckle H, Benn P, Wright D. Down syndrome screening in the first and/or second trimester: model predicted performance using meta-analysis parameters. Semin Perinatol 2005;29:252–7.
2. Wisser J, Dirschedl P, Krone S. Estimation of gestational age by transvaginal sonographic measurements of greatest embryonic length in dated human embryos. Ultrasound Obstet Gynecol 1994;4:457–62.
3. Green JJ, Hobbins JC. Abdominal ultrasound examination of the first trimester fetus. Am J Obstet Gynecol 1988;159:165–75.

4. Rottem S, Bronshtein M, Thaler I, et al. First trimester transvaginal sonographic diagnosis of fetal anomalies. Lancet 1989;1:444–5.
5. Johnson P, Sharland G, Maxwell D, et al. The role of transvaginal sonography in the early detection of congenital heart disease. Ultrasound Obstet Gynecol 1992;2:248–51.
6. Braithwaite JM, Armstrong MA, Economides DL. Assessment of fetal anatomy at 12 to 13 weeks of gestation by transabdominal and transvaginal sonography. Br J Obstet Gynaecol 1996;103:82–5.
7. Hernadi L, Torocsik M. Screening for fetal anomalies in the 12th week of pregnancy by transvaginal sonography in an unselected population. Prenat Diagn 1997;17:753–9.
8. Economides DL, Braithwaite JM. First trimester ultrasonographic diagnosis of fetal structural abnormalities in a low risk population. Br J Obstet Gynaecol 1998;105:53–7.
9. Carvalho MH, Brizot ML, Lopes LM, et al. Detection of fetal structural abnormalities at the 11-14 week ultrasound scan. Prenat Diagn 2002;22:1–4.
10. Souka AP, Pilalis A, Kavalakis I, et al. Screening for major structural abnormalities at the 11- to 14-week ultrasound scan. Am J Obstet Gynecol 2006;194:393–6.
11. Gembruch U, Knopfle G, Bald R, et al. Early diagnosis of fetal congenital heart disease by transvaginal echocardiography. Ultrasound Obstet Gynecol 1993;3:310–7.
12. Achiron R, Rotstein Z, Lipitz S, et al. First-trimester diagnosis of fetal congenital heart disease by transvaginal ultrasonography. Obstet Gynecol 1994;84:69–72.
13. Smrcek JM, Gembruch U, Krokowski M, et al. The evaluation of cardiac biometry in major cardiac defects detected in early pregnancy. Arch Gynecol Obstet 2003;268:94–101.
14. Becker R, Wegner RD. Detailed screening for fetal anomalies and cardiac defects at the 11-13 week scan. Ultrasound Obstet Gynecol 2006;27:613–8.
15. Hyett J, Moscoso G, Papapanagiotou G, et al. Abnormalities of the heart and great arteries in chromosomally normal fetuses with increased nuchal translucency thickness at 11-13 weeks of gestation. Ultrasound Obstet Gynecol 1996;7:245–50.
16. Schwarzler P, Carvalho JS, Senat MV, et al. Screening for fetal aneuploidies and fetal cardiac abnormalities by nuchal translucency thickness measurement at 10-14 weeks of gestation as part of routine antenatal care in an unselected population. Br J Obstet Gynaecol 1999;106:1029–34.
17. Bahado-Singh RO, Wapner R, Thom E, et al. Elevated first-trimester nuchal translucency increases the risk of congenital heart defects. Am J Obstet Gynecol 2005;192:1357–61.
18. Moselhi M, Thilaganathan B. Nuchal translucency: a marker for the antenatal diagnosis of aortic coarctation. Br J Obstet Gynaecol 1996;103:1044–5.
19. Hyett JA, Perdu M, Sharland GK, et al. Increased nuchal translucency at 10-14 weeks of gestation as a marker for major cardiac defects. Ultrasound Obstet Gynecol 1997;10:242–6.
20. Zosmer N, Souter VL, Chan CSY, et al. Early diagnosis of major cardiac defects in chromosomally normal fetuses with increased nuchal translucency. Br J Obstet Gynaecol 1999;106:829–33.
21. Ghi T, Huggon IC, Zosmer N, et al. Incidence of major structural cardiac defects associated with increased nuchal translucency but normal karyotype. Ultrasound Obstet Gynecol 2001;18:610–4.

22. Lopes LM, Brizot ML, Lopes MA, et al. Structural and functional cardiac abnormalities identified prior to 16 weeks' gestation in fetuses with increased nuchal translucency. Ultrasound Obstet Gynecol 2003;22:470–8.
23. Galindo A, Comas C, Martinez JM, et al. Cardiac defects in chromosomally normal fetuses with increased nuchal translucency at 10-14 weeks of gestation. J Matern Fetal Neonatal Med 2003;13:163–70.
24. McAuliffe F, Winsor S, Hornberger L, et al. Fetal cardiac defects and increased nuchal translucency thickness [abstract 571]. Am J Obstet Gynecol 2003;189.
25. Hyett J, Perdu M, Sharland G, et al. Using fetal nuchal translucency to screen for major congenital cardiac defects at 10-14 weeks of gestation: population based cohort study. Br Med J 1999;318:81–5.
26. Mavrides E, Cobian-Sanchez F, Tekay A, et al. Limitations of using first trimester nuchal translucency measurement in routine screening for major congenital heart defects. Ultrasound Obstet Gynecol 2001;17:106–10.
27. Orvos H, Wayda K, Kozinsky Z, et al. Increased nuchal translucency and congenital heart defects in euploid fetuses. The Szeged experience. Eur J Obstet Gynecol Reprod Biol 2002;101:124–8.
28. Hafner E, Schuller T, Metzenbauer M, et al. Increased nuchal translucency and congenital heart defects in a low-risk population. Prenat Diagn 2003;23:985–9.
29. Makrydimas G, Sotiriadis A, Ioannidis JP. Screening performance of first-trimester nuchal translucency for major cardiac defects: a meta-analysis. Am J Obstet Gynecol 2003;189:1330–5.
30. Schemm S, Gembruch U, Germer U, et al. Omphalocele-exstrophy-imperforate anus-spinal defects (OEIS) complex associated with increased nuchal translucency. Ultrasound Obstet Gynecol 2003;22:95–7.
31. Sebire NJ, Snijders RJM, Davenport M, et al. Fetal nuchal translucency thickness at 10-14 weeks of gestation and congenital diaphragmatic hernia. Obstet Gynecol 1997;90:943–7.
32. Smrcek JM, Germer U, Krokowski M, et al. Prenatal ultrasound diagnosis and management of body stalk anomaly: analysis of nine singleton and two multiple pregnancies. Ultrasound Obstet Gynecol 2003;21:322–8.
33. Monteagudo A, Mayberry P, Rebarber A, et al. Sirenomelia sequence: first-trimester diagnosis with both two- and three-dimensional sonography. J Ultrasound Med 2002;21:915–20.
34. Souka AP, Snidjers RJM, Novakov A, et al. Defects and syndromes in chromosomally normal fetuses with increased nuchal translucency at 10-14 weeks of gestation. Ultrasound Obstet Gynecol 1998;11:391–400.
35. Souka A, Heath V. Increased nuchal translucency with normal karyotype. In: Sebire NJ, Snijders RJM, Nicolaides KH, editors. The 11-14 week scan: diagnosis of fetal abnormalities. Carnforth (UK): Parthenon Publishing; 1999. p. 67–88.
36. Souka A, von Kaisenberg C, Hyett J. Increased nuchal translucency with normal karyotype. Am J Obstet Gynecol 2005;192:1005–21.
37. Ben Ami M, Perlitz Y, Haddad S, et al. Increased nuchal translucency is associated with asphyxiating thoracic dysplasia. Ultrasound Obstet Gynecol 1997;10:297–8.
38. Soothill PW, Vuthiwong C, Rees H. Achondrogenesis type 2 diagnosed by transvaginal ultrasound at 12 weeks of gestation. Prenat Diagn 1993;13:523–8.
39. Makrydimas G, Souka A, Skentou H, et al. Osteogenesis imperfecta and other skeletal dysplasias presenting with increased nuchal translucency in the first trimester. Am J Med Genet 2001;98:117–20.

40. Fisk NM, Vaughan J, Smidt M, et al. Transvaginal ultrasound recognition of nuchal oedema in the first-trimester diagnosis of achondrogenesis. J Clin Ultrasound 1991;19:586–90.
41. Meizner I, Barnhard Y. Achondrogenesis type I diagnosed by transvaginal ultrasonography at 13 weeks' gestation. Am J Obstet Gynecol 1995;173:1620–2.
42. den Hollander NS, van der Harten HJ, Vermeij-Keers C, et al. First trimester diagnosis of Blomstrand lethal osteochondrodysplasia. Am J Med Genet 1997;73:345–50.
43. Souka AP, Raymond FL, Mornet E, et al. Hypophosphatasia associated with increased nuchal translucency: a report of three consecutive pregnancies. Ultrasound Obstet Gynecol 2002;20:294–5.
44. Eliyahu S, Weiner E, Lahav D, et al. Early sonographic diagnosis of Jarcho-Levin syndrome: a prospective screening program in one family. Ultrasound Obstet Gynecol 1997;9:314–8.
45. Souter V, Nyberg D, Siebert JR, et al. Upper limb phocomelia associated with increased nuchal translucency in a monochorionic twin pregnancy. J Ultrasound Med 2002;21:355–60.
46. Petrikovsky BM, Gross B, Bialer M, et al. Prenatal diagnosis of pseudothalidomide syndrome in consecutive pregnancies of a consanguineous couple. Ultrasound Obstet Gynecol 1997;10:425–8.
47. Percin EF, Guvenal T, Cetin A, et al. First-trimester diagnosis of Robinow syndrome. Fetal Diagn Ther 2001;16:308–11.
48. Hill LM, Leary J. Transvaginal sonographic diagnosis of short-rib polydactyly dysplasia at 13 weeks' gestation. Prenat Diagn 1998;18:1198–201.
49. Achiron R, Heggesh J, Grisaru D, et al. Noonan syndrome: a cryptic condition in early gestation. Am J Med Genet 2000;92:159–65.
50. Souka AP, Krampl E, Geerts L, et al. Congenital lymphedema presenting with increased nuchal translucency at 13 weeks of gestation. Prenat Diagn 2002;22:91–2.
51. Fincham J, Pandya PP, Yuksel B, et al. Increased first-trimester nuchal translucency as a prenatal manifestation of salt-wasting congenital adrenal hyperplasia. Ultrasound Obstet Gynecol 2002;20:392–4.
52. Souka AP, Skentou H, Geerts L, et al. Congenital nephrotic syndrome presenting with increased nuchal translucency in the first trimester. Prenat Diagn 2002;22:93–5.
53. Hyett J, Noble P, Sebire NJ, et al. Lethal congenital arthrogryposis presents with increased nuchal translucency at 10-14 weeks of gestation. Ultrasound Obstet Gynecol 1997;9:310–3.
54. Rijhsinghani A, Yankowitz J, Howser D, et al. Sonographic and maternal serum screening abnormalities in fetuses affected by spinal muscular atrophy. Prenat Diagn 1997;17:166–9.
55. de Jong-Pleij EA, Stoutenbecek P, van der Mark-Batseva NN, et al. The association of spinal muscular atrophy type II and increased nuchal translucency. Ultrasound Obstet Gynecol 2002;19:312–3.
56. Lam YH, Tang MH, Lee CP, et al. Nuchal translucency in fetuses affected by homozygous a-thalassemia-1 at 12-13 weeks of gestation. Ultrasound Obstet Gynecol 1999;13:238–40.
57. Souka AP, Bower S, Geerts L, et al. Blackfan-Diamond anemia and dyserythropoietic anemia presenting with increased nuchal translucency at 12 weeks of gestation. Ultrasound Obstet Gynecol 2002;20:197–9.

58. Pannier E, Viot G, Aubry MC, et al. Congenital erythropoietic porphyria (Gunther's disease): two cases with very early prenatal manifestation and cystic hydroma. Prenat Diagn 2003;23:25–30.
59. Tercanli S, Miny P, Siebert MS, et al. Fanconi anemia associated with increased nuchal translucency detected by first-trimester ultrasound. Ultrasound Obstet Gynecol 2001;17:160–2.
60. Petrikovsky BM, Baker D, Schneider E. Fetal hydrops secondary to human parvovirus infection in early pregnancy. Prenat Diagn 1996;16:342–4.
61. Markenson G, Correia LA, Cohn G, et al. Parvoviral infection associated with increased nuchal translucency: a case report. J Perinatol 2000;20:129–31.
62. Smulian JC, Egan JF, Rodis JF. Fetal hydrops in the first trimester associated with maternal parvovirus infection. J Clin Ultrasound 1998;26:314–6.
63. Ville Y, Lalondrelle C, Doumerc S, et al. First-trimester diagnosis of nuchal anomalies: significance and fetal outcome. Ultrasound Obstet Gynecol 1992;2:314–6.
64. Brady AF, Pandya PP, Yuksel B, et al. Outcome of chromosomally normal live-births with increased fetal nuchal translucency at 10-14 weeks' gestation. J Med Genet 1998;35:222–4.
65. Souka AP, Krampl E, Bakalis S, et al. Outcome of pregnancy in chromosomally normal fetuses with increased nuchal translucency in the first trimester. Ultrasound Obstet Gynecol 2001;18:9–17.
66. Mangione R, Guyon F, Taine L, et al. Pregnancy outcome and prognosis in fetuses with increased first-trimester nuchal translucency. Fetal Diagn Ther 2001;16:360–3.
67. Bilardo CM, Pajkrt E, de Graaf IM, et al. Outcome of fetuses with enlarged nuchal translucency and normal karyotype. Ultrasound Obstet Gynecol 1998; 11:401–6.
68. Michailidis GD, Economides DL. Nuchal translucency measurement and pregnancy outcome in karyotypically normal fetuses. Ultrasound Obstet Gynecol 2001;17:102–5.
69. Shulman LP, Emerson DS, Grevengood C, et al. Clinical course and outcome of fetuses with isolated cystic nuchal lesions and normal karyotypes detected in the first trimester. Am J Obstet Gynecol 1994;171:1278–81.
70. Cheng C, Bahado-Singh RO, Chen S, et al. Pregnancy outcomes with increased nuchal translucency after routine Down syndrome screening. Int J Gynaecol Obstet 2004;84:5–9.
71. Senat MV, De Keersmaecker B, Audibert F, et al. Pregnancy outcome in fetuses with increased nuchal translucency and normal karyotype. Prenat Diagn 2002; 22:345–9.
72. Cha'Ban FK, van Splunder P, Los FJ, et al. Fetal outcome in nuchal translucency with emphasis on normal fetal karyotype. Prenat Diagn 1996;16:537–41.
73. Monteagudo A, Timor-Tritsch I, Sharma S. Early and simple determination of chorionic and amniotic type in multifetal gestations in the first 14 weeks by high frequency transvaginal ultrasound. Am J Obstet Gynecol 1994;170:824–9.
74. Sepulveda W, Sebire NJ, Hughes K, et al. The lambda sign at 10-14 weeks of gestation as a predictor of chorionicity in twin pregnancies. Ultrasound Obstet Gynecol 1996;7:421–3.
75. Selpuveda W, Sebire NJ, Hughes K, et al. Evolution of the lambda or twin/chorionic peak sign in dichorionic twin pregnancies. Obstet Gynecol 1997;89: 439–41.
76. Noble PL, Snijders RJM, Abraha HD, et al. Maternal serum free beta-hCG at 10 to 14 weeks in trisomic twin pregnancies. BJOG 1997;104:741–3.

77. Spencer K. Screening for trisomy 21 in twin pregnancies in the first trimester using free beta-hCG and PAPP-A, combined with fetal nuchal translucency thickness. Prenat Diagn 2000;20:91–5.

78. Spencer K, Nicolaides KH. Screening for trisomy 21 in twins using first trimester ultrasound and maternal serum biochemistry in a one-stop clinic: a review of three years experience. BJOG 2003;110:276–80.

79. Maiz N, Staboulidou I, Leal AM, et al. Ductus venosus Doppler at 11 to 13 weeks of gestation in the prediction of outcome in twin pregnancies. Obstet Gynecol 2009;113:860–5.

80. Souka AP, Pilalis A, Kavalakis Y, et al. Assessment of fetal anatomy at the 11-14 week ultrasound examination. Ultrasound Obstet Gynecol 2004;24:730–4.

81. van Zalen-Sprock RM, van Vugt JMG, van Geijn HP. First-trimester sonography of physiological midgut herniation and early diagnosis of omphalocele. Prenat Diagn 1997;17:511–8.

82. Snijders RJ, Sebire NJ, Souka A, et al. Fetal exomphalos and chromosomal defects: relationship to maternal age and gestation. Ultrasound Obstet Gynecol 1995;6:250–5.

83. Johnson SP, Sebire NJ, Snijders RMJ, et al. Ultrasound screening for anencephaly at 10-14 weeks of gestation. Ultrasound Obstet Gynecol 1997;9:14–6.

84. Wright D, Kagan KO, Molina FS, et al. A mixture model of nuchal translucency thickness in screening for chromosomal defects. Ultrasound Obstet Gynecol 2008;31(4):376–83.

85. Whitlow BJ, Economides DL. The optimal gestational age to examine fetal anatomy and measure nuchal translucency in the first trimester. Ultrasound Obstet Gynecol 1998;11:258–61.

86. Mulvey S, Baker L, Edwards A, et al. Optimising the timing for nuchal translucency measurement. Prenat Diagn 2002;22:775–7.

87. Snijders RJM, Noble P, Sebire N, et al. UK multicentre project on assessment of risk of trisomy 21 by maternal age and fetal nuchal translucency thickness at 10-14 weeks of gestation. Lancet 1998;351:343–6.

88. Cicero S, Curcio P, Papageorghiou A, et al. Absence of nasal bone in fetuses with Trisomy 21 at 11-14 weeks of gestation: an observational study. Lancet 2001;358:1665–7.

89. Sonek J, Borenstein M, Dagklis T, et al. Fronto-maxillary facial angle in fetuses with Trisomy 21 at 11-13 (+6) weeks'. Am J Obstet Gynecol 2007;196(3):271.

90. Falcon O, Auer M, Gerovassili A, et al. Screening for trisomy 21 by tricuspid regurgitation, nuchal translucency and maternal serum free β-hCG and PAPP-A at 11 +0 to 13 +6 weeks. Ultrasound Obstet Gynecol 2006;27:151–5.

91. Antolin E, Comas C, Torrents M, et al. The role of ductus venosus blood flow assessment in screening for chromosomal abnormalities at 10-16 weeks of gestation. Ultrasound Obstet Gynecol 2001;17:295–300.

92. Liao AW, Snijders R, Geerts L, et al. Fetal heart rate in chromosomally abnormal fetuses. Ultrasound Obstet Gynecol 2000;16:610–3.

93. Rembouskos G, Cicero S, Longo D, et al. Single Umbilical Artery at 11-14 weeks: relation to chromosomal defects. Ultrasound Obstet Gynecol 2003;22:567–70.

94. Sebire NJ, Von Kaisenberg C, Rubio C, et al. Fetal megacystis at 10-14 weeks of gestation. Ultrasound Obstet Gynecol 1996;8:387–90.

95. Liao AW, Sebire NJ, Geerts L, et al. Megacystis at 10-14 weeks of gestation: chromosomal defects and outcome according to bladder length. Ultrasound Obstet Gynecol 2003;21:338–41.

96. Favre R, Kohler M, Gasser B, et al. Early fetal megacystis between 11 and 15 weeks of gestation. Ultrasound Obstet Gynecol 1999;14:402–6.
97. Nicolaides KH, Snijders RJM, Gosden CM, et al. Ultrasonographically detectable markers of fetal chromosomal abnormalities. Lancet 1992;340:704–7.
98. Langdon Down J. Observations on an ethnic classification of idiots. Clin Lectures and Reports, London Hospital 1866;3:259–62.
99. Nicolaides KH, Azar G, Byrne D, et al. Fetal nuchal translucency: ultrasound screening for chromosomal defects in first trimester of pregnancy. Br Med J 1992;304:867–89.
100. Braithwaite JM, Morris RW, Economides DL. Nuchal translucency measurements: frequency, distribution, and changes with gestation in a general population. Br J Obstet Gynaecol 1996;103:1201–4.
101. Whitlow BJ, Chatzipapas IK, Economides DL. The effect of fetal neck position on nuchal translucency measurement at 10-14 weeks. Br J Obstet Gynaecol 1998;105:872–6.
102. Shaefer M, Laurichesse-Delmas H, Ville Y. The effect of nuchal cord on nuchal translucency measurement at 10-14 weeks. Ultrasound Obstet Gynecol 1998;11:271–3.
103. Molina F, Avgidou K, Kagan K, et al. Cystic hygromas, nuchal edema, and nuchal translucency at 11-14 weeks of gestation. Obstet Gynecol 2006;107:678–83.
104. Hewitt BG, de Crespigny L, Sampson AJ, et al. Correlation between nuchal thickness and abnormal karyotype in first trimester fetuses. Med J Aust 1996;165:365–8.
105. Simpson JM, Sharland GK. Nuchal translucency and congenital heart defects: heart failure or not? Ultrasound Obstet Gynecol 2000;16:30–6.
106. Rizzo G, Muscatello A, Angelini E, et al. Abnormal cardiac function in fetuses with increased nuchal translucency. Ultrasound Obstet Gynecol 2003;21:539–42.
107. Hyett JA, Brizot ML, von Kaisenberg CS, et al. Cardiac gene expression of atrial natriuretic peptide and brain natriuretic peptide in trisomic fetuses. Obstet Gynecol 1996;87:506–10.
108. Tsuchimochi H, Kurimoto F, Leki K, et al. Atrial natriuretic peptide distribution in fetal and failed adult human hearts. Circulation 1988;78:920–7.
109. Recalde AL, Landing BH, Lipsey AI. Increased cardiac muscle size and reduced cell number in Down syndrome. Pediatr Pathol 1986;6:47–53.
110. von Kaisenberg CS, Krenn V, Ludwig M, et al. Morphological classification of nuchal skin in fetuses with trisomy 21, 18 and 13 at 12-18 weeks and in a trisomy 16 mouse. Anat Embryol 1998;197:105–24.
111. von Kaisenberg CS, Brand-Saberi B, Christ B, et al. Collagen type VI gene expression in the skin of trisomy 21 fetuses. Obstet Gynecol 1998;91:319–23.
112. Bohlandt S, von Kaisenberg CS, Wewetzer K, et al. Hyaluronan in the nuchal skin of chromosomally abnormal fetuses. Hum Reprod 2000;15:1155–8.
113. Gittenberger-De Groot AC, Bartram U, Oosthoek PW, et al. Collagen type VI expression during cardiac development and in human fetuses with trisomy 21. Anat Rec 2003;275A:1109–16.
114. Carvalhaes LS, Gervásio OL, Guatimosim C, et al. Collagen XVIII/endostatin is associated with the epithelial-mesenchymal transformation in the atrioventricular valves during cardiac development. Dev Dyn 2006;235:132–42.
115. Chitayat D, Kalousek DK, Bamforth JS. Lymphatic abnormalities in fetuses with posterior cervical cystic hygroma. Am J Med Genet 1989;33:352–6.

116. Von Kaisenberg CS, Nicolaides KH, Brand-Siberi B. Lymphatic vessel hypoplasia in fetuses with Turner syndrome. Hum Reprod 1999;14:823.
117. Nicolaides KH, Rodeck CH, Lange I, et al. Fetoscopy in the assessment of unexplained fetal hydrops. Br J Obstet Gynaecol 1985;92:671–9.
118. Sohan K, Carroll S, Byrne D, et al. Parvovirus as a differential diagnosis of hydrops fetalis in the first trimester. Fetal Diagn Ther 2000;15:234–6.
119. Pajkrt E, van Lith JMM, Mol BWJ, et al. Screening for Down's syndrome by fetal nuchal translucency measurement in a general obstetric population. Ultrasound Obstet Gynecol 1998;12:163–9.
120. Spencer K, Souter V, Tul N, et al. A screening program for trisomy 21 at 10-14 weeks using fetal nuchal translucency, maternal serum free ß-human chorionic gonadotropin and pregnancy-associated plasma protein-A. Ultrasound Obstet Gynecol 1999;13:231–7.
121. Spencer K, Spencer DE, Power M, et al. Screening for chromosomal abnormalities in the first trimester using ultrasound and maternal serum biochemistry and in a one-stop clinic: a review of three years prospective experience. BJOG 2003; 110:281–6.
122. Kagan KO, Wright D, Baker A, et al. Screening for trisomy 21 by maternal age, fetal nuchal translucency thickness, free beta human chorionic gonadotropin and pregnancy-associated plasma protein-A. Ultrasound Obstet Gynecol 2008;31:618–24.
123. Kagan KO, Etchegaray A, Zhou Y, et al. Prospective validation of first-trimester combined screening for trisomy 21. Ultrasound Obstet Gynecol 2009;34:14–8.
124. Nicolaides KH, Spencer K, Avgidou K, et al. Multicenter study of first-trimester screening for trisomy 21 in 75 821 pregnancies: results and estimation of the potential impact of individual risk-orientated two-stage first-trimester screening. Ultrasound Obstet Gynecol 2005;25:221–6.
125. Avgidou K, Papageorghiou A, Bindra R, et al. Prospective first-trimester screening for trisomy 21 in 30,564 pregnancies. Am J Obstet Gynecol 2005; 192:1761–7.
126. Kagan KO, Wright D, Valencia C, et al. Screening for trisomies 21,18 and 13 by maternal age, fetal nuchal translucency, fetal heart rate free beta-hCG and pregnancy-associated plasma protein-A. Hum Reprod 2008;23: 1968–75.
127. Kagan KO, Anderson JM, Anwandter G, et al. Screening for triploidy by the risk algorithms for trisomies 21, 18 and 13 at 11-13 weeks and 6 days of gestation. Prenat Diagn 2008;28:1209–13.
128. Kagan KO, Wright D, Maiz N, et al. Screening for trisomy 18 by maternal age, fetal nuchal translucency, free beta-human chorionic gonadotropin and pregnancy-associated plasma protein-A. Ultrasound Obstet Gynecol 2008;4: 488–92.
129. Otano L, Aiello H, Igarzabal L, et al. Association between first trimester absence of fetal nasal bone on ultrasound and Down's syndrome. Prenat Diagn 2002;22: 930–2.
130. Zoppi MA, Ibba RM, Axinan C, et al. Absence of fetal nasal bone and aneuploidies at first-trimester nuchal translucency screening in unselected pregnancies. Prenat Diagn 2003;23:496–500.
131. Viora E, Masturzo B, Errante G, et al. Ultrasound evaluation of fetal nasal bone at 11 to 14 weeks in a consecutive series of 1906 fetuses. Prenat Diagn 2003;23: 784–7.

132. Wong SF, Choi H, Ho LC. Nasal bone hypoplasia: is it a common finding amongst chromosomally normal fetuses of southern Chinese women? Gynecol Obstet Invest 2003;56:99–101.
133. Cicero S, Longo D, Rembouskos G, et al. Absent nasal bone at 11-14 weeks of gestation and chromosomal defects. Ultrasound Obstet Gynecol 2003;22:31–5.
134. Sonek J, Cicero S, Neiger R, et al. Nasal bone assessment in prenatal screening for trisomy 21. Am J Obstet Gynecol 2006;195:1219–30.
135. Cicero S, Bindra R, Rembouskos G, et al. Fetal nasal bone length in chromosomally normal and abnormal fetuses at 11-14 weeks of gestation. J Matern Fetal Neonatal Med 2002;11:400–2.
136. Rembouskos G, Cicero S, Longo D, et al. Assessment of the fetal nasal bone at 11-14 weeks of gestation by three-dimensional ultrasound. Ultrasound Obstet Gynecol 2004;23:232–6.
137. Cicero S, Rembouskos G, Vandecruys H, et al. Likelihood ratio for Trisomy 21 in fetuses with absent nasal bone at the 11-14 weeks scan. Ultrasound Obstet Gynecol 2004;23:218–23.
138. Cicero S, Bindra R, Rembouskos G, et al. Integrated ultrasound and biochemical screening for trisomy 21 using nuchal translucency, absent fetal nasal bone, free beta and PAPP A at 11 to 14 weeks. Prenat Diagn 2003;23:306–10.
139. Cicero S, Avgidu K, Rembouskos G, et al. Nasal bone assessment in prenatal screening for trisomy 21. Am J Obstet Gynecol 2006;195:109–44, 2009.
140. Kagan KO, Cicero S, Staboulidou I, et al. Fetal nasal bone in screening for trisomy 21, 18, 13 and Turner syndrome at 11-13 weeks of gestation. Ultrasound Obstet Gynecol 2009;33:259–64.
141. Plasencia W, Dagklis T, Pachoumi C, et al. Frontomaxillary facial angle at 11 +0 to 13 +6 weeks: effect of plane of acquisition. Ultrasound Obstet Gynecol 2007; 29:660–5.
142. Sonek J, Borenstein M, Downing C, et al. Frontomaxillary facial angles in screening for trisomy 21 at 14-23 weeks' gestation. Am J Obstet Gynecol 2007;197:160.
143. Borenstein M, Persico N, Kaihura C, et al. Frontomaxillary facial angle in chromosomally normal fetuses at 11 +0 to 13 +6 weeks. Ultrasound Obstet Gynecol 2007;30:737–41.
144. Borenstein M, Persico N, Kagan KO, et al. Frontomaxillary facial angle in screening for trisomy 21 at 11 +0 to 13 +6 weeks. Ultrasound Obstet Gynecol 2008;32:5–11.
145. Borenstein M, Persico N, Dagklis T, et al. Frontomaxillary facial angle in fetuses with trisomy 13 at 11 +0 to 13 +6 weeks. Ultrasound Obstet Gynecol 2007;30: 819–23.
146. Borenstein M, Persico N, Strobl I, et al. Frontomaxillary and mandibulomaxillary facial angles at 11 +0 to 13 +6 weeks in fetuses with trisomy 18. Ultrasound Obstet Gynecol 2007;30:928–33.
147. Kiserud T, Eik-Nes SH, Blaas HG, et al. Ductus venosus blood velocity and the umbilical circulation in the seriously growth-retarded fetus. Ultrasound Obstet Gynecol 1994;4:109–14.
148. Hecher K, Campbell S, Doyle P, et al. Assessment of fetal compromise by Doppler ultrasound investigation of the fetal circulation. Arterial, intracardiac, and venous blood flow velocity studies. Circulation 1995;91:129–38.
149. Maiz N, Valencia C, Emmanuel EE, et al. Screening for adverse pregnancy outcome by ductus venosus Doppler at 11-13 +6 weeks of gestation. Obstet Gynecol 2008;112:598–605.

150. Mavrides E, Sairam S, Hollis B, et al. Screening for aneuploidy in the first trimester by assessment of blood flow in the ductus venosus. BJOG 2002; 109:1015–9.
151. Murta CG, Moron AF, Avila MA, et al. Application of ductus venosus Doppler velocimetry for the detection of fetal aneuploidy in the first trimester of pregnancy. Fetal Diagn Ther 2002;1:308–14.
152. Zoppi MA, Putzolu M, Ibba RM, et al. First-trimester ductus venosus velocimetry in relation to nuchal translucency thickness and fetal karyotype. Fetal Diagn Ther 2002;17:52–7.
153. Borrell A, Martinez JM, Seres A, et al. Ductus venosus assessment at the time of nuchal translucency measurement in the detection of fetal aneuploidy. Prenat Diagn 2003;23:921–6.
154. Maiz N, Valencia C, Kagan KO, et al. Ductus venosus Doppler in screening for trisomies 21, 18, and 13 and Turner syndrome at 11-13 weeks of gestation. Ultrasound Obstet Gynecol 2009;33:512–7.
155. Bilardo CM, Muller MA, Zikulnig L, et al. Ductus venosus studies in fetuses at high risk for chromosomal or heart abnormalities: relationship with nuchal translucency measurement and fetal outcome. Ultrasound Obstet Gynecol 2001;17: 288–94.
156. Maiz N, Plasencia W, Daklis T, et al. Ductus venosus Doppler in fetuses with cardiac defects and increased nuchal translucency thickness. Ultrasound Obstet Gynecol 2008;31:256–60.
157. Huggon IC, DeFigueiredo DB, Allan LD. Tricuspid regurgitation in the diagnosis of chromosomal anomalies in the fetus at 11-14 weeks of gestation. Heart 2003; 89:1071–3.
158. Faiola S, Tsoi E, Huggon IC, et al. Likelihood ratio for trisomy 21 in fetuses with tricuspid regurgitation at the 11 to 13 +6 week scan. Ultrasound Obstet Gynecol 2005;26:22–7.
159. Kagan KO, Valencia C, Livanos P, et al. Tricuspid regurgitation in screening for trisomies 21, 18 and 13 and Turner syndrome at 11 +0 to 13 +6 weeks of gestation. Ultrasound Obstet Gynecol 2009;33:18–22.
160. Braithwaite JM, Kadir RA, Pepera TA, et al. Nuchal translucency measurement: training of potential examiners. Ultrasound Obstet Gynecol 1996;8:192–5.
161. Cicero S, Dezerega V, Andrade E, et al. Learning curve for sonographic examination of the fetal nasal bone at 11-14 weeks. Ultrasound Obstet Gynecol 2003; 22:135–7.
162. Maiz N, Kagan KO, Milovanovic A, et al. Learning curve for Doppler assessment of ductus venosus flow at 11-13 +6 weeks' gestation. Ultrasound Obstet Gynecol 2008;31:503–6.

Monitoring Quality Control of Nuchal Translucency

Howard Cuckle, MSc, DPhil

KEYWORDS

• Nuchal • Screening • Down syndrome • Quality • Prenatal

Nuchal translucency (NT) is by far the most discriminatory marker of fetal Down syndrome available today and is the main component of the most effective multi-marker screening strategies. However, the quality control of ultrasound markers is more difficult than that of maternal serum markers, and this leads to practical difficulties. This article discusses the importance of maintaining the quality of NT and the different ways of achieving this quality.

MAIN SCREENING MARKERS

Typically, screening markers have considerable overlap in the distribution of results between affected and unaffected individuals. The potential utility in the screening of a given marker depends on the extent of separation between the 2 distributions, which can be expressed as the absolute difference between the means of the distribution divided by the average standard deviation for the 2 distributions, a form of Mahalanobis distance.

The levels of all commonly used Down syndrome screening markers change with gestation: NT, maternal serum pregnancy-associated plasma protein (PAPP)-A, α-fetoprotein (AFP), and unconjugated estriol (uE_3) increase steadily; human chorionic gonadotropin (hCG) and the free β subunit of hCG decrease rapidly to a plateau; inhibin-A decreases to a nadir and increases thereafter. To allow for these changes with gestation, marker levels are expressed in multiples of the gestation-specific median for unaffected pregnancies, derived by regression. Early ultrasonography studies of NT did not allow for gestation at all, but levels are now being reported in either multiples of median (MoMs) or deviations from the gestation-specific normal median (delta-NT).

Unlike NT, all serum markers have a negative correlation between the MoM level and maternal weight. This negative correlation is largely because of dilution; a fixed mass of chemical produced in the fetoplacental unit is diluted by a variable volume in the

Department of Obstetrics and Gynecology, Columbia University Medical Center, 622 West 168th Street, New York, NY 10032, USA
E-mail address: hsc2121@columbia.edu

Clin Lab Med 30 (2010) 593–604
doi:10.1016/j.cll.2010.04.012
0272-2712/10/$ – see front matter © 2010 Elsevier Inc. All rights reserved.

labmed.theclinics.com

maternal unit. It is standard practice to adjust for this dilution by dividing the observed MoM by the expected value for the maternal weight derived by regression. Many centers also adjust serum MoMs, but not NT, to allow for maternal smoking and ethnicity. The levels of both hCG isoforms are reduced on an average in smokers, and there is a reduction of similar magnitude in PAPP-A levels, whereas inhibin-A levels are increased to an even greater extent. Adjustment is achieved by dividing the observed MoM by the average value reported in the literature among smokers or non-smokers, as approapriate. In women of African Caribbean origin or in African American women, levels of hCG isoforms are increased, whereas those of AFP and inhibin-A are decreased; PAPP-A level is markedly increased in African Caribbeans but not to the same extent in African Americans. In women of South Asian origin, uE_3 and total hCG levels seem to be somewhat higher than those in Caucasian women. In ethnically homogeneous populations, there is no need to make adjustments because the normal median reflects the local ethnicity. In an ethnically mixed population with large enough minorities, MoMs can be calculated with ethnic-specific medians or the observed MoM can be divided by a factor derived from the average in published studies for different ethnic groups, taking account of the local ethnic mix.

MOST DISCRIMINATORY SINGLE MARKER

To calculate the Mahalanobis distance, the most reliable estimates of means and standard deviations are from meta-analyses of all the published literature, as are the correlation coefficients between markers. The advantages of meta-analysis are that it produces the most robust estimate of the mean and by combining the results from a wide range of centers, it reflects the average experience likely to be achieved in practice. Parameters from a single study are subject to considerable sampling error because even the largest study to date includes no more than about 100 affected pregnancies. Nonintervention studies produce estimates of the means for cases that present at term. Intervention studies introduce viability bias that will skew the results toward the extreme. This bias arises because a proportion of those with extreme marker levels who have a termination of pregnancy would have been destined to miscarry anyway, whereas nonviable affected pregnancies with normal screening results will not be known to the investigators.

   Table 1 shows the Mahalanobis distance for the commonly used markers, according to gestation, based on published meta-analyses.[1] NT is by far the single best individual marker, followed by PAPP-A, which is the most discriminatory serum marker, although the Mahalanobis distance declines with gestation. In contrast, the discriminatory power of free β-hCG increases with gestation; intact hCG is less discriminatory than free β-hCG at all gestations, particularly before 13 weeks when it is a poor marker. Inhibin-A is the best second-trimester marker, whereas AFP and uE_3 are much less discriminatory than the hCG isoforms or inhibin-A.

MULTIMARKER SCREENING

None of the individual markers is discriminatory enough to stand alone; a Mahalanobis distance of at least 3 would be required for that. This consideration has led to the development of several multimarker tests based on the estimation of risk for Down syndrome from the marker profile. This estimation is done by modifying the maternal age-specific risk by likelihood ratio (LR) derived from the marker profile. The LR is the relative height of the theoretical marker distribution in Down syndrome compared with that of unaffected pregnancies. Multivariate log Gaussian distributions seem to fit the data well, but some investigators have proposed other distributions for NT.

Table 1
Commonly used Down syndrome screening markers and their Mahalanobis distance according to gestation

Marker	Gestation (wk)	Mahalanobis Distance
NT	11	2.02
	12	1.87
	13	1.65
PAPP-A	10	1.31
	11	1.14
	12	0.90
	13	0.61
Free β-hCG	10	0.76
	11	0.94
	12	1.05
	13	1.11
	14–18	1.33
hCG	10	0.05
	11	0.32
	12	0.68
	13	1.14
	14–18	1.15
Inhibin-A	14–18	1.12
AFP	14–18	0.79
uE_3	14–18	0.83

The Fetal Medicine Foundation (FMF) has promoted the use of an empiric distribution of NT values,[2] but this has been criticized on the grounds that it is likely to overfit the initial data set on which it was based. Moreover, because empiric distribution does not lend itself to a simple statistical description, non-FMF screeners have not had access to software using it. More recently, the FMF has moved to a Gaussian approach, albeit using 2 sets of distributions for Down syndrome pregnancies in which proportions differ according to gestational age (the so-called mixture model).[3] It remains to be seen if this model improves on a simple Gaussian approach.

MULTIMARKER TESTS INCLUDING NT

Until recent years, most experience with Down syndrome screening was in the second trimester. The best test at that period was the so-called quad test, which uses 4 markers: intact hCG or free β-hCG in combination with AFP, uE_3, and inhibin-A. However, better performance is obtainable using first-trimester marker combinations, and in this period, termination of pregnancy, if required, is safer, is more acceptable to religious minorities, is less traumatic, and provides earlier reassurance.

The best first-trimester results are obtained using NT in combination with PAPP-A and either total hCG or free β-hCG, the so-called combined test. There is an important practical constraint influencing the design of such policies, namely, the results of a scan can be reported to the patient immediately, whereas a serum test result is not usually available for several days. The reason for the delay is that biochemical assays are normally done in batches, which, to avoid unnecessary expense, include about 50 to 100 samples. However, new techniques that allow single samples to be tested economically and results to be available in an hour have been developed. This means that if the test equipment is installed close to the ultrasound unit, combined serum test and ultrasonography results can be reported together (sometimes known as OSCAR, one-stop clinic for the assessment of risk). Concurrent screening can also be performed without such equipment, provided a blood sample is obtained a few days before the scheduled scan appointment and arrangements are made to ensure that the serum MoMs are available for risk calculation as soon as the NT is measured (sometimes known as IRA, instant risk assessment).

The combination of first- and second-trimester serum markers yield better results than the combined test. One approach is to measure all markers when they are most discriminatory, that is, to measure NT and PAPP-A in the first trimester but to delay hCG or free β-hCG measurement until the second trimester with other quad markers.[4] This 6-marker combination, known as the integrated test, requires nondisclosure of any intermediate risk based on the levels of NT and PAPP-A. Some regard the nondisclosure to be unethical or at least impractical because of the difficulty for professionals to not act on intermediate findings that would of themselves be abnormal, particularly the NT. Furthermore, any increase in detection is paid for by sacrificing early diagnosis and reassurance. Alternative 2-stage 7-marker strategies have been suggested to overcome these limitations. One approach is the stepwise sequential test in which the first stage is the same as in the combined test, and women with risks less than the cutoff are offered the same second-trimester markers as the in the quad test, with the final risk based on all markers.[5] The first-stage cutoff risk is much higher than usual for the combined test. The contingent test is similar except that only women who are at borderline risk after the first stage are offered the second-stage markers.[6]

MODEL PREDICTIONS

The performance of the different tests in terms of detection rate (DR), which is the proportion of affected pregnancies referred for invasive prenatal diagnosis, and the false-positive rate (FPR), which is the proportion of unaffected pregnancies referred, is predicted from statistical models. Two widely used methods have been adopted: numerical integration and Monte Carlo simulation. Numerical integration uses the theoretical log Gaussian distributions of each marker in Down syndrome pregnancies and unaffected pregnancies. The theoretical range is divided into several equal sections, thus forming a grid in multidimensional space. The Gaussian distributions are then used to calculate for each section (square for 2 markers, cube for 3 markers, and so on) the proportion of Down syndrome pregnancies and unaffected pregnancies and the LR in that section. These values are then applied to a specified maternal population. At each maternal age, the number of Down syndrome pregnancies and unaffected pregnancies is estimated from the age-specific risk curve. The distributions of risks are then calculated from the grid values. Monte Carlo simulation also uses the Gaussian distributions, but instead of rigid summation over a fixed grid, it uses a random sample of points in multidimensional space to simulate the outcome of a population being screened.

The model predictions are highly dependent on the maternal age distribution, and to allow comparison between tests a standard population is used; in this article, it is a Gaussian distribution with mean age 27 years and standard deviation 5.5 years.[7] The relative benefits of different tests can be judged by fixing the FPR (eg, 1% or 5%), and the practical implications of changing test are seen by fixing the risk cutoff (eg, 1 in 250 at term).

Table 2 shows the model predictions for NT alone and for combined tests, according to gestation and the level of hCG isoform. The DR for a fixed FPR declines with

Table 2
Model-predicted performance: NT alone and the Combined test

Test	Gestation (wk)	DR for FPR		1 in 250 Cutoff Risk[a]	
		1% (%)	5% (%)	DR (%)	FPR (%)
NT alone					
	11	64	77	73	2.9
	12	62	75	70	2.7
	13	57	71	66	2.8
Combined test					
NT, free β-hCG & PAPP-A	11	74	87	81	2.4
	12	72	84	79	2.5
	13	66	80	75	2.8
Combined test					
NT, hCG & PAPP-A	11	71	84	79	2.5
	12	70	83	77	2.5
	13	67	81	76	2.7

[a] At term.

advancing gestation, but even with NT alone at 13 weeks, the rate is comparable with that of the quad test, which has a predicted DR of 71% for a 5% FPR using free β-hCG and 67% for intact hCG. The combined test performs considerably better than NT alone at all gestations. The use of free β-hCG improves detection compared with total hCG when a combined test is performed before 13 weeks. Despite this, another modeling exercise claims that there is no material difference in the DR of combined test according to hCG isoform.[8] This model used parameters from the First- and Second-Trimester Evaluation of Risk (FaSTER) trial together with hCG levels based on the retrospective assaying of stored serum samples from only 79 Down syndrome pregnancies and 395 unaffected pregnancies. Larger data sets are needed before concluding that there is no difference.

Table 3 shows the predicted rates for the integrated, stepwise sequential, and contingent tests. The integrated test is predicted to increase detection for a fixed 5% FPR by more than 10%. However, the stepwise sequential and contingent tests have a predicted rate comparable with the integrated test. A retrospective analysis of data from the FaSTER trial has reached the same conclusion.[9] Marker levels from women who completed the first and second stages of the trial—intervention was in the second stage—were used to calculate risks of Down syndrome. For the contingent test, DR was 91% and FPR was 4.5%; the initial DR was 60%, and the initial FPR was 1.2%, and 23% had borderline risks. Stepwise testing had a DR of 92% and an FPR of 5.1%; integrated screening had a DR of 88% and an FPR of 4.9%. These DRs are lower than expected from **Table 3** because some early detected cases, particularly those with cystic hygromas, were excluded. From modeling and the FaSTER results, the practical conclusion is that given the human and practical benefits and lower costs, the contingent test should be the across-trimester strategy of choice.

CONSEQUENCES OF NT ERRORS

The models assume that the parameters in the risk calculator correspond to the distribution of marker levels in the population being screened. Specifically, the mean NT level in the unaffected pregnancies being screened is assumed to be 1.00 MoM,

Table 3
Model-predicted performance: integrated, stepwise sequential, and contingent tests

Test[b]	Gestation (wk)	DR for FPR		1 in 250 Final Cutoff[a]	
		1% (%)	5% (%)	DR (%)	FPR (%)
Integrated					
NT, PAPP-A & Quad[a]	11	85	93	87	1.6
	12	83	92	86	1.7
	13	79	89	84	2.0
Stepwise sequential					
NT, free β-hCG & PAPP-A; Quad if	11	85	94	89	1.7
negative	12	84	93	88	1.9
	13	80	91	86	2.1
NT, hCG & PAPP-A; Quad if	11	86	94	89	1.6
negative	12	83	92	87	1.8
	13	80	91	85	2.0
Contingent					
NT, free β-hCG & PAPP-A; Quad if	11	85	92	88	1.6
borderline	12	83	91	86	1.7
	13	79	88	84	1.9
NT, hCG & PAPP-A; Quad if	11	84	90	86	1.4
borderline	12	82	89	85	1.6
	13	79	88	83	1.8

[a] At term.
[b] Quad: AFP, uE$_3$, free β-hCG, and inhibin-A; initial cutoff for stepwise sequential and contingent, 1 in 50 at term; borderline cutoffs for contingent, 1 in 50–1500 at term.

and in the earlier mentioned modeling, the $\log_{10}$ MoM standard deviations are 0.132, 0.116, and 0.112 at 11, 12, and 13 weeks, respectively; in Down syndrome pregnancies the means are 2.30, 2.10, and 1.92 MoM at each week, and the standard deviation is 0.229.

Table 4 shows what would happen to the Down syndrome risk based on NT alone in a 25-year-old woman, if the accuracy of the NT at 12 weeks' gestation in the screened population is altered by systematically shifting the mean up or down by 10%. At this age, the practical consequences are in NT values that are greater than about 1.50 MoM. For example, using the risk calculator, which assumes complete accuracy and average precision, a value of 1.80 MoM would correspond to a term risk of 1 in 250, exactly on the cutoff used in many countries. But if the operator is overmeasuring by 10%, the true risk would only be 1 in 550, whereas if there is a 10% undermeasurement the risk will be 1 in 95.

Table 4 also shows what would happen in the same circumstances, if the precision was to be changed by a 0.020 reduction or an increase in the standard deviation of $\log_{10}$ MoM in unaffected pregnancies. The corresponding parameter for Down syndrome pregnancies is obtained by reducing or increasing the variance by the same amount it has been changed in unaffected pregnancies. The same observed value of 1.80 MoM with an apparent 1 in 250 term risk would have a much higher 1 in 95 risk, if the operator had greater-than-average precision and a much lower risk, 1 in 430, if the precision was low.

Table 5 shows the consequences of these changes on the model-predicted DR and FPR at 12 weeks' gestation for NT alone and the combined test. As might be expected, a change in accuracy shifts the DR and FPR in the same direction. A change

Table 4
Risk for Down syndrome (1 in x at term) in a 25-year-old woman according to NT level at 12 weeks and the quality of the local NT distribution

NT Level (MoM)	Average Accuracy & Precision	Accuracy[a]		Precision[b]	
		−10%	+10%	−0.02	+0.02
0.50	3700	5700	2300	1300	6000
0.60	7200	9000	5300	4600	8200
0.70	9600	10,000	8300	8900	9000
0.80	10,000	9100	9900	11,000	8500
0.90	9000	7200	9900	11,000	7300
1.00	7200	5100	8800	9100	5900
1.10	5300	3400	7200	6400	4500
1.20	3700	2200	5500	4100	3400
1.30	2500	1300	4000	2400	2400
1.40	1600	800	2800	1300	1800
1.50	1000	470	1900	720	1200
1.60	650	280	1300	370	870
1.70	400	160	840	190	610
1.80	250	95	550	95	430
1.90	150	55	350	45	300
2.00	95	30	230	25	210
2.10	55	19	150	12	140
2.20	35	11	95	10	100
2.30	20	10	60	10	70
2.40	14	10	40	10	50
2.50	10	10	25	10	35

[a] Change in the median NT MoM.
[b] Change in the $\log_{10}$ standard deviation.

in precision mainly affects the FPR; a tighter distribution reduces the FPR, whereas a broader distribution increases it. The effect of changes in accuracy or precision is less for the combined test than for NT alone because any loss of performance is cushioned to some extent by the other markers in the combined test. This effect is even more marked for the integrated, stepwise sequential, and contingent tests because of more markers, and hence, this is another argument for adopting one of these 2-stage approaches.

EVIDENCE FOR SUBOPTIMAL PERFORMANCE

Examination of the results from prospective intervention studies of Down syndrome screening is a means of determining whether or not there is substantial reason for concern about the quality of NT measurement. However, the observed DR in such studies is necessarily an overestimation of the true rate because of the nonviability bias described earlier. To overcome this, an unbiased estimate can be derived from the observed numbers of Down syndrome cases using the formula $(n1 \times p + n2)/(n1 \times p + n2 + n3 \times p + n4)$, where n1, n2, n3, and n4 are the observed numbers of screen detected and terminated, screen detected but not terminated, missed by screening but terminated subsequently, and missed by screening and born cases of

Table 5 Model-predicted performance at 12 weeks according to the quality of the local NT distribution				
	Accuracy[a]		Precision[b]	
Average Accuracy & Precision (%)	−10% (%)	+10% (%)	−0.02 (%)	+0.02 (%)
NT alone				
70 & 2.7	63 & 1.2	76 & 5.4	71 & 1.3	70 & 4.7
Combined: NT, free β-hCG, & PAPP-A				
79 & 2.5	73 & 1.4	83 & 4.3	80 & 1.6	78 & 3.8
Combined: NT, hCG, & PAPP-A				
77 & 2.5	72 & 1.3	82 & 4.5	78 & 1.5	77 & 3.9

[a] Change in the median NT MoM.
[b] Change in the $\log_{10}$ standard deviation.

Down syndrome, respectively, and p is the intrauterine survival rate for Down syndrome at the time of prenatal diagnosis.

Twenty-five large second-trimester intervention studies have been analyzed in this way, and the results have been found to be consistent with model predictions.[1] But when the same was done for studies using NT, the results seemed to be suboptimal. For the 6 studies of NT alone that expressed the results in terms of risk, there were a total of 142,000 screened women of whom 643 were observed to have a fetus with Down syndrome. This finding yielded an observed DR of 84%, equivalent to 72% after allowance for bias, and an FPR of 8.4%. When 15 studies of the combined test were analyzed, with a total of 145,000 women including 638 with Down syndrome pregnancies, the observed DR was 89% and the unbiased DR was 81% with an FPR of 5.9%. There have been 4 prospective intervention studies of the integrated test,[10–13] totaling 50,000 pregnancies, 135 with Down syndrome; observed and unbiased DRs of 88% and 85%; and FPR of 2.8%. Some of the shortfall in detection was because of a failure of all women to complete both stages of the screening protocol. The completion rates ranged from 75% to 92%. On the other hand, the largest study also acted on a high NT alone,[11] a type of stepwise sequential protocol. There has so far been only 1 published intervention study of the stepwise sequential test and it was small.[14] The test was performed on 1528 women, and there were only 3 Down syndrome cases, all of which were identified with an FPR of 6.9%. No contingent test results have been published yet.

QUALITY CONTROL METHODS

NT is visualized in the midsagittal section used for crown-rump length (CRL) measurement, and the FMF has published a standardized technique to be adopted for CRL measurement.[15] This technique relates to the position of the fetus, the ultrasound section chosen, the separation of the fetus from the amnion, the placement of the calipers, and the magnification of the image. Various methods have been described for scoring the quality of the image per se.[16–18]

In addition to ensuring that the aforementioned guidelines on measurement are understood by all sonographers taking part in a particular screening program and, if possible, to having senior staff oversee new trainees, it is necessary to carry out epidemiologic monitoring of results.

A direct approach is to compare the observed positive rate, excluding any known cases of aneuploidy, with the expected rate for the maternal age distribution in the population being screened. The incidence of Down syndrome is not high enough for the observed DR to be a practical indicator of performance.

Using NT alone, a particularly high positive rate may indicate an upward shift in values, a broader spread of results, or both. A low rate could relate to a downward shift in values but could also mean that NT is being measured more precisely than expected. For a combined test or the 2 trimester policies, an excess or a deficit may be contributed to by the biochemical marker distributions. There may be a problem with NT even when the positive rate is consistent with the expected rate, if the biochemical markers are performing particularly well. In these circumstances, indirect indicators of performance are preferable, specifically the median MoM and the standard deviation, on a logarithmic scale, of the MoM values.

This concept is no different from quality assessment of biochemical screening markers. The median MoM value should be calculated on a regular basis for the overall program and for each sonographer. The observed median, excluding only known cases of fetal aneuploidy, is the best estimator of the unaffected mean because it is not subject to distortion by occasional outliers. Similarly, the overall and operator-specific standard deviations of $\log_{10}$ MoM should be calculated. The nonparametric estimator based on the difference between the 90th and 10th percentiles, in $\log_{10}$ MoM, divided by 2.563 is relatively unaffected by outliers.

A value for the median, which is outside the range 0.90 to 1.10 MoM, is a matter of concern. Depending on the number of scans included in the calculation, it is possible to exceed these limits by chance alone, and a statistically significant deviation would be a more compelling evidence of a problem. If deviant results are obtained for an individual or with all operators, some form of retraining will be required. But if this has no effect, one possibility is to use operator- or center-specific normal median curves for calculating MoMs.[19] Such adjustment was used by the Serum, Urine and Ultrasound Screening Study and the FaSTER trial.

For the model prediction in this article, the NT standard deviations were obtained from 4 large prospective studies combined.[2] Because this involved several different centers and operators, the values are necessarily wider than should be obtained for a single operator or even center. From the author's personal experience, the target for an individual operator should be a $\log_{10}$ standard deviation of 0.09 with an acceptable range of 0.07 to 0.11; for a whole center a realistic value might be 0.10, with range 0.08 to 0.12. An individual with an NT value less than the range might have a particularly precise technique, but another possibility is that the different NTs may not be discriminated sufficiently, which could be as serious as measuring imprecisely. The use of MoMs implies multiplicative accuracy, which for biochemical markers is equivalent to having a good recovery in doubling dilutions. One way of assessing accuracy for NT is to observe the rate of change in median NT according to CRL. As the MoM equation is curved, the rate of change is not uniform, but as a guide, the median NT should increase by about one-third for a 20-mm span of CRL at 11 to 12 weeks and by about 10% at 12 to 13 weeks. A shallower increase in an operator with a low standard deviation would be a concern.

FMF has an external quality assessment scheme for NT, which has branches in different countries. Sonographers receive training, initial credentialing, and remediation by sending images and data to the scheme. The Nuchal Translucency Quality Review scheme in the United States also performs a similar function.

Whatever the external scheme involved, the import step is for those who are out of target to be assessed by experienced colleagues in the same center. When biochemical screening was the norm, it was possible for an individual laboratory to manage its own quality, but with the newer tests incorporating NT, the laboratory needs to have good working relationships with those in each participating ultrasound unit who can take responsibility for NT results. In some settings, this can be logistically difficult.

QUALITY MONITORING RESULTS

It is common for inexperienced sonographers to underestimate NT. In one study of NT quality in 19 trainees, the criterion was the proportion of results less than the normal median derived by experienced sonographers. Only after a minimum of 50 scans were half the results less than the median, and on an average, it took 131 scans.[20] Similar results were found in a Danish training study.[17] Among the inexperienced, an excess of low values is particularly seen at the low end of the NT range,[21] and in these circumstances, a moderately reduced median MoM together with a moderately increased standard deviation may be the grounds for reviewing the individual's technique.

In the initial half year of the BUN (**B**iochemical, **U**ltrasound, **N**uchal translucency) trial, NT quality was assessed using an FMF protocol.[15] Of the 5 sonographers fulfilling training requirements, 4 had NT values on average significantly less than the mean expected by FMF and 1 was significantly greater than the mean based on 23 to 136 images reviewed. In the next half year, the situation had not materially changed based on a further 24 to 153 images reviewed, but when feedback was given on the quality of their images, the next half year saw a considerable convergence of results (41–370 new images).

Undermeasurement is not just a problem for the inexperienced. An audit of 264 sonographers providing results for a large laboratory in Belgium found widespread undermeasurement.[22] One of the sonographers was FMF trained and had a median delta-NT of 0.03 mm but the rest had a median of −0.14 mm.

An insight into the extent of poor performance in routine practice can be found in a study of 14,210 NT scans by 140 sonographers providing at least 50 results for 6 laboratories in the United States.[23] Three epidemiologic indicators were used: median, 0.9 to 1.1 MoM; standard deviation, 0.08 to 0.13; and slope, 15% to 35% per week. Only 56% of operators were within all 3 targets.

In the FaSTER trial, high NT quality was maintained in a 3-level approach. A total of 102 participating sonographers received training, and a minimum of 50 images were assessed by a single external reviewer before active screening began. Thereafter, each sonographer used a checklist to confirm adherence to the protocol and a within-center assessor reviewed all that was imaged. Using center-specific medians, epidemiologic monitoring was performed with median MoM, standard deviation, and slope as the indicators. A recent analysis of these results has shown that despite this intensive review, some 7% of NT measurements were inadequate and changes in the NT measurements occurred over time.[24]

In the Netherlands, a retrospective analysis was performed on 27,738 NT measurements recorded centrally in the National Institute for Public Health and the Environment.[25] A single published MoM curve was used.[26] The 42 sonographers credentialed by FMF got a mean NT value of 0.98 MoM, whereas the remaining 64 got a mean of 0.92 MoM. Of even greater concern was the upward trend in values over the 2-year study period from a mean of 0.86 MoM increasing to 0.96 MoM.

SUMMARY

Current best practice for Down syndrome screening involves the use of NT measurement in combination with maternal serum markers. Differences in the distribution of NT levels between the theoretical values in the risk calculator and the actual practice lead to changes in performance. The observed positive rate is a direct indicator of performance, but the essential indicators are the median MoM and standard deviation of log MoM. Operators need to be credentialed and monitored by external schemes using this approach. Laboratories should also monitor the sonographers performing NTs as part of tests for which they are responsible.

REFERENCES

1. Cuckle H, Benn P. Multianalyte maternal serum screening for chromosomal defects. In: Milunsky A, editor. Genetic disorders and the fetus: diagnosis, prevention and treatment. 6th edition. Baltimore (MD): Johns Hopkins University Press; 2009. p. 771–818.
2. Spencer K, Bindra R, Nix AB, et al. Delta-NT or NT MoM, which is the most appropriate method for calculating accurate patient-specific risks for trisomy 21 in the first trimester? Ultrasound Obstet Gynecol 2003;22:142–8.
3. Wright D, Kagan KO, Molina FS, et al. A mixture model of nuchal translucency thickness in screening for chromosomal defects. Ultrasound Obstet Gynecol 2008;31(4):376–83.
4. Wald NJ, Rodeck C, Hackshaw AK, et al. First and second trimester antenatal screening for Down's syndrome: the results of the Serum, Urine and Ultrasound Screening Study (SURUSS). Health Technol Assess 2003;7(11):1–88.
5. Malone FD, Canick JA, Ball RH, et al, First- and Second-Trimester Evaluation of Risk (FASTER) Research Consortium. First trimester or second-trimester screening, or both, for Down's syndrome. N Engl J Med 2005;353(19):2001–11.
6. Wright D, Bradbury I, Benn P, et al. Contingent screening for Down's syndrome is an efficient alternative to non-disclosure sequential screening. Prenat Diagn 2004;24(10):762–6.
7. Cuckle H, Aitken D, Goodburn S, et al, UK National Down's Syndrome Screening Programme, Laboratory Advisory Group. Age-standardisation when target setting and auditing performance of Down syndrome screening programmes. Prenat Diagn 2004;24(11):851–6.
8. Canick JA, Lambert-Messerlian GM, Palomaki GE, et al, First and Second Trimester Evaluation of Risk (FASTER) Trial Research Consortium. Comparison of serum markers in first-trimester Down syndrome screening. Obstet Gynecol 2006;108:1192–9.
9. Cuckle HS, Malone FD, Wright D, et al, FaSTER Research Consortium. Contingent screening for Down syndrome—results from the FaSTER trial. Prenat Diagn 2008;28:89–94.
10. Weisz B, Pandya PP, David AL, et al. Ultrasound findings after screening for Down syndrome using the integrated test. Obstet Gynecol 2007;109:1046–52.
11. Okun N, Summers A, Hoffman B, et al. Prospective experience with integrated prenatal screening and first trimester combined screening for trisomy 21 in a large Canadian urban center. Prenat Diagn 2008;8:987–92.
12. Wald NJ, Huttly WJ, Murphy KW, et al. Antenatal screening for Down's syndrome using the Integrated test at two London hospitals. J Med Screen 2009;16(1):7–10.
13. Rodrigues LC, Ramos-Dias AM, Carvalho V, et al. Evaluation of four years of prenatal screening for aneuploidies in Hospital S. Francisco Xavier using the integrated test. J Med Screen 2009;16(1):46–7.
14. Benn PA, Campbell WA, Zelop CM, et al. Stepwise sequential screening for fetal aneuploidy. Am J Obstet Gynecol 2007;197(3):312, e1–5.

15. Snijders RJ, Thom EA, Zachary JM, et al. First-trimester trisomy screening: nuchal translucency measurement training and quality assurance to correct and unify technique. Ultrasound Obstet Gynecol 2002;19(4):353–9.
16. Herman A, Maymon R, Dreazen E, et al. Nuchal translucency audit: a novel image-scoring method. Ultrasound Obstet Gynecol 1998;12:398–403.
17. Wøjdemann KR, Christiansen M, Sundberg K, et al. Quality assessment in prospective nuchal translucency screening for Down syndrome. Ultrasound Obstet Gynecol 2001;18(6):641–4.
18. Fries N, Althuser M, Fontanges M, et al. Quality control of an image-scoring method for nuchal translucency ultrasonography. Am J Obstet Gynecol 2007; 196(3):272, e1–5.
19. Logghe H, Cuckle H, Sehmi I. Centre-specific ultrasound nuchal translucency medians needed for Down's syndrome screening. Prenat Diagn 1995;23(5): 389–92.
20. Frey Tirri B, Troeger C, Holzgreve W, et al. Quality management of nuchal translucency measurement in residents. Ultraschall Med 2007;28(5):484–8.
21. Evans MI, Van Decruyes H, Nicolaides KH. Nuchal translucency measurements for first-trimester screening: the 'price' of inaccuracy. Fetal Diagn Ther 2007;22: 401–4.
22. Gyselaers WJ, Vereecken AJ, Van Herck EJ, et al. Audit on nuchal translucency thickness measurements in Flanders, Belgium: a plea for methodological standardization. Ultrasound Obstet Gynecol 2004;24(5):511–5.
23. Palomaki GE, Neveux LM, Donnenfeld A, et al. Quality assessment of routine nuchal translucency measurements: a North American laboratory perspective. Genet Med 2008;10(2):131–8.
24. D'Alton ME, Cleary-Goldman J, Lambert-Messerlian G, et al. Maintaining quality assurance for sonographic nuchal translucency measurement: lessons from the FASTER Trial. Ultrasound Obstet Gynecol 2009;33(2):142–6.
25. Koster MP, Wortelboer EJ, Engels MA, et al. Quality of nuchal translucency measurements in The Netherlands: a quantitative analysis. Ultrasound Obstet Gynecol 2009;34(2):136–41.
26. Nicolaides KH, Snijders RJ, Cuckle HS. Correct estimation of parameters for ultrasound nuchal translucency screening. Prenat Diagn 1998;18(5):519–23.

Clinical Implications of First-Trimester Screening

Stephen T. Chasen, MD

KEYWORDS

- First-trimester screening • Pregnancy
- Prenatal screening • Aneuploidy risk assessment

It is well established that first-trimester aneuploidy risk assessment, when performed by appropriately credentialed practitioners in a quality setting, is associated with very high detection rates for Trisomy 21, Trisomy 18, Trisomy 13, and triploidy.[1,2] What is less clear is the clinical impact of first-trimester screening. The information obtained during risk assessment has the potential to change the rate of invasive prenatal diagnosis (amniocentesis or chorionic villus sampling [CVS]) and the gestational age of prenatal diagnosis and abortion, and to lead to earlier prenatal diagnosis of certain major structural abnormalities. With more research focusing on the association between abnormal nuchal translucency and biochemistry and adverse outcomes in chromosomally normal fetuses, first trimester screening could also conceivably impact the diagnosis and management of pregnancies with these complications.

PHYSICIAN EDUCATION

Any positive impact of first-trimester screening would depend on availability and use of quality testing, and the appropriate interpretation of results. A key component of this is physician education. Before 2007, the American College of Obstetricians and Gynecologists (ACOG) described first-trimester screening as investigational and recommended against its use outside of research trials.[3] In 2007, however, an ACOG Practice Bulletin recommended that first-trimester screening be offered to all pregnant women, and indicated that the practice of maternal age–based risk categorization (ie, age ≥35 y considered high-risk) should be discontinued.[4]

Based on a recent survey administered to ACOG Fellow and Junior Fellows, most general obstetricians now offer first-trimester screening to all patients. Those who reported the 2007 Practice Bulletin more closely were more likely to report that their practice had changed, and appeared more knowledgeable about screening.[5] In Europe, most countries have incorporated first-trimester screening in national

Department of Obstetrics and Gynecology, Weill Medical College of Cornell University, Room J130, 525 East 68th Street, New York, NY 10065, USA
E-mail address: stchasen@med.cornell.edu

Clin Lab Med 30 (2010) 605–611
doi:10.1016/j.cll.2010.04.014
0272-2712/10/$ – see front matter © 2010 Elsevier Inc. All rights reserved.

labmed.theclinics.com

screening policies for Down syndrome, and women in Denmark and Switzerland are routinely offered early screening.[6]

Physicians are expected to become more knowledgeable about first-trimester testing and more comfortable in interpreting results. As this happens, early testing will be increasingly used to guide clinical management. Although certain benefits of first-trimester screening have been identified in single centers in the United States or regionally in other countries, broad-based clinical benefits are likely to be increasingly recognized over time.

RATE OF INVASIVE PRENATAL DIAGNOSIS

It is intuitive that the addition of screening tests will result in an increase in the rate of diagnostic testing. Clearly, the use of mammography, cervical cytology (Papanicolau test), and prostate-specific antigen (PSA) for cancer screening has resulted in higher rates of breast, cervical, and prostate biopsies than in unscreened populations. With implementation of first-trimester screening, one might also expect a corresponding increase in the rate of invasive prenatal diagnosis. To evaluate the impact of first-trimester screening on the rate of invasive testing, it is useful to review the history of prenatal diagnosis.

Invasive testing to determine fetal karyotype has been performed for several decades. Amniocentesis in the second trimester was introduced in the 1970s,[7] and CVS was described in the 1980s.[8] These tests were initially restricted to an older obstetric population (commonly defined as age ≥ 35 years) and women with a history of prior fetuses or newborns diagnosed with chromosomal abnormalities.

When low maternal serum alfa-fetoprotein was identified as a marker of fetal Down syndrome, a screening test was made available women older than 35 years.[9] With the recognition of additional biochemical markers, second-trimester multiple-marker screening became common, leading to higher rates of amniocentesis in younger women.[10] Although serum screening was initially recommended only in younger women, its benefits in those aged 35 years or older were subsequently documented.[11] In addition to second-trimester biochemistry, multiple ultrasound markers associated with Down syndrome were identified, providing another useful tool for evaluating risk.[12]

The recognition that biochemistry and ultrasound could provide valuable information about risk in women of all ages led to a more efficient use of amniocentesis. Women aged 35 years or older could now choose to learn more about their particular risk than the age-related risk before deciding whether to undergo amniocentesis. In many countries, this led to changes in the use of amniocentesis, with a higher proportion of affected pregnancies identified.[13,14]

With the widespread availability of first-trimester ultrasound and biochemical screening, women have been provided a similar opportunity to obtain information regarding risk when CVS is an option. Many studies have shown that first-trimester risk assessment using biochemistry and nuchal translucency provides superior screening performance compared with second-trimester biochemistry.[1,2,4,15]

The Maternal-Fetal Medicine division at the Weill-Cornell Medical Center implemented the first-trimester screening program in 2000, estimating risk based on nuchal translucency and maternal age.[16] The authors evaluated the rates of invasive testing over successive 6-month intervals in women aged 35 years or older, and found that the rate of screening increased from 0% to 42% from 2000 to 2002. During this period, the overall rate of CVS declined from 7% to 2%, resulting in an overall lower rate of invasive testing. In women aged 40 years or older, a decline in the rate of CVS was accompanied by an increased rate of amniocentesis, and no net change in the overall rate of invasive testing. In contrast, the overall rate of invasive testing was significantly lower in women aged 35 to 39 years.[17]

Based on these data, the authors concluded that the availability of first-trimester screening significantly reduced the rate of CVS. In women at highest age-related risk, first-trimester screening seemed to help them decide whether to undergo CVS or amniocentesis, rather than determine whether they would undergo invasive testing.[17]

The authors' experience seems to be consistent with Maternal-Fetal Medicine specialists in the United States. A recent study compared responses to surveys among members of the Society for Maternal-Fetal Medicine (SMFM) from 2001 and 2007, and evaluated trends in the use of screening tests and diagnostic procedures for Down syndrome. Performance of first-trimester screening more than doubled from 2001 to 2007, with an estimated 20% decrease in invasive testing.[18]

A population-based study from Australia evaluated trends in use of first- and second-trimester screening, invasive testing, and prenatal detection of Down syndrome from 1995 to 2005. That 10-year period showed a significant decrease in the use of second-trimester serum screening from 75% to 25%, and a corresponding increase in the rate of first-trimester combined screening from 1% to 49%. In the population, the rate of invasive testing decreased from 9.3% to 7.6%. Although no significant change occurred in the high proportion of Down syndrome cases detected, the number of invasive procedures for each prenatal diagnosis declined from 86 to 40 over the 10-year interval.[19]

Based on these studies, it is reasonable to conclude that the availability of first-trimester screening has led to a more efficient use of invasive prenatal testing. Clearly, early risk assessment does not represent a new effort to screen for Down syndrome in the first trimester. Instead, for many it has replaced the less-accurate and inefficient use of maternal age to identify candidates for invasive testing. Because first-trimester screening with nuchal translucency and biochemistry provides high detection rates with low screen-positive rates, women can make informed decisions with better information, exposing fewer pregnancies to the risks associated with invasive testing.

GESTATIONAL AGE AT ABORTION

In the United States and elsewhere, many women will choose abortion after the prenatal diagnosis of Down syndrome.[20–22] Although both first- and second-trimester abortions are safe when performed by experienced practitioners, the rate of complications increases with advancing gestational age.[23] There are also fewer providers of second trimester abortion, thereby limiting access in many parts of the country.[24] Finally, abortion earlier in pregnancy may be more private, because women are less likely to be visibly pregnant. For these reasons, early Down syndrome screening has the potential to improve care by minimizing the number of abortions performed in the second trimester.

The authors' department examined gestational age at abortion for chromosomal abnormalities for which first-trimester risk assessment has high sensitivity, including Down syndrome, Trisomy 18, Trisomy 13, Triploidy, and Turner syndrome. From 1999 to 2005, as first-trimester screening became more prevalent, the median gestational age at abortion for these chromosomal abnormalities was significantly reduced from 19 to 15 weeks. Although only 6% of these cases were diagnosed with CVS in 1999, 40% were diagnosed with CVS in 2005. Similar trends were observed when gestational age at abortion was examined for Down syndrome only.[25]

A recent study analyzed a European registry of congenital anomalies and examined the correlation between national Down syndrome screening policies and gestational age at prenatal diagnosis. The two countries (Denmark and Switzerland) with a policy of routinely offering first-trimester screening had a higher proportion of cases identified during the prenatal period than the countries with a policy of offering first- or second-trimester screening. These two countries had lower median gestational ages at prenatal diagnosis (11 weeks for Denmark, and 15 weeks for Switzerland) than the remaining countries, with high rates of abortion reported (86% for Denmark and 91% for Switzerland). Although data on gestational age at abortion were not provided, it is reasonable to infer that earlier prenatal diagnosis would lead to earlier abortion.[6]

As first-trimester screening becomes more widely incorporated into clinical practice, the gestational age at prenatal diagnosis will likely continue to decline. In populations in which many women choose abortion after prenatal diagnosis of chromosomal abnormalities, this practice has the potential to reduce the need for second-trimester abortion.

ADDITIONAL BENEFITS OF ULTRASOUND AT 11 TO 14 WEEKS

Although nuchal translucency as part of the first-trimester screening process may be the main indication for ultrasound, it has other major benefits at 11 to 14 weeks, including improved gestational dating, early diagnosis and evaluation of multiple pregnancy, and early diagnosis of major structural abnormalities.

Measurement of crown-rump length (CRL) at 11 to 14 weeks has an error range of +/−5 days, based on evaluation of a cohort of in vitro fertilization pregnancies with known date of conception.[26] This assessment is more accurate than second-trimester ultrasound, and a significant proportion of pregnancies may have the gestational age changed based on CRL when nuchal translucency is measured. More precise gestational dating is associated with a lower rate of labor induction at term,[27] and may improve the diagnosis of fetal growth disorders and evaluation and management of preterm labor.

Evaluation of multiple pregnancies at 11 to 14 weeks results in improved assessment of amnionicity and chorionicity compared with second-trimester ultrasound.[28] Early and accurate identification of monochorionic/diamniotic and monochorionic/monoamniotic twin pregnancies is crucial, because more intensive fetal surveillance is required to identify and manage complications, such as twin–twin transfusion syndrome.

Ultrasound at 11 to 14 weeks cannot replace second-trimester evaluation of fetal anatomy, because some structures are not well visualized in the first trimester. Nevertheless, some major malformations, including anencephaly, holoprosencephaly, limb reduction defects, and ventral wall defects, can be identified with confidence when nuchal translucency is measured.[29] In addition, some findings at 11 to 14 weeks, although not diagnostic, can lead to earlier second-trimester diagnosis of structural abnormalities. A strong correlation exists between abnormal nuchal translucency and cardiac abnormalities in euploid fetuses, and fetal echocardiography early in the second trimester can lead to earlier diagnosis of cardiac malformations.[30] At Cornell, more than one-third of patients who underwent abortion for structural abnormalities had prenatal diagnosis in the third trimester, or early in the second trimester after suspicious findings at 11 to 14 weeks.[31]

ADDITIONAL BENEFITS OF BIOCHEMISTRY AT 9 TO 14 WEEKS

In pregnancies unaffected by chromosomal abnormalities, ample evidence shows that abnormal levels of pregnancy-associated plasma protein A (PAPP-A) and the beta subunit of human chorionic gonadotropin (beta-hCG) are correlated with complications in pregnancies. Aside from increasing the probability of autosomal trisomy, a low serum level of PAPP-A is associated with higher rates of fetal loss, stillbirth, growth restriction, and preeclampsia.[32] Low levels of beta-hCG have also been associated with an increased rate of fetal loss.[32,33] In the authors' population of twin pregnancies, low PAPP-A was associated with discordant fetal growth and preeclampsia.[34]

Currently, no consensus exists on how to manage pregnancies with low PAPP-A. Close monitoring of fetal health in the third trimester is reasonable, although no prospective studies have evaluated its impact on obstetric outcomes. Although fetal surveillance may improve obstetric outcomes, it is not clear that recognizing the association between abnormal first-trimester biochemistry and adverse outcomes will ultimately be beneficial.

SUMMARY

Evidence from single centers and surveys and regional data already suggests that first-trimester screening is associated with lower rates of invasive testing while achieving high rates of prenatal diagnosis. More efficient use of invasive testing would result in fewer procedure-related complications. Available evidence also suggests that first-trimester screening can lower the gestational ages at prenatal diagnosis of and abortion for chromosomal abnormalities and some structural anomalies. The use of abnormal first-trimester biochemistry values, such as low PAPP-A, to predict adverse obstetric outcomes could also be beneficial. Currently, however, it is not clear that changes in clinical management, such as more fetal surveillance or earlier delivery, improve outcomes.

The clinical benefits of first-trimester screening are likely to become more apparent as screening becomes more prevalent. To maximize these benefits, obstetric providers must become comfortable interpreting the results, and appropriate management protocols must be implemented. Prospective studies are needed evaluating the management of patients with abnormal first-trimester biochemistry in the absence of chromosomal abnormalities.

REFERENCES

1. Avgidou K, Papageorghiou A, Bindra R, et al. Prospective first-trimester screening for Trisomy 21 in 30,564 pregnancies. Am J Obstet Gynecol 2005; 192:1761–7.
2. Malone FD, Canick JA, Ball RH, et al. First-trimester or second-trimester screening, or both, for Down's syndrome. N Engl J Med 2005;353:2001–11.
3. ACOG Committee on Practice Bulletins—Obstetrics. Screening for fetal chromosomal abnormalities. ACOG Practice Bulletin #27. Washington, DC: The American College of Obstetricians and Gynecologists; 2001.
4. ACOG Committee on Practice Bulletins—Obstetrics. Screening for fetal chromosomal abnormalities. ACOG Practice Bulletin #27. Washington, DC: The American College of Obstetricians and Gynecologists; 2007.
5. Driscoll DA, Morgan MA, Schulkin J. Screening for Down syndrome: changing practice of obstetricians. Am J Obstet Gynecol 2009;200:459, e1–9.

6. Boyd PA, Devigan C, Khoshnood B, et al. Survey of prenatal screening policies in Europe for structural malformations and chromosome anomalies, and their impact on detection and termination rates for neural tube defects and Down's syndrome. BJOG 2008;115:689–96.

7. Nadler HL, Gerbie AB. Role of amniocentesis in the intrauterine detection of genetic disorders. N Engl J Med 1970;282:596–9.

8. Simoni G, Brambati B, Danesino C, et al. Efficient direct chromosome analyses and enzyme determinations from chorionic villi samples in the first trimester of pregnancy. Hum Genet 1983;63:349–57.

9. Merkatz IR, Nitowsky HM, Macri JN, et al. An association between low maternal serum alpha-fetoprotein and fetal chromosomal abnormalities. Am J Obstet Gynecol 1984;148:886–94.

10. Phillips OP, Elias S, Shulman LP, et al. Maternal serum screening for fetal Down syndrome in women less than 35 years of age using alpha-fetoprotein, hCG, and unconjugated estriol: a prospective 2-year study. Obstet Gynecol 1992;80: 353–8.

11. Haddow JE, Palomaki GE, Knight GJ, et al. Reducing the need for amniocentesis in women 35 years of age or older with serum markers for screening. N Engl J Med 1994;330:1114–8.

12. Benacerraf BR, Frigoletto FD Jr, Laboda LA. Sonographic diagnosis of Down syndrome in the second trimester. Am J Obstet Gynecol 1985;153:49–52.

13. Cheffins T, Chan A, Haan EA, et al. The impact of maternal serum screening on the birth prevalence of Down's syndrome and the use of amniocentesis and chorionic villus sampling in South Australia. BJOG 2000;107:1453–9.

14. Benn PA, Fang M, Egan JF. Trends in the use of second trimester maternal serum screening from 1991 to 2003. Genet Med 2005;7(5):328–31.

15. Perni SC, Predanic M, Kalish RB, et al. Clinical use of first-trimester aneuploidy screening in a United States population can replicate data from clinical trials. Am J Obstet Gynecol 2006;195:236–9.

16. Chasen ST, Sharma G, Kalish RB, et al. First-trimester screening for aneuploidy with fetal nuchal translucency in a United States population. Ultrasound Obstet Gynecol 2003;22:149–51.

17. Chasen ST, McCullough LB, Chervenak FA. Is nuchal translucency screening associated with different rates of invasive testing in an older obstetric population? Am J Obstet Gynecol 2004;190:769–74.

18. Fang YM, Benn P, Campbell W, et al. Down syndrome screening in the United States in 2001 and 2007: a survey of maternal-fetal medicine specialists. Am J Obstet Gynecol 2009;201:97, e1–5.

19. Muller PR, Cocciolone R, Haan EA, et al. Trends in state/population-based Down syndrome screening and invasive prenatal testing with the introduction of first-trimester combined Down syndrome screening, South Australia, 1995–2005. Am J Obstet Gynecol 2007;196:315, e1–7.

20. Mansfield C, Hopfer S, Marteau TM. Termination rates after prenatal diagnosis of Down syndrome, spina bifida, anencephaly, and Turner and Klinefelter syndromes: a systematic literature review. Prenat Diagn 1999;19:808–12.

21. Morris JK, Alberman E. Trends in Down's syndrome live births and antenatal diagnoses in England and Wales from 1989 to 2008: analysis of data from the National Down Syndrome Cytogenetic Register. BMJ 2009;339:b3794.

22. Jou HJ, Kuo YS, Hsu JJ, et al. The evolving national birth prevalence of Down syndrome in Taiwan. A study on the impact of second-trimester maternal serum screening. Prenat Diagn 2005;25:665–70.

23. Pazol K, Gamble SB, Parker WY, et al, Centers for Disease Control and Prevention (CDC). Abortion surveillance—United States, 2006. MMWR Surveill Summ 2009; 58:1–35.
24. Jones RK, Zolna MR, Henshaw SK, et al. Abortion in the United States: incidence and access to services, 2005. Perspect Sex Reprod Health 2008;40:6–16.
25. Chasen ST, Kalish RB, Chervenak FA. Gestational age at abortion: the impact of first-trimester risk assessment for aneuploidy. Am J Obstet Gynecol 2006;195: 839–42.
26. Kalish RB, Thaler HT, Chasen ST, et al. First- and second-trimester ultrasound assessment of gestational age. Am J Obstet Gynecol 2004;191:975–8.
27. Ewigman BG, Crane JP, Frigoletto FD, et al. Effect of prenatal ultrasound screening on perinatal outcome. RADIUS Study Group. N Engl J Med 1993; 329:821–7.
28. Lee YM, Cleary-Goldman J, Thaker HM, et al. Antenatal sonographic prediction of twin chorionicity. Am J Obstet Gynecol 2006;195:863–7.
29. Timor-Tritsch IE, Fuchs KM, Monteagudo A, et al. Performing a fetal anatomy scan at the time of first-trimester screening. Obstet Gynecol 2009;113:402–7.
30. Clur SA, Ottenkamp J, Bilardo CM. The nuchal translucency and the fetal heart: a literature review. Prenat Diagn 2009;29:739–48.
31. Chasen ST, Kalish RB. Abortion for structural anomalies: the impact of early ultrasound. Am J Obstet Gynecol 2009;201:S156.
32. Dugoff L, Hobbins JC, Malone FD, et al. First-trimester maternal serum PAPP-A and free-beta subunit human chorionic gonadotropin concentrations and nuchal translucency are associated with obstetric complications: a population-based screening study (the FASTER Trial). Am J Obstet Gynecol 2004;191:1446–51.
33. Goetzl L, Krantz D, Simpson JL, et al. Pregnancy-associated plasma protein A, free beta-hCG, nuchal translucency, and risk of pregnancy loss. Obstet Gynecol 2004;104:30–6.
34. Chasen ST, Martinucci S, Perni SC, et al. First-trimester biochemistry and outcomes in twin pregnancy. J Reprod Med 2009;54(5):312–4.

Adverse Pregnancy Outcomes After Abnormal First-Trimester Screening for Aneuploidy

Laura Goetzl, MD, MPH

KEYWORDS

- First trimester screening • Congenital heart disease
- Intrauterine growth restriction • Intrauterine fetal demise

Although the primary aim of first trimester screening is to identify pregnancies at risk of aneuploidy, first trimester findings may give insight into other adverse pregnancy outcomes. This article outlines a practical approach to interpreting abnormal first trimester findings and reviews what further testing may be indicated. Abnormalities discussed include (1) a thickened nuchal translucency, (2) abnormal fetal anatomy detected at first trimester screening, and (3) abnormal levels of serum analytes.

THICKENED NUCHAL TRANSLUCENCY

A thickened nuchal translucency (NT) was originally described as an NT greater than 95th percentile for a given crown rump length. However, recent data have suggested that adverse outcomes are much more common with an NT that exceeds a set threshold of 3.5 mm (ie, ≥3.5 mm), a measurement that essentially represents 99th percentile or more throughout the gestational age window for first trimester screening.[1–3] Given that it can be difficult to distinguish between a thickened NT and a cystic hygroma, all NTs greater than 3.5 mm are grouped together whenever possible. In some investigations, cystic hygromas were excluded, and this is noted where appropriate.

A thickened NT has been associated with a myriad of syndromes; however, most of these have only been reported once or twice in the literature.[4] Therefore, unless there is a specific family history that points to an increased likelihood of a specific disorder, it

No reprints will be available.

Division of Maternal Fetal Medicine, Department of Obstetrics and Gynecology, Medical University of South Carolina, 96 Jonathan Lucas Street, Suite CSB 635, Charleston, SC 29425, USA

E-mail address: goetzl@musc.edu

Clin Lab Med 30 (2010) 613–628
doi:10.1016/j.cll.2010.04.003
0272-2712/10/$ – see front matter © 2010 Elsevier Inc. All rights reserved.

is unlikely to be clinically feasible to counsel patients regarding all these rare possibilities. Further, in most cases, it is not certain whether or not the finding of a thickened NT is specifically associated with the syndrome or if the association was incidental. Therefore, this article focuses on the most likely risks and abnormalities associated with this finding. Given the strong association between thickened NT and abnormal karyotype, it is presumed that definitive diagnosis for chromosomal abnormalities has been offered or performed. The following sections pertain to management of a thickened NT where a normal karyotype has been determined. In cases where karyotype determination has been declined, risks of adverse pregnancy outcome are likely to be increased given the 20% to 60% risk superimposed by undetected chromosomal abnormalities.

Miscarriage or Fetal Death

A thickened NT has been associated with an increased risk of miscarriage or fetal death. The risk increases with increasing NT thickness (**Table 1**). Counseling in the setting of thickened NT should include an increased risk of miscarriage or fetal loss before chorionic villus sampling or amniocentesis and again when a normal karyotype is established. In most cases, fetal loss occurs before 20 weeks and is heralded by progressive fetal hydrops. Therefore, perinatal management should include some surveillance for fetal miscarriage before 20 weeks. However, given that further anatomic and cardiac evaluation of fetuses with thickened NT is warranted, additional sonographic evaluation for the primary aim of detecting inevitable fetal loss is redundant (see later discussion).

Cardiac Defects

Multiple reports have described an association between fetal cardiac defects and a thickened NT. This association is likely due to the effects of reduced diastolic cardiac function, although this finding may not be present in all fetuses with a thickened NT and a cardiac defect. **Table 2** presents the risk of cardiac defects in the setting of a thickened NT. For simplification, studies were only included where sample size exceeded 100 and where specific data could be abstracted for NT of 3.5 mm or more. In cases where outcomes were reported as greater than 99th percentile, this cutoff was used as equivalent to 3.5 mm. At present, the American College of Obstetricians and Gynecologists recommends offering fetal echocardiography following an NT of 3.5 mm or more.[12] The cost-effectiveness of offering fetal screening echocardiography at NT measurements of 2.5 to 3.4 mm has not been established. However, consideration should be given to referring patients with an NT between 2.5 and 3.4

Table 1 Risk of miscarriage in the setting of thickened NT		
Nuchal Translucency (mm)	**Fetal Death[a] (%)**	**Live Birth Without Abnormality[b] (%)**
3.5–4.4	2.7	70
4.5–5.4	3.4	50
5.6–6.4	10.1	30
>6.5	19.0	15

[a] Fetal death in the absence of chromosomal abnormalities.
[b] Residual rate excluding fetal death, major abnormalities, or chromosomal abnormalities.
Data from Refs.[1–4]

Table 2
Incidence of cardiac abnormalities with thickened NT

Study	≥3.5 (all)	3.5–4.4 mm	>4.5 mm
Hyett et al,[5] 1997	18/287	5/188	13/99
Hyett et al,[6] 1999	20/315	6/208	14/107
Ghi et al,[7] 2001	42/597	12/384	30/213
Aztei et al,[8] 2005	64/1087	23/654	41/423
Simpson et al,[9] 2007[a]	12/310		
Clur et al,[10] 2008[b]	28/374	6/199	22/175
Zosmer et al,[11] 1999	19/398		
Totals	203/3368	52/1633	120/1017
Rates (95% CI)	6.0% (5.2%–6.8%)	3.2% (2.3%–4.1%)	11.8% (9.8%–13.8%)

Abbreviation: CI, confidence interval.
[a] Cystic hygromas excluded. Greater than 99.4th percentile (2.5MOM) reported as greater than or equal to 3.5-mm category.
[b] Calculated from data presented in another format.

mm for a level II anatomic ultrasonography at a referral center. Although some investigators have reported diagnosing fetal heart defects on transvaginal ultrasonography at the time a thickened NT is identified, caution should be used in counseling patients based on these results.[13] The rate of false-positive results in one study was 33% (ie, 1 in 3 of suspected abnormalities later was found to have normal fetal heart structure). Others have described an increased risk of cardiac anomalies with the finding of an absent or reversed A wave in the ductus venosus.[14]

Fetal Infections

A thickened NT has been associated with parvovirus infection[15–18] but not with other TORCH infections.[19] The finding of thickened NT in the setting of first trimester parvovirus infection is associated with an adverse outcome in 20% of cases. However, the accuracy of this rate is likely to be poor because of small numbers and the lack of prospective studies evaluating parvovirus status in all women with a thickened NT. If there is a history of an affected contact or maternal symptoms then it is reasonable to evaluate maternal quantitative IgG and IgM for parvovirus. If thickened NT progresses to signs of fetal hydrops at 20 to 22 weeks, parvovirus screening is recommended as well as consideration of evaluation for the standard infections associated with fetal hydrops, such as toxoplasmosis and cytomegalovirus.

Other Fetal Abnormalities

Fetal abnormalities that have been associated with a thickened NT are listed in **Table 3**. This list is by no means exhaustive; however, it serves to focus additional testing as needed and to provide additional guidance for subsequent targeted ultrasound examinations or genetic testing. Attention should be given to potential genetic sources of severe fetal anemia. If anomalies are found on subsequent sonographic evaluation, which are associated with other known syndromes, they should prompt additional counseling, evaluation, or testing. Conversely, some of the genetic disorders in **Table 3** have variable rates of abnormal findings on prenatal ultrasonography. Therefore, the absence of sonographic markers may not be sufficient to exclude the presence of a genetic syndrome. Few studies have evaluated long-term developmental outcomes in neonates born following a NT measurement of 3.5 mm or more.

Table 3
Abnormalities associated with thickened NT with normal karyotype

Abnormality	Defect	Potential Ultrasound Findings
Dandy Walker[2,20]	Developmental	Cerebellar hypoplasia
Holoprosencephaly[2,21,22]	Developmental	Alobar: monoventricle, fused thalami
Facial Cleft[2,23–26]	Developmental	Facial cleft
Diaphragmatic Hernia[2,22,24,27–30]	Developmental	Cardiac axis shift, viscera in thorax
Omphalocele[2,22–25,28,31–36]	Developmental	Abdominal wall defect
Megacystis[2,27,28,37–43]	Developmental	Bladder >7 mm at <14 weeks
Multicystic Dysplastic Kidneys[2,22,23,27,32,40,44,45]	Developmental	Enlarged, cystic kidneys, oligohydramnios
Achondrogenesis[46–48]	Autosomal recessive	Severe limb shortening Hypomineralization
Jarcho-Levin Syndrome[2,49–52]	Autosomal recessive	Scoliosis/spine disorganization
Fetal Akinesia Deformation Sequence[2,22–24,53]	Autosomal recessive	Arthrogryposis
Spinal Muscular Atrophy[2,20,27,54–56]	Autosomal recessive	Decreased fetal activity
Mucopolysaccharidosis Type VII[57–59]	Autosomal recessive	Hydrops, ascites, hepatomegaly
Smith-Lemli-Opitz Syndrome[2,22,60–62]	Autosomal recessive	Polydactyly, cardiac defects, ambiguous genitalia in males
Zellweger Syndrome[20,63–65]	Autosomal recessive	Hypertelorism, cardiac defects, brain defects, hepatomegaly, growth restriction
Body Stalk Anomaly[2,22,66–68]	Developmental	Large abdominal wall defect, kyphoscoliosis
Noonan Autosomal Dominant Pulmonary Stenosis, Syndrome[2,20,31,37,38,40,44,69,70]	Developmental	Large abdominal wall defect, kyphoscoliosis, hypertrophic cardiomyopathy, polyhydramnios, hydrothorax, skin edema

The optimal timing of follow-up sonographic evaluations is also not well established. Some researchers have suggested a targeted sonographic evaluation at 14 to 16 weeks for preliminary evaluation of the fetal anatomy and to evaluate whether or not the thickened NT has resolved.[4] Resolution is associated with a more favorable prognosis, whereas progressive hydrops is associated with a poor prognosis. Subsequent evaluation at 20 to 22 weeks can be performed to complete the anatomic evaluation as needed and to evaluate the fetal cardiac anatomy. These recommendations are based on expert opinion and do not reflect any systematic prospective comparison of the utility of various strategies. Therefore, the exact schedule of evaluation should be based on a combination of factors including provider preference, patient preference, and maternal body habitus. If fetal karyotype and anatomic evaluation at 20 to 24 weeks is normal, then patients can be reassured that the likelihood of a positive pregnancy outcome has been reported as 96% (95% confidence interval, 94%–98%).[71] Further, the one controlled study examining developmental outcome following isolated NT thickening reported no significant increase in rates of developmental delay.[72]

ABNORMAL FIRST TRIMESTER ANATOMY

Although a complete fetal anatomic survey is not feasible in fetuses between 11 and 13 6/7 weeks' gestation, detection of some structural abnormalities is possible, especially using a transvaginal approach.[73,74] Studies in this gestational age range report sensitivities in the detection of fetal anatomic abnormalities ranging from 16% to 65%, although some of these studies included cystic hygroma as one of the abnormalities, boosting detection rates.[73–77]

Table 4 provides a list of some of the abnormalities that can be detected in the first trimester. Although some of these abnormalities may be associated with a thickened NT (see **Table 3**), many are not. Fetal abnormalities identified concurrent with a thickened NT, especially suspected cardiac defects, increase the risk of chromosomal abnormality. It is reasonable to attempt evaluation of the fetal anatomy transvaginally following the finding of a thickened NT. Although any anatomic abnormalities that are detected at the time of nuchal evaluation should be incorporated into patient counseling, early evaluation of fetal heart anatomy and other structural abnormalities is probably most efficient at 14 to 16 weeks.

EXTREMES OF FIRST TRIMESTER MATERNAL SERUM ANALYTES AND ADVERSE PREGNANCY OUTCOMES

Levels of first trimester analytes are thought to reflect in part placental function. Therefore, it is logical that abnormalities would be associated with an increased risk of pregnancy complications related to placental function. This section reviews the associations between depressed levels of pregnancy-associated plasma protein (PAPP)-A and elevated levels of the free β subunit of human chorionic gonadotrophin (HCG) and adverse pregnancy outcomes related to abnormal first trimester placentation, including miscarriage, stillbirth, and intrauterine growth restriction. The association between abnormal levels of first trimester analytes and other pregnancy

Table 4 Structural abnormalities that may be seen in the first trimester	
Abnormality	**Ultrasound Finding**
Acrania-Anencephaly Sequence	Absent cranial vault, echogenic amniotic fluid[78]
Holoprosencephaly	Single ventricle
Cerebellar Defects	Ventriculomegaly
Hydranencephaly	Fluid-filled cranium
Encephalocele	Cranial defect, usually posterior
Spina Bifida	Irregularities of the bony spine, bulging posterior contour of the fetal back
Body Stalk Abnormality	Large abdominal wall defect, kyphoscoliosis
Omphalocele	Bowel herniation beyond 12 weeks gestation
Gastroschisis	Bowel herniation lateral to cord insertion
Cleft Lip	Cleft lip
Cardiac Abnormalities	Various, abnormal ductus venosus flow
Prune Belly Syndrome	Megacystis
Diaphragmatic Hernia	Mediastinal shift, stomach visible in chest
Skeletal Abnormalities	Absent long bones, significantly decreased calcification, joint contractures

complications that may also be related to first trimester placentation, namely preeclampsia and preterm birth, are also reviewed. A possible association between abnormal levels of analytes and other abnormalities have also been reviewed. Although the exact multiple of the median (MOM) cutoff for PAPP-A less than the 1st and 5th percentiles varies slightly by study, this value can easily be obtained from the reference laboratory used in each clinical center.

Early Fetal Loss

Multiple large cohort studies have established a relationship between depressed levels of PAPP-A and early pregnancy loss. **Table 5** reviews the screen positive rates and positive predictive values (PPVs) for PAPP-A levels less than the 5th and 1st percentiles. Overall, the PPV of PAPP-A is relatively low, as the majority of pregnancy loss precedes first trimester screening. HCG less than 1st percentile has also been associated with a 2.8% to 4.1% PPV for early fetal loss.[80,81] Combining depressed PAPP-A levels with maternal characteristics, maternal serum α-fetoprotein (MSAFP) level, and unconjugated estriol level increases the detection rate of early loss to 39%.[81] However, ultrasound examination to evaluate the fetal anatomy is already planned between 16 (in cases of abnormal results in overall first trimester screening) and 18 to 20 weeks (in cases of normal testing) in most cases. Therefore, no additional intervention is indicated in the asymptomatic patient. The maternal risks of a short delay in diagnosis of fetal loss are low as disseminated intravascular coagulation after early pregnancy loss is rare. Further, because there are no proven effective interventions to prevent previable pregnancy loss related to poor placentation, the cost-effectiveness of repeated screening to detect pregnancy loss is likely to be poor. Given that normal first trimester testing is associated with rates of pregnancy loss of 0.36%, clinicians should use normal first trimester as an opportunity to reassure patients regarding subsequent risk of miscarriage.[80]

Late Fetal Loss

Table 5 reviews the screen positive rates and PPVs for PAPP-A levels below the 5th and 1st percentiles for stillbirth or late fetal loss. Even at PAPP-A levels less than 1st percentile, the PPV for stillbirth is only 0.84% to 2.0%. Depressed levels of HCG are not significantly related to the risk of stillbirth.[81] In one report, 7 of the 8 stillbirths that occurred in women with PAPP-A levels less than 5th percentile were related to signs of abnormal placentation, that is, placental abruption or growth restricted fetuses. Given that a PAPP-A level less than 1st percentile is a strong predictor of growth restriction (see later discussion), it is likely that screening strategies to detect small-for-gestational-age (SGA) fetuses will identify the fetuses at highest risk of stillbirth following a depressed PAPP-A level. Although regular fetal surveillance in this population is likely to be accompanied by some reduction in the risk of stillbirth, the ability of fetal surveillance in a population with normal fetal growth to prevent unexplained stillbirth or fetal demise associated with placental abruption is far from certain.

Intrauterine Growth Restriction

Multiple studies have established a correlation between abnormal first trimester analyte levels, especially PAPP-A, and birth weight. One strength of the research in this area is that first trimester screening ensures accurate pregnancy dating. In contrast, many reports are weakened by a poor definition of growth restriction. A definition of growth restriction based on an overall birth weight of less than 10th percentile for gestational age is likely to include a large proportion of constitutionally small neonates that do not have a significantly increased risk of adverse outcome. The most robust studies include a more extreme definition of growth restriction (SGA<5th percentile); therefore studies with growth restriction defined as SGA less than 10th percentile are only included as related to PAPP-A levels less than 1st percentile (see **Table 5**).

Overall as a single marker, a PAPP-A level less than 1st percentile has a strong PPV for SGA less than 5th percentile (15.8%)[81] and SGA less than 10th percentile (24.1%–26.3%)[81,83,87] and appears to be sufficient indication as a single marker to recommend subsequent sonographic evaluation of fetal growth. Further, the cost-effectiveness is likely to be favorable as few women would require screening ($\leq$1%), but 1 in 6 women screened would have a fetus with SGA less than 5th percentile and 1 in 4 would have a fetus with SGA less than 10th percentile.

The strength of PAPP-A levels less than 5th percentile as a single marker is less certain, as the observed rates of SGA less than 5th percentile are only 1.5- to 2-fold higher than expected. Therefore many researchers have used PAPP-A levels less than 5th percentile in combination with other indicators of increased risk of SGA to increase the sensitivity and specificity of testing. One approach is to use parameters obtained at routine second trimester ultrasound evaluations, including fetal growth parameters (routinely obtained) and uterine artery Doppler measurements (not routinely obtained at all centers). Another approach is to combine first trimester measures with second trimester measurements of MSAFP levels that are routinely obtained after 15 weeks to screen for neural tube defects. A third approach is to combine first trimester screening with maternal risk factors.

Of these methods, combining MSAFP values is the most straightforward and reproducible. Smith and colleagues[89] evaluated this approach in a cohort of 8483 women.

In this cohort, a PAPP-A level less than 5th percentile was associated with a 10.9% rate of SGA, whereas an MSAFP level greater than 95 percentile was associated with a 4.9% rate of SGA. There was no association between a test result of a PAPP-A level less than 5th percentile and a subsequent MSAFP level greater than 95 percentile. Of the small proportion of women with both a PAPP-A level less than 5th percentile and an MSAFP level greater than 95 percentile, the subsequent rate of SGA was 32.1%. Therefore, it seems reasonable to perform surveillance for SGA in women whose test results are outside the usual bounds. This study also reported an increased risk of stillbirth in women with both abnormal test values; however, it was not clear how many of these stillbirths occurred in the absence of growth restriction.

The utility of second trimester ultrasound markers is less clear. Fox and colleagues[90] reported that 10.5% of women with a PAPP-A level less than 5th percentile have evidence of fetal growth disturbances defined as (1) estimated fetal weight less than 25 percentile, (2) a greater than 7 day growth discrepancy with established dates or (3) a measurement of greater than 90th percentile for head or abdominal circumference. In this group, the rate of birth weight less than 10th percentile was 47.8% and the rate of birth weight less than 5th percentile was 21.7%. Although these results are provocative, the study was relatively small and these rates are based on only 25 fetuses with both PAPP-A levels less than 5th percentile and growth disturbances seen on second trimester ultrasonography. Cooper and colleagues[91] performed uterine artery Doppler examination at 18 and 22 weeks on all women with a PAPP-A level less than 0.4 MOM (n = 289). In pregnancies with a pulsatility index (PI) of more than 1.45, the subsequent incidence of SGA was 36% at 18 weeks and 64% at 22 weeks. Further prospective studies are needed to evaluate this exploratory cutoff for PI to determine if measuring PI at the midtrimester is an effective strategy. Others have investigated the addition of maternal serum placental growth factor (PlGF) at 11 to 13 6/7 weeks to increase the sensitivity and specificity of first trimester analytes in the prediction of SGA[92]; however, this work is preliminary. Depressed

Table 5
Adverse pregnancy outcomes with low levels of PAPP-A

Outcome	PPV (%) <5th Percentile[a]	Screen Positive Rate (%)	PPV (%) <1st Percentile[a]	Screen Positive Rate (%)
Pregnancy Loss <20–24 Weeks				
Ong et al[79] (n = 5297)	1.4	5.3		
Goetzl et al[80] (n = 7932)	1.4	5.1	2.7	1.05
Dugoff et al[81] (n = 34,271)	2.2	5.1	4.5	1.03
Brameld et al[82] (n = 22,125)	0.6	4.1		
Scott et al[83] (n = 44,535)			8.0	0.44
Stillbirth (>20–24)				
Smith et al[84] (n = 7934)	2.0	5.0		
Brameld et al[82] (n = 22,125)	1.3	4.1		
Smith et al[85] (n = 8839)	0.9	5.2		
Dugoff et al[81] (n = 34,271)	0.6	.58	0.84	1.06
Scott et al[83] (n = 44,535)			2.0	0.44
Birth weight <5th%ile				
Ong et al[79] (n = 5297)	7.9	5.3		
Smith et al[85] (n = 8839)	10.0	5.2		
Spencer et al[86] (n = 46,262)	9.7–12.2[a]	4–5.0[a]		
Dugoff et al[81] (n = 34,271)	9.5	4.8	15.8	0.9

Birth weight<10%ile				
Krantz et al[87] (n = 8012)			24.1	0.8
Dugoff et al[81] (n = 34,271)			26.3	0.8
Scott et al[83] (n = 44,535)			25.0	0.44
Preterm Birth<32 weeks				
Brameld et al[82] (n = 22,125)	4.3	4.1		
Smith et al[85] (n = 8839)	2.6	5.2		
Dugoff et al[81] (n = 34,271)	1.4	5.1	2.4	1.0
Scott et al[83] (n = 44,535)			10.0	0.44
Preterm Birth <34 weeks				
Ong et al[79] (n = 5297)[81]	2.5	5.3		
Krantz et al[87] (n = 8012)	2.5	4.6	2.8	0.9
Spencer et al[88] (n = 54,722)	2.2–2.8[a]	4–5.0[a]		
Preeclampsia				
Ong et al[79] (n = 5297)	5.4	5.3		
Brameld et al[82] (n = 22,125)	7.9	4.2		
Smith et al[85] (n = 8839)	7.6	5.2		
Dugoff et al[81] (n = 34,271)	3.5	5.2	4.2	1.05

Abbreviation: PPV, positive predictive value.

PAPP-A 5th percentile cutoffs where reported: 0.4 MOM,[82,84] 0.45 MOM,[80,87] 0.42 MOM.[81,86]

PAPP-A 1st percentile cutoffs where reported: 0.29 MOM,[80,87] 0.28 MOM.[81]

MOM of 0.2 reported as approximation of PAPP-A at 1st percentile.[83]

[a] Screen positive rates were not reported in this study; we estimated a screen positive rate of 4% to 5.0% and then calculated a range of possible PPV as reported.

levels of HCG less than 1st percentile were related to an increased risk of SGA less than 10th percentile in one report (PPV, 14.3%)[87] but were not related to an increased risk of SGA less than 5th percentile in another report.[81]

Preterm Birth

Overall, the ability of PAPP-A levels to predict spontaneous preterm birth before 34 weeks is low (see **Table 5**). Some of the risk of preterm delivery associated with low levels of PAPP-A is likely due to indicated preterm birth due to the association between PAPP-A and SGA. Therefore, the likelihood that PAPP-A levels can be used to identify a clinical population who are good candidates for preterm birth interventions is low. The sensitivity of PAPP-A levels less than 5th percentile for preterm delivery 32 weeks or less is 9.4%.[81,87] Therefore, if additional tests could increase the sensitivity and specificity, it would be of interest. It is also not know if preterm births associated with depressed levels of PAPP-A would be reduced by currently available treatments, such as 17-OH progesterone. Depressed or elevated levels of HCG are not associated with an increased risk of preterm delivery.[81,87]

Preeclampsia

Overall, a PAPP-A level less than 5th or 1st percentile as a single marker has a poor PPV for preeclampsia. Given the low rates of preeclampsia in a population with depressed PAPP-A levels and the lack of effective preventative strategies in women at relatively low risk, it is unlikely that first trimester analytes used to screen for aneuploidy are useful at this time. In women with abnormal uterine artery Doppler in the second trimester, the retrospective addition of the test results of first trimester serum analytes appears to have only a small effect on ROC curves (area under the curve, 0.818 vs 0.853).[93] However, active research is ongoing regarding other potential first trimester markers of preeclampsia, including the addition of first trimester uterine artery PI,[94] level of maternal plasma inhibin A at 11 to 13 weeks,[95] and a combination of uterine artery PI and level of maternal serum placental protein 13.[96]

Most recently, Poon and colleagues[97] have proposed a multivariate prediction model for early-onset preeclampsia that includes maternal parity, history of prior preeclampsia, uterine artery PI at 11 to 13 weeks, maternal mean arterial pressure, PAPP-A level, and PIGF level. At a rate of 5% false-positive results, 93% of preeclampsia before 34 weeks was detected. Limitations include a very low rate of overall preeclampsia (2%) in the population used to derive the model, the cumbersome nature of the model, and the fact that the model for early onset preeclampsia was based on only 34 cases. Prospective evaluation of this model will be needed in the US population, as well as the availability of effective interventions, before this model can be adopted into clinical practice.

Other Abnormalities

A recent report from Hoffman and colleagues[98] links inhibin A levels greater than or equal to 2.0 MOM with structural abnormalities including multicystic dysplastic kidney (MCDK) and 2-vessel umbilical cord. An HCG level greater than or equal to 2.0 MOM was associated with MCDK and hydrocele and a PAPP-A level greater than or equal to 2.0 MOM was associated with hydrocele. This report is largely of interest because of the questions it raises about the mechanism through which certain structural abnormalities might interact with maternal serum analytes. MCDK and a 2-vessel cord are easily detected on ultrasound examination, and hydrocele is generally not clinically significant. Uccella and colleagues[99] have recently linked a PAPP-A level of less than 0.52 MOM to an increased risk of cesarean delivery for nonreassuring fetal status in labor. Although this result has some biologic plausibility, this information should not be incorporated into clinical practice until this exploratory cutoff is validated.

SUMMARY

A thickened NT in the setting of a normal karyotype is associated with adverse pregnancy outcomes. At first trimester screening, as detailed an anatomic survey as feasible should be performed and definitive diagnosis for aneuploidy should be offered. Patients should be counseled regarding the increased risk of fetal loss before amniocentesis or chorionic villus sampling. Once a normal karyotype has been established, screening for parvovirus and/or targeted genetic testing should be offered if appropriate. An early anatomic survey should be offered at 14 to 16 weeks, followed by repeat ultrasonography with fetal echocardiography at 20 to 22 weeks. Counseling regarding prognosis should be based on these evaluations. Fetal outcome is favorable in the absence of any identified abnormalities and with resolution of the thickened NT. Progression to fetal hydrops is associated with a poor prognosis.

Women with PAPP-A levels less than 1st percentile are at high risk for growth restriction of the fetus and should undergo subsequent evaluation. Those fetuses with suspected intrauterine growth restriction should undergo further evaluation with serial umbilical artery Doppler examinations as well as surveillance for fetal well-being. This stepwise strategy is likely to identify those pregnancies at highest risk for stillbirth in women with a PAPP-A level less than 1st percentile.

Women with a PAPP-A level less than 5th percentile in combination with an MSAFP level greater than 95 percentile should also undergo subsequent screening for intrauterine growth restriction. It is reasonable to consider adding uterine artery PI to the midtrimester anatomic ultrasonography results in women with a PAPP-A level less than 5th percentile. Women with normal results in the first trimester testing should be reassured that their risk of subsequent pregnancy loss is very low and that their risk of other adverse pregnancy outcomes is reduced.

REFERENCES

1. Souka AP, Snijders RJM, Novakov A, et al. Defects and syndromes in chromosomally normal fetuses with increased nuchal translucency at 10–14 weeks of gestation. Ultrasound Obstet Gynecol 1998;11:391–400.
2. Souka AP, Krampl E, Bakalis S, et al. Outcome of pregnancy in chromosomally normal fetuses with increased nuchal translucency in the first trimester. Ultrasound Obstet Gynecol 2001;18:9–17.
3. Michailidis GD, Economides DL. Nuchal translucency measurement and pregnancy outcome in karyotypically normal fetuses. Ultrasound Obstet Gynecol 2001;17:102–5.
4. Souka AP, von Kaisenberg CS, Hyett JA, et al. Increased nuchal translucency with normal karyotype. Am J Obstet Gynecol 2005;192:1005–21.
5. Hyett JA, Perdu M, Sharland GK, et al. Increased nuchal translucency at 10–14 weeks of gestation as a marker for major cardiac defects. Ultrasound Obstet Gynecol 1997;10:242–6.
6. Hyett J, Perdu M, Sharland G, et al. Using fetal nuchal translucency to screen for major congenital heart defects at 10–14 weeks gestation: population based cohort study. BMJ 1999;318:81–5.
7. Ghi T, Huggon IC, Zosmer N, et al. Incidence of major structural cardiac defects associated with increased nuchal translucency but normal karyotype. Ultrasound Obstet Gynecol 2001;18:610–4.

8. Aztei A, Gajewska K, Huggon IC, et al. Relationship between nuchal translucency thickness and prevalence of major cardiac defects in fetuses with normal karyotype. Ultrasound Obstet Gynecol 2005;26:154–7.

9. Simpson LL, Malone FD, Bianchi DW, et al. Nuchal translucency and the risk of congenital heart disease. Obstet Gynecol 2007;109:376–83.

10. Clur SA, Mathijsssen IB, Pajkrt E, et al. Structural heart defects associated with an increased nuchal translucency: 9 years experience in a referral center. Prenat Diagn 2008;28:347–54.

11. Zosmer N, Souter VL, Chan CSY, et al. Early diagnosis of major cardiac defects in chromosomally normal fetuses with increased nuchal translucency. BJOG 1999; 106:829–33.

12. American College of Obstetricians and Gynecologists (ACOG). Screening for fetal chromosomal abnormalities. ACOG Practice Bulletin No. 77. Washington, DC: American College of Obstetricians and Gynecologists; 2007.

13. Weiner Z, Weizman B, Beloosesky R, et al. Fetal cardiac scanning performed immediately following abnormal nuchal translucency examination. Prenat Diagn 2008;28:934–8.

14. Maiz N, Plasencia W, Dagklis T, et al. Ductus venosus Doppler in fetuses with cardiac defects and increased nuchal translucency thickness. Ultrasound Obstet Gynecol 2008;31:256–60.

15. Petrikovsky BM, Baker D, Schneider E. Fetal hydrops secondary to human parvovirus infection in early pregnancy. Prenat Diagn 1996;16:342–4.

16. Markenson G, Correia LA, Cohn G, et al. Parvoviral infection associated with increased nuchal translucency: a case report. J Perinatol 2000;20:129–31.

17. Smulian JC, Egan JF, Rodis JF. Fetal hydrops in the first trimester associated with maternal parvovirus infection. J Clin Ultrasound 1998;26:314–6.

18. Sohan K, Carroll S, Byrne D, et al. Parvovirus as a differential diagnosis of hydrops fetalis in the first trimester. Fetal Diagn Ther 2000;15:234–6.

19. Sebire NJ, Bianco D, Snijders RJM, et al. Increased fetal nuchal translucency thickness at 10–14 weeks: is screening for maternal-fetal infection necessary? BJOG 1997;104:212–5.

20. Bilardo CM, Pajkrt E, de Graaf IM, et al. Outcome of fetuses with enlarged nuchal translucency and normal karyotype. Ultrasound Obstet Gynecol 1998;11:401–37.

21. Salvesen DR, Goble O. Early amniocentesis and fetal nuchal translucency in women requesting karyotyping for advanced maternal age. Prenat Diagn 1995;15:971–4.

22. Pandya PP, Kondylios A, Hilbert L, et al. Chromosomal defects and outcome in 1015 fetuses with increased nuchal translucency. Ultrasound Obstet Gynecol 1995;5:15–9.

23. Ville Y, Lalondrelle C, Doumerc S, et al. First-trimester diagnosis of nuchal anomalies: significance and fetal outcome. Ultrasound Obstet Gynecol 1992;2:314–6.

24. Nadel A, Bromley B, Benacerraf BR. Nuchal thickening or cystic hygromas in first- and early second-trimester fetuses: prognosis and outcome. Obstet Gynecol 1993;82:43–8.

25. Senat MV, De Keersmaecker B, Audibert F, et al. Pregnancy outcome in fetuses with increased nuchal translucency and normal karyotype. Prenat Diagn 2002;22:345–9.

26. Markov D, Jacquemyn Y, Leroy Y. Bilateral cleft lip and palate associated with increased nuchal translucency and maternal cocaine abuse at 14 weeks of gestation. Clin Exp Obstet Gynecol 2003;30:109–10.

27. Van Vugt JM, Tinnemans BW, Van Zalen-Sprock RM. Outcome and early childhood follow-up of chromosomally normal fetuses with increased nuchal translucency at 10–14 weeks' gestation. Ultrasound Obstet Gynecol 1998;11:407–9.

28. Mangione R, Guyon F, Taine L, et al. Pregnancy outcome and prognosis in fetuses with increased first-trimester nuchal translucency. Fetal Diagn Ther 2001;16:360–3.
29. Sebire NJ, Snijders RJM, Davenport M, et al. Fetal nuchal translucency thickness at 10–14 weeks of gestation and congenital diaphragmatic hernia. Obstet Gynecol 1997;90:943–7.
30. Varlet F, Bousquet F, Clemenson A, et al. Congenital diaphragmatic hernia. Two cases with early prenatal diagnosis and increased nuchal translucency. Fetal Diagn Ther 2003;18:33–5.
31. Adekunle O, Gopee A, El-Sayed M, et al. Increased first-trimester nuchal translucency: pregnancy and infant outcomes after routine screening for Down's syndrome in an unselected antenatal population. Br J Radiol 1999;72:457–60.
32. Cha'Ban FK, van Splunder P, Los FJ, et al. Fetal outcome in nuchal translucency with emphasis on normal fetal karyotype. Prenat Diagn 1996;16:537–41.
33. Snijders RJM, Brizot ML, Faria M, et al. Fetal exomphalos at 11–14 weeks of gestation. J Ultrasound Med 1995;14:569–74.
34. van Zalen-Sprock RM, van Vugt JMG, van Geijn HP. First trimester sonography of physiological midgut herniation and early diagnosis of omphalocele. Prenat Diagn 1997;17:511–8.
35. Schemm S, Gembruch U, Germer U, et al. Omphalocele-exstrophy-imperforate anus-spinal defects (OEIS) complex associated with increased nuchal translucency. Ultrasound Obstet Gynecol 2003;22:95–7.
36. Snijders RJ, Sebire NJ, Souka A, et al. Fetal exomphalos and chromosomal defects: relationship to maternal age and gestation. Ultrasound Obstet Gynecol 1995;6:250–5.
37. Johnson MP, Johnson A, Holzgreve W, et al. First-trimester simple hygroma: cause and outcome. Am J Obstet Gynecol 1993;168:156–61.
38. Trauffer ML, Anderson CE, Johnson A, et al. The natural history of euploid pregnancies with first trimester cystic hygromas. Am J Obstet Gynecol 1994;170: 1279–84.
39. Maymon R, Jauniaux E, Cohen O, et al. Pregnancy outcome and infant follow-up of fetuses with abnormally increased first trimester nuchal translucency. Hum Reprod 2000;15:2023–7.
40. van Zalen-Sprock RM, van Vugt JMG, van Geijn HP. First trimester diagnosis of cystic hygroma; course and outcome. Am J Obstet Gynecol 1992;167:94–8.
41. Sebire NJ, Von Kaisenberg C, Rubio C, et al. Fetal megacystis at 10–14 weeks of gestation. Ultrasound Obstet Gynecol 1996;8:387–90.
42. Favre R, Kohler M, Gasser B, et al. Early fetal megacystis between 11 and 15 weeks of gestation. Ultrasound Obstet Gynecol 1999;14:402–6.
43. Liao AW, Sebire NJ, Geerts L, et al. Megacystis at 10–14 weeks of gestation: chromosomal defects and outcome according to bladder length. Ultrasound Obstet Gynecol 2003;21:338–41.
44. Reynders CS, Pauker SP, Benacerraf BR. First trimester isolated fetal nuchal lucency: significance and outcome. J Ultrasound Med 1997;16:101–5.
45. Hewitt B. Nuchal translucency in the first trimester. Aust N Z J Obstet Gynaecol 1993;33:389–91.
46. Fisk NM, Vaughan J, Smidt M, et al. Transvaginal ultrasound recognition of nuchal oedema in the first-trimester diagnosis of achondrogenesis. J Clin Ultrasound 1991;19:586–90.
47. Soothill PW, Vuthiwong C, Rees H. Achondrogenesis type 2 diagnosed by transvaginal ultrasound at 12 weeks of gestation. Prenat Diagn 1993;13:523–8.

48. Meizner I, Barnhard Y. Achondrogenesis type I diagnosed by transvaginal ultrasonography at 13 weeks' gestation. Am J Obstet Gynecol 1995;173:1620–2.

49. Eliyahu S, Weiner E, Lahav D, et al. Early sonographic diagnosis of Jarcho-Levin syndrome: a prospective screening program in one family. Ultrasound Obstet Gynecol 1997;9:314–8.

50. Lam YH, Eik-Nes SH, Tang MHY, et al. Prenatal sonographic features of spondylocostal dysostosis and diaphragmatic hernia in the first trimester. Ultrasound Obstet Gynecol 1999;13:213–5.

51. Hull AD, James G, Pretorius DH. Detection of Jarcho-Levin syndrome at 12 weeks' gestation by nuchal translucency screening and three-dimensional ultrasound. Prenat Diagn 2001;21:390–4.

52. Clementschitsch G, Hasenohrl G, Steiner H, et al. Early diagnosis of a fetal skeletal dysplasia associated with increased nuchal translucency with 2D and 3D ultrasound. Ultraschall Med 2003;24:349–52.

53. Hyett J, Noble P, Sebire NJ, et al. Lethal congenital arthrogryposis presents with increased nuchal translucency at 10–14 weeks of gestation. Ultrasound Obstet Gynecol 1997;9:310–3.

54. Rijhsinghani A, Yankowitz J, Howser D, et al. Sonographic and maternal serum screening abnormalities in fetuses affected by spinal muscular atrophy. Prenat Diagn 1997;17:166–9.

55. Stiller RJ, Lieberson D, Herzlinger R, et al. The association of increased fetal nuchal translucency and spinal muscular atrophy type I. Prenat Diagn 1999;19:587–9.

56. de Jong-Pleij EA, Stoutenbecek P, van der Mark-Batseva NN, et al. The association of spinal muscular atrophy type II and increased nuchal translucency. Ultrasound Obstet Gynecol 2002;19:312–3.

57. van Eyndhoven HWF, Ter Brugge HG, van Essen AJ, et al. Beta-glucuronidase deficiency as cause of recurrent hydrops fetalis: the first early prenatal diagnosis by chorionic villus sampling. Prenat Diagn 1998;18:959–62.

58. den Hollander NS, Kleijer WJ, Schoonderwaldt EM, et al. In-utero diagnosis of mucopolysaccharidosis type VII in a fetus with an enlarged nuchal translucency. Ultrasound Obstet Gynecol 2000;16:87–90.

59. Geipel A, Berg C, Germer U, et al. Mucopolysaccharidosis VII (Sly disease) as a cause of increased nuchal translucency and non-immune fetal hydrops: study of a family and technical approach to prenatal diagnosis in early and late pregnancy. Prenat Diagn 2002;22:493–5.

60. Hobbins JC, Jones OW, Gottesfeld S, et al. Transvaginal sonography and transabdominal embryoscopy in the first-trimester diagnosis of Smith-Lemli-Opitz syndrome, type 2. Am J Obstet Gynecol 1994;171:546–9.

61. Hyett JA, Clayton PT, Moscoso G, et al. Increased first trimester nuchal translucency as a prenatal manifestation of Smith-Lemli-Opitz syndrome. Am J Med Genet 1995;58:374–6.

62. Sharp P, Haant E, Fletcher JM, et al. First trimester diagnosis of Smith-Lemli-Opitz syndrome. Prenat Diagn 1997;17:355–61.

63. de Graaf IM, Pajkrt E, Keessen M, et al. Enlarged nuchal translucency and low serum protein concentration as possible markers for Zellweger syndrome. Ultrasound Obstet Gynecol 1999;13:268–70.

64. Christiaens GC, de Pater JM, Stoutenbeek P, et al. First trimester nuchal anomalies as a prenatal sign of Zellweger syndrome. Prenat Diagn 2000;20:517–25.

65. Johnson JM, Babul-Hirji R, Chitayat D. First-trimester increased nuchal translucency and fetal hypokinesia associated with Zellweger syndrome. Ultrasound Obstet Gynecol 2001;17:344–6.

66. Cheng C, Bahado-Singh RO, Chen S, et al. Pregnancy outcomes with increased nuchal translucency after routine Down syndrome screening. Int J Gynaecol Obstet 2004;84:5–9.
67. Daskalakis G, Sebire NJ, Jurkovic D, et al. Body stalk anomaly at 10–14 weeks of gestation. Ultrasound Obstet Gynecol 1997;10:416–8.
68. Smrcek JM, Germer U, Krokowski M, et al. Prenatal ultrasound diagnosis and management of body stalk anomaly: analysis of nine singleton and two multiple pregnancies. Ultrasound Obstet Gynecol 2003;21:322–8.
69. Hiippala A, Eronen M, Taipale P, et al. Fetal nuchal translucency and normal chromosomes: a long-term follow-up study. Ultrasound Obstet Gynecol 2001;18: 18–22.
70. Achiron R, Heggesh J, Grisaru D, et al. Noonan syndrome: a cryptic condition in early gestation. Am J Med Genet 2000;92:159–65.
71. Bilardo CM, Muller MA, Pajkrt E, et al. Increased nuchal translucency thickness and normal karyotype: time for parental reassurance. Ultrasound Obstet Gynecol 2007;30:11–8.
72. Brady AF, Pandya PP, Yuksel B, et al. Outcome of chromosomally normal live births with increased fetal nuchal translucency at 10–14 weeks' gestation. J Med Genet 1998;35:222–4.
73. Timor-Tritsch IE, Fuchs KM, Monteagudo A, et al. Performing a fetal anatomy scan at the time of first-trimester screening. Obstet Gynecol 2009;113:402–7.
74. Achiron R, Tadmor O. Screening for fetal anomalies during the first trimester of pregnancy: transvaginal versus transabdominal sonography. Ultrasound Obstet Gynecol 1991;1:186–91.
75. Carvalho MH, Brizot ML, Lopes LM, et al. Detection of fetal structural abnormalities at the 11–14 week ultrasound scan. Prenat Diagn 2002;22:1–4.
76. McAuliffe FM, Fong KW, Toi A, et al. Ultrasound detection of fetal anomalies in conjunction with first-trimester nuchal translucency screening: a feasibility study. Am J Obstet Gynecol 2005;193:1260–5.
77. Drysdale K, Ridley D, Walker K, et al. First trimester pregnancy scanning as a screening tool for high-risk and abnormal pregnancies in a district general hospital setting. J Obstet Gynaecol 2002;22:159–65.
78. Cafici D, Sepulveda W. First-trimester echogenic amniotic fluid in the acrania-anencephaly sequence. J Ultrasound Med 2003;22:1075–9.
79. Ong CYT, Liao AW, Spencer K, et al. First trimester maternal serum free β human chorionic gonadotrophin and pregnancy associated plasma protein A as predictors of pregnancy complications. BJOG 2000;107:1265–70.
80. Goetzl L, Krantz D, Simpson JL, et al. Pregnancy-associated plasma protein A, free beta-hCG, nuchal translucency, and risk of pregnancy loss. Obstet Gynecol 2004;104:30–6.
81. Dugoff L, Cuckle HS, Hobbins JC, et al. Prediction of patient-specific risk for fetal loss using maternal characteristics and first- and second-trimester maternal serum Down syndrome markers. Am J Obstet Gynecol 2008;199:290, e1–6.
82. Brameld KJ, Dickinson JE, O'Leary P, et al. First trimester predictors of adverse pregnancy outcomes. Aust N Z J Obstet Gynaecol 2008;48:529–35.
83. Scott F, Coates A, McLennan A. Pregnancy outcome in the setting of extremely low first trimester PAPP-A levels. Aust N Z J Obstet Gynaecol 2009;49:258–62.
84. Smith GC, Crossley JA, Aitken DA, et al. First-trimester placentation and the risk of antepartum stillbirth. JAMA 2004;292:2249–54.
85. Smith GC, Stenhouse EJ, Crossley JA, et al. Early pregnancy levels of pregnancy-associated plasma protein A and the risk of intrauterine growth

restriction, premature birth, preeclampsia, and stillbirth. J Clin Endocrinol Metab 2002;87:1762–7.

86. Spencer K, Cowans NJ, Avgidou K, et al. First-trimester biochemical markers of aneuploidy and the prediction of small-for-gestational age fetuses. Ultrasound Obstet Gynecol 2008;31:15–9.

87. Krantz D, Goetzl L, Simpson JL, et al, First Trimester Maternal Serum Biochemistry and Fetal Nuchal Translucency Screening (BUN) Study Group. Association of extreme first-trimester free human chorionic gonadotropin-beta, pregnancy-associated plasma protein A, and nuchal translucency with intrauterine growth restriction and other adverse pregnancy outcomes. Am J Obstet Gynecol 2004;191:1452–8.

88. Spencer K, Cowans NJ, Molina F, et al. First-trimester ultrasound and biochemical markers of aneuploidy and the prediction of preterm or early preterm delivery. Ultrasound Obstet Gynecol 2008;31:147–52.

89. Smith GC, Shah I, Crossley JA, et al. Pregnancy-associated plasma protein A and alpha-fetoprotein and prediction of adverse perinatal outcome. Obstet Gynecol 2006;107:161–6.

90. Fox NS, Shalom D, Chasen ST. Second-trimester fetal growth as a predictor of poor obstetric and neonatal outcome in patients with low first-trimester serum pregnancy-associated plasma protein-A and a euploid fetus. Ultrasound Obstet Gynecol 2009;33:34–8.

91. Cooper S, Johnson JA, Metcalfe A, et al. The predictive value of 18 and 22 week uterine artery Doppler in patients with low first trimester maternal serum PAPP-A. Prenat Diagn 2009;29:248–52.

92. Poon LC, Zaragoza E, Akolekar R, et al. Maternal serum placental growth factor (PlGF) in small for gestational age pregnancy at 11(+0) to 13(+6) weeks of gestation. Prenat Diagn 2008;28:1110–5.

93. Spencer K, Yu CK, Cowans NJ, et al. Prediction of pregnancy complications by first-trimester maternal serum PAPP-A and free beta-hCG and with second-trimester uterine artery Doppler. Prenat Diagn 2005;25:949–53.

94. Poon LC, Maiz N, Valencia C, et al. First-trimester maternal serum pregnancy-associated plasma protein-A and pre-eclampsia. Ultrasound Obstet Gynecol 2009;33:23–33.

95. Akolekar R, Minekawa R, Veduta A, et al. Maternal plasma inhibin A at 11–13 weeks of gestation in hypertensive disorders of pregnancy. Prenat Diagn 2009; 29:753–60.

96. Nicolaides KH, Bindra R, Turan OM, et al. A novel approach to first-trimester screening for early pre-eclampsia combining serum PP-13 and Doppler ultrasound. Ultrasound Obstet Gynecol 2006;27:13–7.

97. Poon LC, Kametas NA, Maiz N, et al. First-trimester prediction of hypertensive disorders in pregnancy. Hypertension 2009;53:812–8.

98. Hoffman JD, Bianchi DW, Sullivan LM, et al. Down syndrome serum screening also identifies an increased risk for multicystic dysplastic kidney, two-vessel cord, and hydrocele. Prenat Diagn 2008;28:1204–8.

99. Uccella S, Colombo GF, Bulgheroni CM, et al. First-trimester maternal serum screening and the risk for fetal distress during labor. Am J Obstet Gynecol 2009;201(2):166, e1–6.

Cost-Effectiveness of Down Syndrome Screening Paradigms

Aaron B. Caughey, MD, MPP, MPH, PhD[a,b,*],
Anjali J. Kaimal, MD, MAS[b,c], Anthony O. Odibo, MD, MSCE[b,d]

KEYWORDS

- Cost-benefit analysis • Cost-effectiveness analysis
- Economics • Prenatal diagnosis • Down syndrome

Increases in health care costs continue to outpace inflation.[1] In 2007, total expenditures on health care were greater than $2.2 trillion dollars, or 16% of the gross domestic product (GDP) in the United States.[2–4] In this setting, health care systems, health insurance providers, health care providers, the government, and patients themselves are increasingly aware of rising costs and interested in controlling them. However, although payers are primarily interested in reigning costs in, other stakeholders, such as providers and patients, are also concerned with maintaining access to quality health care.

Efforts to balance health care quality with expenditure have led to a new emphasis on comparative effectiveness research, which examines the differences in outcomes and the costs of health care interventions. To compare the marginal benefits to be gained from new procedures, medications, and screening tests to their often increased costs, economic evaluations of such innovations are now commonly used.[5,6] These analyses may help guide health care providers, organizations, professional societies, and policy makers to determine how and to whom particular health care services are provided.[7]

Economic analyses have been used for at least 30 years to inform the development of prenatal screening and diagnosis guidelines. Prenatal diagnosis has several attributes that make such analyses challenging.[8,9] These features include trade-offs of the risks

---

[a] Department of Obstetrics and Gynecology, Oregon Health and Science University, L466,3181 SW Sam Jackson Park Road, Portland, OR 97239-3098, USA
[b] Decision and Economic Analysis in Reproduction and Women's Health Group, USA
[c] Department of Obstetrics and Gynecology, Massachusetts General Hospital, Harvard Medical School, Boston, MA, USA
[d] Division of Maternal-Fetal Medicine, Department of Obstetrics and Gynecology, Washington University, St Louis, MO, USA
* Corresponding author. Department of Obstetrics and Gynecology, Oregon Health and Science University, L466,3181 SW Sam Jackson Park Road, Portland, OR 97239-3098.
E-mail address: abcmd@berkeley.edu

Clin Lab Med 30 (2010) 629–642
doi:10.1016/j.cll.2010.04.007
0272-2712/10/$ – see front matter © 2010 Elsevier Inc. All rights reserved.

and benefits to the mother and fetus; redundancy of screening and diagnostic tests in the current pregnancy and in subsequent pregnancies; balancing short- and long-term outcomes; ethical issues regarding termination of pregnancy; and the incorporation of patient preferences, which can range widely for the possible outcomes. The following review discusses the different types of economic analyses commonly used in health care with a particular focus on the diagnosis of Down syndrome (DS).

ECONOMIC ANALYSES IN HEALTH CARE

The simplest economic analysis in health care takes into account only the costs. Such a cost analysis or cost-only analysis may be limited to just the direct costs of the provision of health care or may be expanded to incorporate the indirect costs of patients' travel time and lost work productivity. A *cost-benefit analysis* (CBA) assumes that the health outcomes from two or more strategies are essentially equal and makes a comparison between multiple programs or strategies on a purely financial level. In a CBA, all direct and indirect costs of health care are included as well as economic valuations of the outcomes. For example, if one of the possible outcomes is the loss of use of the lower extremities, this is converted into the costs of treatment (surgery, assisted living, wheelchair, and so forth) plus the lost productivity experienced by someone who no longer has the use of the lower extremities. In this purely financial analytic tool, only economic distinctions are made between the value to society and individuals having particular health outcomes.

The term *cost-effectiveness analysis* (CEA) is often used loosely to describe many types of economic analyses in health care. However, it specifically refers to an analysis in which costs and outcomes between two or more health care programs or strategies are compared. A cost-effectiveness ratio is composed of a numerator, which is the difference between the costs of two programs, and a denominator, which is the difference between the outcomes of two programs. The denominator in a CEA can be any of a variety of outcomes, including the commonly used years of life saved (life-years), number of diagnoses made, and number of cases prevented. Within a particular clinical arena, these may all be reasonable outcomes to compare. However, attempts to compare the outcomes from disparate procedures, such as routine dental care and cardiothoracic surgery, are more difficult, suffering from the apples-to-oranges problem. Comparing the cost-effectiveness of different programs is not particularly important if the new program is cheaper and leads to better outcomes (*a dominant strategy*), in which case the new program should be adopted. A careful comparison is also less important if the new program costs more and leads to worse outcomes (*a dominated strategy*). However, for new strategies that cost more and lead to better outcomes or cost less but lead to worse outcomes, CEA is a useful tool to evaluate differences between programs.

It is straightforward to make comparisons between programs in different clinical arenas using CBA. By converting all of the outcomes into financial ones, they become comparable. However, CBA is limited when considering outcomes that lead not to financial burdens but rather to burdensome morbidities. A way to compare such outcomes is by quality adjusting the value of one's life using utilities. *Utility* is the unit of value that some product or outcome, or in this case, health state, brings to an individual's life. It is the common valuation given to consumption of goods and services in economics and is defined as ranging from 0 (no utility or death) to 1 (perfect happiness). In CEAs, these valuations are defined as 0 for death and 1 for perfect health, with all other health states falling between these two. There is occasionally debate about whether there are certain health states that should be scored as worse than death, but most analyses use death as the bottom anchor of utilities, which is assigned the value 0. Once utilities are assigned to particular health states they can be multiplied by the time spent in that particular health state to generate *quality-adjusted life-years* (QALYs). When QALYs are used as the outcome measure in the denominator of a CEA, the analysis is considered a *cost-utility analysis* (CUA).

Estimation of utilities has been done in many ways, but the two most commonly used are the standard gamble and time trade-off metrics.[10] In the standard gamble, patients are asked what probability of death they would be willing to take to avoid a particular health outcome and live in perfect health.[11] For example, if an individual is willing to take a 5% chance of death to avoid losing their sight, then the sightless state has a utility of 0.95 (1.0–0.05). In the time trade-off, an individual is asked how many years of life they would give up to avoid a particular health outcome and live in perfect health.[12] Thus, if a 25 year-old individual has a life expectancy of 50 additional years and is willing to give up 5 years of life to avoid losing their sight, a valuation of 0.9 (1–5/50) would be the estimated utility. Methodologic concerns with these metrics include realism and avoidance of loss of life in a standard gamble and different valuations for different times of life in time trade-offs. Despite these problems, their estimation allows comparison between different clinical outcomes.

Given the importance of estimating the benefits from different interventions in health care, these economic analytic techniques can be quite useful. However, like any research approach, rigorous methodology is important to obtain robust estimates of the outcomes in these analyses. The US Public Health Service convened a panel in 1996 to establish strict criteria for the effective application of CEA.[13] These criteria have been used to analyze the methodologic quality of published CEAs in health care[14,15] and specifically in obstetrics and gynecology.[16,17] These criteria should be carefully considered when either performing or evaluating a CEA.

COST-EFFECTIVENESS ANALYSIS METHODOLOGY

Ten principles for CEA have been derived from guidelines established by the Panel on Cost-Effectiveness in Health and Medicine convened by the US Public Health Service.[13] These principles, summarized later with examples from prenatal diagnosis, comprise an appropriate minimum standard for performing and reporting CEAs (**Box 1**). In any CEA study, each principle should be explicitly addressed.

1. *Research question:* The research question must be clearly stated and appropriate for CEA. It must involve a comparison of at least two different health care programs or strategies resulting in different costs and health outcomes.
2. *Time frame:* The period of time over which costs and benefits are estimated should be long enough to capture future health outcomes and the economic impact of an intervention. In prenatal diagnosis, analyses will vary substantially in the short- and long-term when lifetime costs and outcomes are included.
3. *Perspective:* The viewpoint from which the analysis is conducted is called the perspective. Commonly used perspectives are societal, payer, and patient. If the intent of an analysis is to estimate the overall costs and benefits of a prenatal screening or diagnostic program, then the societal perspective should be used. However, the payer and patient perspectives can provide information regarding incentives and effectiveness that the societal viewpoint may miss.
4. *Analytic framework*: CEAs may be clinical studies or explicitly modeled with a decision tree, Markov chain, or Monte Carlo simulation. Because of the expense of prospective clinical studies, the latter two are more commonly used for CEA.

Box 1
Ten methodologic principles for cost-effectiveness analysis

Research question: interesting, novel, clearly stated

Time frame: incorporates all outcomes in reasonable fashion

Perspective: commonly societal, also payer or patient

Analytic framework: decision analytic, Markov, Monte Carlo, clinical trial

Probabilities: obtained from systematic reviews or clinical trials, feasible ranges

Costs: direct and indirect costs from studies, or adjusted charges or reimbursements

Outcome measure: life years saved, diagnoses made, quality adjusted life years (QALYs)

Incremental analysis: comparison between two programs, not average

Sensitivity analysis: variation of inputs over feasible ranges

Discounting: commonly exponential, 3% to 5%

Regardless, in either method, the specific intervention needs to be carefully described, possible courses of events identified, and specific outcomes described (eg, in prenatal diagnosis of DS these might include diagnoses made, termination of pregnancy, procedure-related miscarriage, or normal live birth as shown in **Fig. 1**).

5. *Probabilities:* In the modeling approaches, probabilities are abstracted from the existing literature for each event described in the analytic model. The most accurate point estimates and a reasonable range of probabilities for each event in the model should be included with documentation of sources.

6. *Costs:* Costs are identified and estimated for each of the interventions and outcomes in a CEA. The term *costs* refers to the actual resources used to provide

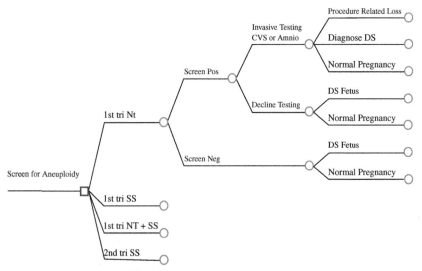

Fig. 1. Decision tree for noninvasive screens for DS. 1st tri NT, nuchal translucency, performed in first trimester; 1st tri SS, first trimester serum screen, PAPP-A + free beta; 1st tri NT + SS, combined screen regimen; 2nd SS, current second trimester serum screen used (MSAFP, unconjugated estriol, beta-hCG); DS, Down syndrome.

health care rather than what is charged or paid. However, resource allocation is not commonly available and in many cases charges or reimbursements are used. Cost estimates should include direct and indirect costs. In prenatal diagnosis examples of direct costs include the costs of screening tests; costs of performing diagnostic procedures, such as amniocentesis or chorionic villus sampling; and costs of performing diagnostic tests, such as karyotype or polymerase chain reaction. Indirect costs include patient travel costs and time spent undergoing screening, counseling, and diagnosis.

7. *Outcome measure:* Measures of effectiveness depend on the type and objectives of a particular analysis and should be expressed in the most appropriate natural units. In prenatal diagnosis, common outcomes used in these analyses are diagnoses made, cases averted, normal live births, and QALYs.

8. *Incremental analysis:* One common mistake in CEAs is the use and comparison of average cost-effectiveness ratios. There is a difference between comparing the costs divided by outcomes from two separate strategies and dividing the difference in costs by the difference in outcomes. It is important to make an incremental comparison in these analyses because this provides information regarding the marginal benefits obtained from marginal increases in cost.

(Costs1/Outcomes1) − (Costs2/Outcomes2) ≠ (Costs1 − Costs2)/(Outcomes1 − Outcomes2)
Average cost-effectiveness comparison   Incremental cost-effectiveness

9. *Sensitivity analysis:* Evaluation of the effects of uncertainty inherent in CEA requires the performance of sensitivity analysis. Data in the model are varied over plausible ranges and the cost-effectiveness ratio is recalculated. Sensitivity analysis demonstrates whether a conclusion is robust over a reasonable range of estimates. One-way analyses examine the cost-effectiveness ratio as one input varies. Two-way analyses vary two inputs simultaneously to evaluate changes in the cost-effectiveness ratio. Multiway analyses increase the number of inputs changed simultaneously and most commonly examine maximum and minimum effects to the cost-effectiveness ratio with variation in the inputs. Threshold analysis can be used to determine beyond what point in the range of an input a strategy remains cost-effective. A particularly rigorous sensitivity analysis is the Monte Carlo simulation, which incorporates the distributions of the different point estimates. The results of such a simulation give probabilities that a particular strategy will be cost-effective.

10. *Discounting:* Because the value of a given monetary value and time are decreased in future time periods over the current one, discounting is used to calculate the present value of money that will be spent and health states that will occur in the future. Exponential discounting is most commonly used. This method allows future costs and utilities to be discounted at rates of usually 3% to 5% per year.

COST-EFFECTIVENESS ANALYSIS OF THE PRENATAL DIAGNOSIS

CEAs of prenatal diagnosis have been performed for more than 30 years and have informed the development of guidelines surrounding particular screening and diagnostic strategies. The analyses have considered questions regarding screening and diagnosis of fetal aneuploidy; screening and diagnosis of single gene disorders, such as cystic fibrosis and hemoglobinopathies; and screening and diagnosis of congenital abnormalities, such as neural tube defects, congenital cardiac anomalies, and other fetal anomalies. The majority of these strategies have been deemed to be cost-effective. However, even the more recent analyses could be improved with careful consideration of several methodologic issues particular to prenatal diagnosis.

The benefits of prenatal screening and diagnosis include diagnosing a problem that can be treated prenatally (eg, fetal anemia in cases of alloimmunization); diagnosing a problem that can be treated postnatally (eg, cardiac anomalies); diagnosing severe genetic disorders, anomalies, and syndromes so that termination of pregnancy can be performed (eg, cystic fibrosis, renal agenesis, or DS); and reassurance of women and their partners that their fetus has either a low risk for or is without any of the more common diagnosable conditions (eg, reassuring nuchal translucency or normal karyotype). Unfortunately, how each of these benefits is accounted for in CEAs is inconsistent at best. For example, all of the studies in the literature examining the cost-effectiveness of screening for DS look specifically at the benefits to the woman undergoing prenatal diagnosis. None of the studies to date have included benefits to either her partner or her other children. When considering the benefits from screening for neural tube defects, the biggest financial gain is achieved by society when a diagnosed fetus is terminated.[18] However, with increased interest in fetal surgery programs, costs from diagnosis may actually be increased by screening for this anomaly. Although the largest economic gains in many of the strategies come from not having to treat a chronically physically or mentally challenged person, one recent study showed that the primary reason for the cost-effectiveness of amniocentesis was the reassurance gained by patients undergoing the test.[19]

Down Syndrome Screening and Diagnosis

Although amniocentesis and karyotype for fetal aneuploidy was described almost 40 years ago,[20] it is still not made widely available to all pregnant women.[21] Part of the justification for the National Institute of Child Health and Human Development (NICHD) guidelines limiting routine access to amniocentesis to women aged 35 and older[22] was a CBA of DS screening.[23] Unfortunately, this analysis simply compared costs of a program of receiving amniocentesis to not receiving amniocentesis and determined that beyond 35 years of age, amniocentesis was cost saving. As previously discussed, this is a much stricter threshold than is commonly used to determine whether an intervention is cost-effective. In fact, a recent CUA demonstrated that routinely offering amniocentesis to women of all ages was cost-effective when compared with using an age-35 threshold.[19]

Screening for DS is one of the most common topics for CEAs in prenatal diagnosis. One reason is the development of many different screening strategies beginning with maternal age followed by maternal serum alpha-fetoprotein (MSAFP); the triple screen, which adds estriol and beta human chorionic gonadotropin to MSAFP; and the quad screen, which adds inhibin A to the triple screen. More recently, a battery of first-trimester and either sequential or integrated screening tests have been developed and studied, including the nuchal translucency (NT), free beta hCG and pregnancy-associated plasma protein A (PAPP-A).[24,25] The vast majority of these CEAs demonstrate that screening for DS is cost-effective. In the first cost-utility analysis of DS screening, first-trimester screening was cost-effective when compared with second-trimester screening.[26] However, it may be that with an increasing number of screens, eventually the marginal gains of an improved screen will be too small to be justified on a cost-effective basis. However, it does not appear that threshold has been reached. Next, the authors review 4 of the more recent CEA studies of DS screening, all of which include first-trimester screening for DS.

ECONOMIC ANALYSES OF FIRST-TRIMESTER SCREENING FOR DOWN SYNDROME

In 2004, Biggio and coworkers compared the cost-effectiveness of 5 prenatal screening options for DS[25]:

1. Triple screen
2. Quad screen
3. Integrated (NT/PAPP-A/Free-beta hCG + Quad)
4. Sequential (NT/PAPP-A/Free-beta hCG, then Quad screen)
5. First trimester only (NT/PAPP-A/Free-beta hCG).

The analysis was limited to women younger than 35 years of age and was not from a societal perspective. The denominator or effectiveness was measured in DS cases diagnosed. Key probability and cost estimates are listed in **Box 2**. Importantly, spontaneous losses of DS pregnancies were accounted for in this analysis.

Clinical outcomes are shown in **Table 1**. All strategies were less costly and more effective than no screening; thus, screening for DS is economically justified. Sequential was the least costly strategy and integrated the most costly. The most effective

---

Box 2
Key probabilities and costs in cost-effectiveness analysis

Down syndrome prevalence at 10 weeks: 1 of 595

    Down syndrome loss rate at 10 to 14 weeks: 25%; at 15+ weeks: 23%

    Euploid loss rate at 10 to 14 weeks: 1%; at 15+ weeks: 1%

Acceptance of diagnostic test: 70%

Post amniocentesis loss: 0.9%

Post-CVS loss: 1.6%

Triple screen: 60% sensitivity; 95% specificity

Quad screen: 70% sensitivity; 95% specificity

First trimester: 80% sensitivity; 95% specificity

Integrated: 85% sensitivity; 99% specificity

Sequential: 95% sensitivity; 90% specificity

Triple/Quad: $59 to $76

First trimester: $130

Integrated: $206

Amniocentesis: $191

Chorionic villus sampling: $235

Counseling: $60

Karyotype: $384

Curettage: $375

Midtrimester termination: $2000

Lifetime Down syndrome cost: $677,000

Data from Biggio JR Jr, Morris TC, Owen J, et al. An outcomes analysis of five prenatal screening strategies for trisomy 21 in women younger than 35 years. Am J Obstet Gynecol 2004;190:721–9.

Strategy	Cost ($Millions)	T21 Live Births Averted	Euploid Losses	T21 Live Birth Averted/Euploid Loss
No screen	662	0	0	NA
Triple	497	366	311	1.3
Quad	472	427	311	1.5
First trimester	486	490	559	0.97
Integrated	521	520	62	9.3
Sequential	455	678	859	0.87

Table 1
Costs and outcomes in CEA

Abbreviations: NA, not applicable; T21, trisomy 21.
Data from Biggio JR Jr, Morris TC, Owen J, et al. An outcomes analysis of five prenatal screening strategies for trisomy 21 in women younger than 35 years. Am J Obstet Gynecol 2004;190:721–9.

strategy, in DS detection, was sequential screening, followed by integrated and first trimester. Sequential screening was associated with the highest number of procedure related losses, whereas integrated had the lowest number. DS births averted per procedure-related loss is another way to express the trade-off between efficacy and safety of DS screening.[27] A loss ratio more than 1.0 indicated that more DS births will be averted per loss, whereas a loss ratio less than 1.0 suggests that there will be more procedure-related losses than DS cases averted. From the Biggio analysis, the most favorable loss ratio was integrated (loss ratio = 9.3), followed by quad screen (loss ratio = 1.5) and triple screen (loss ratio = 1.3). Sequential screening had the least favorable loss ratio (loss ratio = 0.87).

Incremental analysis is a way to assess the cost for increased clinical benefit when comparing two strategies. This is employed when a more effective strategy is also more expensive, which is often the case. Several incremental comparisons from the Biggio and coworkers analysis are described next.

Quad Screen Versus Integrated Screen

A total of 93 additional DS live births will be averted if we move from quad screen to integrated screen, at a cost of $526,000 per additional DS averted, and 249 euploid losses would be prevented.

First Trimester Versus Integrated Screen

A total of 30 additional DS live births will be averted if we move from first trimester to integrated screen, at a cost of $1,200,000 per additional DS averted, and 497 euploid losses would be prevented.

It is difficult to judge which strategy is most favorable, because there is clearly a trade-off between efficacy, safety, and cost. The authors' interpretation of the Biggio study would include the following points. First, DS screening is economically justified compared with no screening. Second, the use of sequential screening may be questionable because of the extremely high number of procedure-related losses compared with other strategies.

Another analysis was published in 2005 by Odibo and colleagues.[28] This analysis included the following 8 screening strategies

1. No screening
2. NT only

3. First trimester combined screen (NT/PAPP-A/Free-beta hCG)
4. First trimester serum only (PAPP-A, Free-beta hCG)
5. Quad screen
6. Integrated screening (NT/PAPP-A/Free-beta hCG + quad)
7. Integrated serum screen (PAPP-A/Free-beta hCG + quad)
8. Sequential screening (NT/PAPP-A/Free-beta hCG → quad).

This analysis was from a societal perspective. Outcomes analyzed include number of DS cases detected and prevented by each strategy, procedure-related pregnancy losses, and costs. The estimates used were from a systematic review of the literature and the costs were based on Medicare charges from the United States when available (only direct medical costs are included). These probabilities and costs were similar, although not identical, to those used by Biggio and colleagues. All strategies are less costly than no screening, suggesting that DS screening is justified (**Table 2**). The model results confirmed that sequential screening averts the highest number of DS cases compared with the other strategies, corroborating the report by Biggio and colleagues. The price for this high detection rate is the highest rate of procedure-related losses. Most loss ratios were positive, although the most favorable loss ratios were achieved by integrated and integrated serum testing. The strategies with the most favorable trade-offs between cost, detection, and safety seem to be first trimester, integrated serum screening, and integrated. Several incremental analyses were also performed.

Quad Screen Versus Integrated Screen

A total of 1344 additional DS live births will be averted if we move from quad screen to integrated screen, at a cost of $270,000 per additional DS averted, and 2331 euploid losses would be prevented.

Integrated Serum Versus Integrated

A total of 504 additional DS live births will be averted if we move from integrated serum to integrated, at a cost of $607,000 per additional DS averted, and 55 euploid losses would be prevented.

Table 2
Cost-effectiveness of screening strategies for Down syndrome

Strategy	Cost ($Millions)	T21 Live Birth Averted	Euploid Losses	T21 Live Birth/ Euploid Loss
No screen	2382	0	0	—
NT	698	4620	1525	1.4
Quad	1024	3920	2855	3.0
First trimester	968	4920	1082	4.5
First trimester (serum)	739	3600	2088	1.7
Integrated serum	1248	4760	524	9.1
Integrated	1554	5264	579	9.1
Sequential	1715	5320	3767	1.4

Abbreviation: T21, trisomy 21.
Data from Odibo AO, Stamilio DM, Nelson DB, et al. A cost-effectiveness analysis of prenatal screening strategies for Down syndrome. Obstet Gynecol 2005;106:562–8.

The authors' interpretation of the analysis of Odibo and coworkers would support the following conclusions. First, screening for DS is economically justified. Second, first trimester, integrated, and integrated serum seem to be the most favorable strategies. There is only small incremental gain when comparing integrated serum to integrated testing.

COST EFFECTIVENESS OF CONTINGENT SCREENING

Although the studies by Biggio and colleagues and Odibo and colleagues represent an exhaustive exploration of the comparisons one can make between a wide range of screening regimens, neither considered contingent screening. Contingent screening operates under the assumption that one will use a 3-pronged approach in the first-trimester screening test: (1) positive screen: those women with a high risk (commonly 1 in 50) would proceed to invasive prenatal diagnosis; (2) negative screen: those with a very low risk (perhaps <1 in 1500 or <1 in 2000) would not obtain a second-trimester test, thus saving on the additional testing; and (3) intermediate screen: those women with a risk between these thresholds would go on to be screened in the second trimester.

In the first cost-effectiveness study to include contingent screening as a strategy, a cost-utility analysis by Ball and colleagues[29] based on clinical data from the First and Second Trimester Evaluation of Risk (FASTER) trial[30] found that contingent screening was a dominant strategy (**Table 3**). This analysis conducted incremental comparisons, analysis from the societal perspective, and used QALYs as its effectiveness measure.

An important component of the contingent screening protocol is the choice of the risk thresholds of low and high risk. A recent analysis by Gekas and colleagues[31] examined just that. Similar to the study by Ball and colleagues, they too found contingent screening to be a dominant strategy. Further, in their exploration of risk thresholds, using a cost-effectiveness ratio of dollars per additional cases of DS averted, they found that at a risk threshold of 1 in 58, the cost per additional DS case averted is $64,000, but it jumps to $260,000 per case averted at a risk threshold of 1 in 114

Table 3
Costs and cost-utility analysis of Down syndrome screening strategies

Screen Method	Costs in 2006 ($Millions)	Quality-Adjusted Life Years	Incremental Cost-Utility Ratio Versus Quad Screen
Triple screen	37.5	—	Dominated[a]
Quad	32.8	980,774	—
Combined first	35.2	980,777	$500,560/QALY
Integrated	34.5	980,820	$33,385/QALY
Serum integrated	33.6	980,790	$42,188/QALY
Stepwise sequential	34.4	980,823	$29,524/QALY
Contingent sequential	32.3	980,832	Dominant[b]

[a] Dominated = costs more with worse outcomes.
[b] Dominant = costs less with better outcomes.
Data from Ball RH, Caughey AB, Malone FD, et al. First- and second-trimester evaluation of risk for Down syndrome. Obstet Gynecol 2007;110:10–7.

(**Table 4**). In the end, as this is not a CUA, there are no particular defined levels of what should be considered a cost-effectiveness threshold, but this analysis points out that determining the optimal levels for contingent screening is a worthwhile endeavor.

METHODOLOGIC ISSUES AND CONCERNS

Although CEA is a useful tool in the evaluation of prenatal screening and diagnostic programs, there are several important methodologic issues that need to be emphasized. The first issue, which we see in 3 of the analyses previously mentioned, is the problem of a useful denominator. From a societal perspective, if we are to compare investment in various programs we have to have a comparable denominator. For better or worse, this is commonly life years or QALYs. However, this can be challenging in prenatal diagnosis where the outcomes do not affect maternal life expectancy and the valuation of utilities is limited. Fortunately, there have been several studies that evaluate maternal preferences toward DS by Kuppermann and colleagues.[32,33] Therefore, studies of prenatal diagnosis of DS benefit from including these values, as was done in the study by Ball and colleagues.

Another methodologic issue that arises is the use of cost-benefit analysis. Although a CBA can demonstrate whether a program will cost more than it will save, it cannot be used to assess whether a program is cost-effective. If the benefits in quality of life are worth the additional expenditures, the program may be cost-effective despite its expense. For example, one study of population-based fragile X screening demonstrated that it would not be cost-beneficial,[34] because the costs of such a program would be greater than savings from the reduced number of fragile X individuals in the population. However, from a cost-effectiveness standpoint, the best way to analyze this question is to determine whether the additional costs are worth the outcomes achieved. A recent cost-utility analysis demonstrated that such a screening program would be cost-effective when measures of patients' quality of life were included.[35] Further, even if a program is not cost-effective from a societal perspective, the screening test may be desirable to a subset of individuals based on their particular preferences. In this setting, at the very least, patients should be given information about such screening or diagnostic tests and be allowed to determine for themselves whether they wish to bear the costs and risks of such tests.

Table 4			
Costs and incremental cost-effectiveness analysis of varying the contingent high-risk screening threshold			
Contingent Screen First-Trimester Threshold	Costs ($Millions)	Down Syndrome Cases Averted	Incremental Cost Per Down Syndrome Cases Averted[a]
1 in 6	2.75	101.4	baseline
1 in 9	2.76	102.5	$9,091
1 in 30	2.86	106.5	$25,000
1 in 58	3.00	108.7	$63,636
1 in 114	3.26	109.7	$260,000
1 in 237	3.85	111.6	$310,526

[a] Calculated using values from **Table 3**.
Data from Gekas J, Gagné G, Bujold E, et al. Comparison of different strategies in prenatal screening for Down's syndrome: cost effectiveness analysis of computer simulation. BMJ 2009;338:b138.

The assumption regarding the termination of affected pregnancies is another key methodologic concern in prenatal diagnosis. Although many programs may be cost-effective based on the costs of affected fetuses being averted, if a large proportion of women decide to continue affected pregnancies, these costs may remain. Another important aspect of CEA in prenatal diagnosis is the reassurance gained by women with normal results, which should be accounted for in the outcomes analyzed. How this and other outcomes are valued by other members of the family should also be incorporated into analyses, although they have not been addressed in such analyses to date.

The majority of CEAs in prenatal diagnosis have been modeling studies. Although the insight gained from such analyses is important, before screening programs are made universal, clinical trials or prospective studies to assess the true costs and benefits should be performed. How patients use the information from prenatal screening and diagnosis may differ from the intended design, leading to different outcomes from those modeled. Similar to the differences between effectiveness and efficacy that are seen in clinical trials, different cost-effectiveness results may occur when a clinical evaluation of a screening program is performed. Thus, any new screening or diagnostic program bears close follow-up from its inception to determine what the true costs and outcomes are. As new programs are analyzed, economies of scale from volume effects and economies of scope from the redundancy of prenatal diagnostic and screening tests should be estimated as an aspect of these studies. With the recent programmatic change in the state of California and the introduction of a variety of screening strategies around the United States and other countries, prospective analysis of these programs is merited.

SUMMARY

It appears in several studies that first-trimester screening for DS is cost effective. In particular, contingent screening appears to be dominant as compared with other forms of screening. One aspect of contingent screening that should be considered closely is individualizing where the optimal thresholds of low and high risk may vary from person to person, which is easy to accommodate but requires patient counseling. From a societal perspective, the risk threshold at which contingent screening is optimized has not been fully characterized and deserves further research.

REFERENCES

1. Chernew ME, Hirth RA, Cutler DM. Increased spending on health care: how much can we afford? Health Aff 2003;22:15–25.
2. US Bureau of the Census. Statistical abstract of the United States. Washington, DC: Government Printing Office; 2009.
3. Heffler S, Smith S. Health spending projections for 2001–2011: the latest outlook. Health Aff 2002;21:207–18.
4. Kaplan E, Rodgers MA. The costs and benefits of a public option in health care reform: an economic analysis. Policy brief. Berkeley (CA): Berkeley Center on Health, Economics, and Security; 2009.
5. Weinstein MC, Stason WB. Foundations of cost-effectiveness analysis for health and medical practices. N Engl J Med 1979;296:716–21.
6. Eisenberg JM. Clinical economics: a guide to the economic analysis of clinical practices. JAMA 1989;262:2879–86.
7. Cutler DM, McClellan M. Is technological change in medicine worth it? Health Aff 2001;20:11–29.

8. Shackley P. Economic evaluation of prenatal diagnosis: a methodological review. Prenat Diagn 1996;16:389–95.
9. Caughey AB. Cost-effectiveness analysis of prenatal screening and diagnosis: methodologic issues. Gynecol Obstet Invest 2005;60:11–8.
10. Gold MR, Siegal JE, Russell LB, et al. Cost-effectiveness in health and medicine. New York: Oxford University Press; 1996.
11. Torrance GW. Measurement of health state utilities for economic appraisal. J Health Econ 1986;5:1–30.
12. Torrance GW, Thomas WH, Sacket DL. A utility maximization model for evaluation of health care programs. Health Serv Res 1972;7:118–33.
13. Weinstein MC, Siegel JE, Gold MR, et al. Russell LB for the panel on cost-effectiveness in health and medicine. Recommendations of the panel on cost-effectiveness in health and medicine. JAMA 1996;276(15):1253–8.
14. Detsky AS, Naglie IG. A clinician's guide to cost-effectiveness analysis. Ann Intern Med 1990;113:147–54.
15. Drummond MF, Jefferson TO. Guidelines for authors and peer reviewers of economic submissions to the BMJ. The BMJ Economic Evaluation Working Party. BMJ 1996;313:275–83.
16. Subak LL, Caughey AB, Washington AE. Cost-effectiveness analyses in obstetrics & gynecology. Evaluation of methodologic quality and trends. J Reprod Med 2002;47(8):631–9.
17. Smith WJ, Blackmore CC. Economic analyses in obstetrics and gynecology: a methodologic evaluation of the literature. Obstet Gynecol 1998;91(3):472–8.
18. Layde PM, von Allmen SD, Oakley GP Jr. Maternal serum alpha-fetoprotein screening: a cost-benefit analysis. Am J Public Health 1979;69:566–73.
19. Harris RA, Washington AE, Nease RF Jr, et al. Cost utility of prenatal diagnosis and the risk-based threshold. Lancet 2004;363:276–82.
20. Steele MW, Breg WR Jr. Chromosome analysis of human amniotic fluid cells. Lancet 1966;1(7434):383–5.
21. Kuppermann M, Goldberg JD, Nease RF Jr, et al. Who should be offered prenatal diagnosis? The 35-year-old question. Am J Public Health 1999;89:160–3.
22. National Institute of Child Health and Human Development. Antenatal diagnosis: report of a consensus development conference. Bethesda (MD): US Department of Health, Education and Welfare, Public Health Service, National Institutes of Health; 1979.
23. Hagard S, Carter FA. Preventing the birth of infants with Down's syndrome: a cost-benefit analysis. Br Med J 1976;1(6012):753–6.
24. Wapner R, Thom E, Simpson JL, et al. First-trimester screening for trisomies 21 and 18. N Engl J Med 2003;349:1405–13.
25. Biggio JR Jr, Morris TC, Owen J, et al. An outcomes analysis of five prenatal screening strategies for trisomy 21 in women younger than 35 years. Am J Obstet Gynecol 2004;190:721–9.
26. Caughey AB, Kuppermann M, Norton ME, et al. Nuchal translucency and first trimester biochemical markers for Down syndrome screening: a cost-effectiveness analysis. Am J Obstet Gynecol 2002;187:1239–45.
27. Caughey AB, Lyell DJ, Filly R, et al. The impact of the use of echogenic intracardiac focus as a screen for Down syndrome in women under the age of 35. Am J Obstet Gynecol 2001;85:1021–7.
28. Odibo AO, Stamilio DM, Nelson DB, et al. A cost-effectiveness analysis of prenatal screening strategies for Down syndrome. Obstet Gynecol 2005;106:562–8.

29. Ball RH, Caughey AB, Malone FD, et al. First- and second-trimester evaluation of risk for Down syndrome. Obstet Gynecol 2007;110:10–7.

30. Malone FD, Canick JA, Ball RH, et al. A comparison of first trimester screening, second trimester screening, and the combination of both for evaluation of risk for Down syndrome. N Engl J Med 2005;353:2001–11.

31. Gekas J, Gagné G, Bujold E, et al. Comparison of different strategies in prenatal screening for Down's syndrome: cost effectiveness analysis of computer simulation. BMJ 2009;338:b138.

32. Kuppermann M, Feeny D, Gates E, et al. Preferences of women facing a prenatal diagnostic choice: long-term outcomes matter most. Prenat Diagn 1999;19:711–6.

33. Kuppermann M, Nease RF, Learman LA, et al. Procedure-related miscarriages and Down syndrome affected births: implications for prenatal testing based on women's preferences. Obstet Gynecol 2000;96:511–6.

34. Vintzileos AM, Ananth CV, Fisher AJ, et al. Economic evaluation of prenatal carrier screening for fragile X syndrome. J Matern Fetal Med 1999;8:168–72.

35. Musci TJ, Caughey AB. Cost-effectiveness analysis of prenatal population-based fragile X carrier screening. Am J Obstet Gynecol 2004;189:S117.

Screening and Testing in Multiples

Mark I. Evans, MD[a,b,c,*], Stephanie Andriole, MS, CGC[b]

KEYWORDS
- Multiple pregnancy • Screening • Testing • Safety

MULTIPLE PREGNANCIES

In the past 30 years, treatment of infertility has gone from fundamentally little more than providing encouragement to highly sophisticated, pharmacologic, and surgical interventions allowing literally millions of couples to have their own children.[1] However, of all babies born following in vitro fertilization (IVF), more than half are part of multiple pregnancies. In the United States the twin pregnancy rate, commonly quoted for decades to be 1 in 90, has more than doubled to more than 1 in 40. About 65% of all twins in the United States emanate from infertility treatments. Furthermore, the rate of spontaneous monozygotic (MZ) twinning and as part of higher-order multiples has continued to increase with its associated dramatically increased risks of anomalies, loss, and prematurity.[1]

The increasing rate of multiple pregnancies associated with advanced maternal age has expanded the need for prenatal diagnosis in twins and higher-order gestations.[2] The same principles for diagnosis and screening in singleton pregnancies apply to multiples. However, there can be significant differences in the safety and efficacy of all approaches.[3] Furthermore, screening for aneuploidy in multiple gestations with the possibility of discordant karyotypes involves significant clinical, technical, and ethical issues:

1. Lower performance of serum screening protocols compared with singleton pregnancies[4]
2. The complexity of the invasive diagnostic procedures
3. The risk of loss of an unaffected twin caused by the sequelae of the invasive procedures.

Risks of Anomalies

It has long been recognized that the incidence of certain structural abnormalities such as neural tube defects and cardiac defects are more commonly seen in twin

[a] Fetal Medicine Foundation of America, New York, NY, USA
[b] Comprehensive Genetics, 131 East 65th Street, New York, NY 10065, USA
[c] Department of Obstetrics and Gynecology, Mount Sinai School of Medicine, 131 East 65th Street, New York, NY 10065, USA
* Corresponding author. Comprehensive Genetics, 131 East 65th Street, New York, NY 10065.
E-mail address: evans@compregen.com

Clin Lab Med 30 (2010) 643–654
doi:10.1016/j.cll.2010.05.005
0272-2712/10/$ – see front matter © 2010 Elsevier Inc. All rights reserved.

gestations than in singletons.[5] Chromosomal risks are the same per fetus, but given that there are 2 chances per dizygotic (DZ) pregnancy, the effective rate seems double (**Table 1**). MZ twins are especially prone to defects of laterality such as situs inversus, but they are identical for chromosomal or Mendelian disorders.

For DZ twins the risk of either twin being aneuploid is essentially an independent probability. For example, the risk of having a baby with a chromosome abnormality at maternal age 35 years is approximately 1 in 190. If there are 2 fetuses, the risk is essentially doubled (ie, 2 in 190 or 1 in 95). A 1 in 95 risk corresponds to the risk of a singleton for a 38-year-old woman. Similarly, the risk for a 30-year-old woman with a singleton is 1 in 380. With twins the risk is approximately 2 in 380 (ie, 1 in 190) which is the risk of a 35-year-old woman. Overall, the risk of at least 1 DZ twin having a serious problem is about 7%, but for an MZ twin, the number is about 10%. Monoamniotic twins have an even higher incidence of structural abnormalities than monochorionic (MC)/diamniotic (DA) fetuses.

Counseling

Counseling for prenatal diagnosis should include appreciation of the differences between screening and diagnosis, and the risks and benefits of each. For multiple pregnancies, most of which are conceived after long-standing infertility and treatment, patients' attitudes and choices regarding invasive prenatal diagnosis might differ from patients conceiving naturally.[6,7] Likewise, because of the high percentage of patients using donor eggs from women much younger than them, the difference between the numerically greater risk based on egg age and the patient's tolerance of risk are often at odds. Many patients in their 40s and 50s specifically state they would rather take the risk of diagnostic procedures even with a low abnormality incidence to avoid the chance of being in their 70s and having a child with special needs. This emphasizes the special issues in counseling such a selected population.

Evaluation of the risks of definitive diagnosis (eg, chorionic villus sampling [CVS] and amniocentesis) in twins have varied widely but are usually quoted as a risk of procedure-associated fetal loss of 0.5% to 2% for CVS and 0.3% to 1% for amniocentesis.[8–10] A recent meta-analysis showed no differences in risk between amniocentesis and CVS done by experienced operators.[11] Patients considering whether to have any invasive test in twin pregnancies would benefit from data comparing outcome of twins having CVS or amniocentesis with outcome of twin pregnancies without having any invasive diagnostic procedure (ie, natural history of twin pregnancies). Most of the studies conclude that the spontaneous total pregnancy loss rate is about 6% to 7%.[12] Patients considering which diagnostic test to have should be counseled regarding the specific risks (and benefits) of such procedures in twins (eg, the

Table 1
Incidence of chromosomal abnormalities in at least 1 fetus in a multifetal gestation

Maternal Age (Years)	Singleton	Twin	Triplet
20	1/526	1/263 (age 34)	1/175 (age 36)
25	1/476	1/238 (age 34)	1/150 (age 36)
30	1/385	1/192 (age 35)	1/128 (age 37)
35	1/192	1/96 (age 38)	1/64 (age 40)
40	1/66	1/33 (age 43)	1/22 (age 45)

Risk numbers in parentheses are comparable age for singletons.

risk of fetal loss after having CVS compared with amniocentesis, specifically in twin pregnancies). Moreover, as a result of sampling errors, the certainty of concordant or discordant results in each test should be addressed during counseling. The need for a second procedure because of placental mosaicism, inappropriate sampling and laboratory failures, or for selective fetocide should also be discussed. In our experience. in the most experienced of hands, the procedure risks are equal and therefore we strongly favor CVS for the privacy available and the lower risk of fetal reduction in appropriate circumstances.[3]

Documentation and Identification

The initial step before any diagnostic procedure in multifetal pregnancies is evaluation and documentation of the chorionicity, preferably at 10 to 12 weeks, followed by identification of each specific fetus and placenta (**Fig. 1**). Although chorionicity is best evaluated during the first trimester,[13] second trimester scanning can detect chorionicity with accuracy of 94% to 100%.[14] The location of both (or more) sacs, fetuses, placentas, cord insertions, and fetal genders should be evaluated and clearly documented using text and diagrams. Because any woman undergoing genetic amniocentesis or CVS is unfortunately a potential candidate for selective termination, incorrect documentation, sampling or labeling might bring about a disastrous termination of the wrong fetus.[3]

Aneuploidy Screening

Screening for genetic disorders in pregnancies has evolved over multiple decades.[15] Space does not permit a comprehensive approach here or even citing an appropriate number of references, but many aspects are covered in other chapters by Bahado-Singh and Argoti elsewhere in this issue and other publications. This article focuses on those issues specifically related to multiple pregnancies. Maternal carrier detection of Mendelian disorders is unaffected by multiple gestation, but those conditions (eg, aneuploidy) in which fetal status is key are subject to the uncertainty of determination of which fetus contributed what component to the observed value in the mother. Those assessments, such as nuchal translucency (NT), that are fetus specific are less likely to be influenced by the presence of multiples than those that depend on maternal serum blending of multiple fetal contributions.

Several investigators proposed the use of pseudo risks for Down syndrome from second trimester screening, recognizing that differentiation between 1 normal and 1 abnormal twin was problematic.[16,17] It was believed was that maternal serum levels

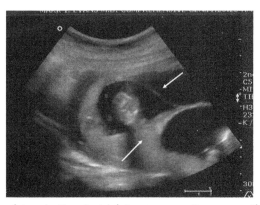

Fig. 1. Chorionicity determination in triplet pregnancy. Top arrow, thin monochorionic membrane; bottom arrow, thick lambda sign of dichorionic twins.

in a twin gestation should be essentially double that of singleton pregnancies. However, it was appreciated even in the 1980s and 1990s that that was not exactly the case for second trimester biochemical screening. Obrien and colleagues[18] showed in more than 4000 twins that α-fetoprotein levels were more than doubled, human chorionic gonadotropin (hCG) was slightly less than doubled, and estriol considerably less than doubled. Thus, using a mere doubling as expected would bias the data and be suboptimal. Furthermore, the well-appreciated ethnic and racial differences known for second trimester screening still need to be evaluated by ethnic group in multiples. The same questions regarding the usefulness of maternal serum values still remain in the first trimester.

NT measurements have also been used extensively in multiple pregnancies. The general conclusion is that in DZ twins and higher, there is effectively no influence of 1 fetus on the other. In MZ twins, which, by definition, are genetically the same, how to interpret differences in NT is problematic. The general consensus has been to use the largest value for communication to the patient.[19]

The interpretation of biochemistry in multiples is even more problematic for reasons exactly paralleling those in the second trimester, that is, what is the contribution of each fetus to the overall value? There is no clear answer to that question. Overall data suggest that screening efficiency is decreased at least 10% in twins and is essentially useless in triplets or higher. Furthermore, several studies suggest that the pattern of normal biochemistry in natural versus IVF pregnancies differs with assisted cases having higher free β-hCG and lower pregnancy-associated plasma protein A levels, thus building in an increased risk for Down syndrome when actuarial data do not show an increase.[19]

The tremendous growth of first trimester screening has had 2 conflicting effects on the preference for early prenatal diagnosis and its use. Many cytogenetic laboratories have noticed a 20% to 40% drop in karyotypes requested for prenatal diagnosis as more and more patients are relying on first and second trimester screening methods.[20] Although some centers have reported high detection rates with reduced use of invasive procedures, other reports have suggested that the net detection has not improved, and in fact in some cases even worsened.[20] A major caveat in the interpretation of much of the data is that several centers continually publish modeled expected outcomes that in many cases to not correlate with their actual published results, but then continue to use the modeled numbers in future publications.[21]

There is a large literature on the competing methods for determining genetic risks on which patients make decisions about whether to have definitive results by diagnostic tests or to rely on screening methods that provide odds adjustments only.[22] These have examined issues concerning the measurements, quality control, and statistical manipulation of NT measurements, and the interpretation of the laboratory results.[23] These issues are beyond the scope of this article but form an important aspect of the overall picture of risks and benefits of diagnostic procedures that cannot be completely separated from the procedure-specific results.

DIAGNOSTIC PROCEDURES
Amniocentesis

Amniocentesis has been the mainstay of diagnostic procedures since the late 1960s. Its use in twin pregnancies has been established for about 30 years,[24] but the exact methodology varies between centers. Furthermore, different views are held on specific issues such as using dye to mark the sampled sac and the need for 2 punctures in monochorionic (MC) pregnancies.

Three techniques have been described for amniocentesis in twins. The most common technique is the use of 2 different needles (usually 20- or 22-gauge spinal needles) inserted separately and sequentially into each amniotic cavity under ultrasound guidance. After the insertion of the first needle, about 2 mL are drawn into a small syringe to clear out any maternal cell contamination. Then 20 mL of fluid are aspirated for cytogenetic evaluation. We then reattach the discard syringe, draw back to fill about 5 mL, and then plunge the contents back into the uterine cavity. This produces a snowstorm of the debris already lying in the cavity (**Fig. 2**). The pattern outlines the cavity very nicely. The other sac is clear. A second needle is then inserted into 1 of the clear areas. In earlier years, some investigators advocated the use of Methylene Blue, but this is now considered contraindicated because of the associated risks of small bowel atresia, hemolytic anemia, and fetal death.[25] Indigo Carmine has been widely used and has not been related to any adverse effects.[26,27] Using the plunge technique, we believe that dye is essentially unnecessary with twins. In triplets or more, there are not enough data to be certain. Dye could be reserved for cases in which it is difficult to clearly demonstrate the septum (such as in amniotic fluid volume discordance).

Two other approaches have been used occasionally: using the same needle and going directly from 1 sac to the other, and using 2 needles simultaneously into both sacs. We have discussed these topics elsewhere, and these are relatively rarely used.[27]

Amniocentesis in monochorionic twins

MC pregnancies can be diagnosed with reasonably high specificity and sensitivity even in later stages of pregnancy. Such pregnancies are by definition monozygotic, and carry identical sets of chromosomes (and are referred to as identical twins). Therefore, to karyotype MC/DA pregnancies, generally only 1 sac needs be tapped. However, many case reports have described identical twins with discordant phenotype and karyotype. The causes of the phenotypic discordance are varied and include rare karyotypic differences, mosaicism, skewed X-inactivation, differential gene-imprinting, and

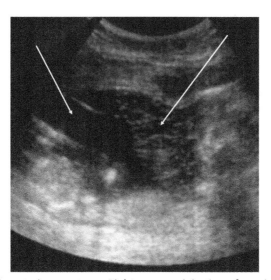

Fig. 2. Twin amniocentesis snowstorm. Right arrow, reinjection of amniotic fluid creating bubbles of debris; left arrow, clear side.

small scale mutation.[28] Cases of MC twins with discordant phenotype include mosaicism for Turner syndrome, Down syndrome, Patau syndrome, trisomy 1, and 22q11 deletion syndrome.[29] The exact prevalence of heterokaryotypic MZ pregnancies is unknown, but it is a rare phenomenon. Our opinion, and that of others,[30] is that if 1 or both of the fetuses has an ultrasound abnormality (or marker of aneuploidy), both sacs should be sampled, even if the twins are apparently MC. When chorionicity is certain, both fetuses do not have any anatomic abnormality, and fetal growth is not severely discordant, sampling a single amniotic sac is sufficient. Although the risk of a single puncture in twins should theoretically be lower than tapping both amniotic cavities, data regarding such a comparison in MC twins are limited.

Fetal loss rate

The natural history of twin pregnancies carries a pregnancy loss rate up to 24 weeks of about 6.3% and severe prematurity (24–28 weeks) rate of about 8%.[12] The data regarding the pregnancy loss rate after amniocentesis are comparable with these background loss rates.

Evans and Wapner[31] analyzed the literature and found a general consensus of amniocenteses risks of about 1/300 to 1/350 when done by experienced operators and much higher rates for occasional operators. Eddlemen and colleagues[32] from the FASTER consortium suggested a 1/1600 procedure risk, but there were multiple methodologic problems with their conclusions. Wapner and colleagues[33] reported that with proper design, their loss rates were actually close to the 1/300 figure. For example, the loss rate in Eddleman's high-risk unsampled group was 3.76%, whereas in the high-risk sampled group it was only 1.06%. No one actually believes that performing amniocentesis is protective. The same inverse ratio is seen with advanced maternal age in which the amniocentesis group had a lower loss rate than the control group. Alfirevic and Tabor[10] showed that had the original Tabor study[34] used the same loss classifications (only counting losses and deaths before 24 weeks) as the Eddleman study, then Tabor would have concluded a loss rate difference of 0.21%, which would have been statistically not significant.

CVS

Multiple studies over 25 years, including national and collaborative trials, have shown that CVS in singleton pregnancies is safe with an acceptable rate of fetal loss of about 0.5% to 3%.[8] The advantages of early prenatal diagnosis by CVS in twin pregnancies (providing rapid karyotyping, enzyme and DNA analysis) are similar to those related to singleton pregnancies; for example, early diagnosis allowing earlier termination of pregnancy, if indicated. However, in multifetal pregnancies, early diagnosis by CVS also facilitates early selective reduction of the affected fetus with fewer psychological and medical complications.[35,36]

Specific issues concerning CVS in multifetal pregnancies include (1) the methodology and safety of CVS in these pregnancies, (2) the sampling error rates for twins, and (3) issues concerning the effect of CVS on subsequent procedures (eg, selective termination).

The technique of CVS in multiple pregnancies is considerably more complicated than in singletons and should be done by experienced operators to ensure accurate mapping of the fetuses and placentas and correct ultrasound-guided placement of the instruments into each specific placenta (**Fig. 3**). It is crucial to evaluate and document the chorionicity (based on first trimester ultrasound using the lambda sign), location of the fetuses, their related placentas, and the location of the cord insertions. The description of the fetal and placental locations should be detailed in a manner that

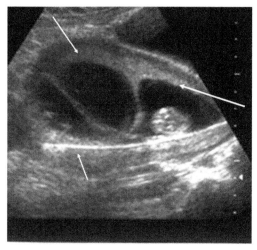

Fig. 3. Triplet CVS approach. Arrow at bottom shows catheter in posterior fundal placenta. Arrow at right shows path for catheter in low anterior placenta. Arrow at left shows path for needle to anterior fundal placenta.

allows proper identification of the affected fetus, especially when fetocide might be considered.

The contamination rate (of one sample with villi from the other fetus) reported in the literature is based usually on cases with incorrect gender determination or XX/XY mosaicism (which is later ruled out). With experience and careful methodology, the sampling error rates reported earlier[37] of about 4% to 5% have dropped down to almost none.[32] DNA fingerprinting can be used to determine zygocity when required in same sex twins with placental findings that are not conclusive.

CVS in multifetal pregnancies can be achieved by either a transabdominal or transcervical approach.[3] Operators must be facile with both approaches. Technique is even more critical in multiples, as the operator must make sure that a needle or catheter does not go through one placenta to reach another.

Fetal loss rate
The estimated risk of spontaneous abortion and fetal loss after CVS in singletons has varied widely over the years (0.5–4.3%). Early studies suggested that 2 or more samplings during 1 procedure might be associated with an increased risk of fetal loss.[38] The mean number of samplings per twin pregnancy reported in the literature ranges between 2.02 and 2.2 but some cases underwent up to 5 needle insertions.[37] However, those studies that have compared fetal loss rates in singletons and twins within the same institution found that CVS was not associated with an increased risk of either total pregnancy losses or single fetal losses.[39] Several papers have addressed the questions of procedure risks and reached different conclusions. Caughey and colleagues[40] from University of California San Francisco performed a retrospective cohort study of nearly 10,000 CVS and 30,000 amniocenteses with normal cytogenetic results in a 30-year period and documented lowered complication rates in both groups over time but a much greater decrease in CVS losses. When the data were adjusted for maternal age, indication for procedure, provider, year of procedure, gestational age at procedure, race, ethnicity, and parity, the ratio of losses for CVS to amniocentesis decreased from 4.23 based on a cohort from 1983 to 1987, to 1.03 based on a cohort from 1998 to 2003.

In the most experienced of hands, CVS on multiples is fundamentally no different than in singletons and no different than amniocentesis. Furthermore, because of the clear advantage of doing fetal reductions in the first trimester compared with the second, we believe CVS has clear advantages for patients who desire definitive answers.

In an attempt to coordinate the published data, Mujezinovic and Alfirevic[11] performed a meta-analysis of CVS and amniocentesis complications. They found 29 studies since 1995 that met their criteria for amniocentesis performed after 14 weeks and 16 studies for CVS (performed up to 13 weeks?). Pooled total pregnancy losses were classified as being (1) within 14 days of procedure, (2) before 24 weeks of gestation, or (3) total. For amniocentesis the results were 0.6%, 0.9%, and 1.9%. For CVS the corresponding rates were virtually identical at 0.7%, 1.3%, and 2.0% (**Table 2**). For all these studies, it needs to be remembered that the earlier gestational age at which CVS is performed translates into higher likely rates at all data points, because more destined-to-die cases will still be in the viable pool at the time of CVS that would be lost before amniocentesis.

From our experience, however, the transcervical procedure requires considerably more skill and experience for the operator to become competent, but for optimal outcomes, both procedures need to be in the armamentarium of the prenatal diagnostic center.

Multifetal Pregnancy Reduction

Multifetal pregnancy reduction (MFPR) has been used for more than 2 decades to improve the clinical outcome of high-order multiple pregnancies. In multiple collaborative publications from around the world, the most experienced centers have shown that with multiples, if success is defined as a healthy mother and a healthy family, fewer is always better. The specifics depend on the actual starting and finishing numbers (**Fig. 4**). Furthermore, recent data suggest that for the woman who starts with twins, using the same definition of success, it is safer to reduce to a singleton than keep the twins. The improvement is not as great as going down from quintuplets, but the improvement is real.

The selection process in experienced hands is hierarchical. In inexperienced hands, it is essentially empiric/technical criteria (such as fetal location). Some operators use sonographic screening either by NT measurement, presence of nasal bone, or complete anatomic survey (by transvaginal or transabdominal scanning).[1,36]

CVS AND MFPR

Our approach in most cases is to offer CVS before reduction. Typically we sample 1 more fetus than we are planning on keeping, that is, if we are keeping 2 we sample

Table 2 Loss rates after procedures		
	Meta-Analysis	
	Amniocentesis (%)	**CVS (%)**
14 days	0.6	0.7
24 weeks	0.9	1.0
Total	1.9	2.0

Data from Mujezinovic F, Alfirevic Z. Procedure related complications of amniocentesis and chorionic villus sampling. Obstet Gynecol 2007;110: 687–94.

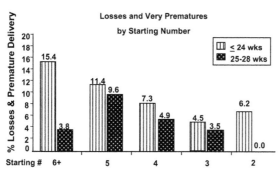

Fig. 4. Multifetal pregnancy reduction. (*Data from* Evans MI, Berkowitz R, Wapner R, et al. Multifetal pregnancy reduction (MFPR): improved outcomes with increased experience. Am J Obstet Gynecol 2001;184:97–103.)

all 3 triplets or 3 of 4 quadruplets. We then run a fluorescence in situ hybridization analysis overnight and use that data in the overall evaluation of which fetuses to preserve. We use the following hierarchy:

1. A documented abnormality
2. Suspicion and concern such as smaller crown-rump length or larger NT
3. Other technical factors of serious concern
4. If nothing else matters, then gender differences can be considered.

The last criteria is new, and was only added in the past several years when it became apparent that patients' wishes for gender information now no longer include the significant preference for male fetuses seen in earlier decades. For couples reducing to twins, the most common preference is for one of each gender.[1,36]

Several reports have shown that genetic analysis by CVS before selective early fetal reduction does not increase the risk of miscarriage or early delivery (compared with reduction without CVS). As expected, Brambati and colleagues[41] have shown that the preterm delivery rate was associated with the final number of fetuses; having CVS did not increase the risk of fetal losses (including perinatal losses) or early deliveries. Furthermore, in a review by Jenkins and Wapner,[42] the rate of miscarriage in a group that had CVS and fetal reduction (5.5% total pregnancy loss) was similar to a group that did not have CVS (5.6%).

SUMMARY

The choice of screening or diagnostic procedure in twin pregnancies depends on several factors but ultimately comes down to a personal choice of where the patient wishes to put her risk; that is, take a small risk of having a baby with a serious disorder versus a small risk of having a complication because she wishes to avoid that. The advantages in early diagnosis are clear.[9,37,38] In our experience how patients process information (framing) involves many factors, and there is no clear answer that applies to every patient.[43]

Given that the past 20 years have not settled the question of the true risks of amniocentesis and CVS or the differences between them, how such risks are interpreted has profound effects on the perceived value of invasive techniques, either leading to a decision to choose a screening test or go directly to CVS. There are profound practical, economic, and patent issues surrounding the data and the implications of the interpretation of the data. No one short review can possibly examine all of the issues exhaustively.

REFERENCES

1. Evans MI, Britt DW. Selective reduction in multifetal pregnancies In: Paul M, Grimes D, Stubblefield P. et al, editors. Management of unintended and abnormal pregnancy. London: Blackwell-Wiley; 2009. p. 312–8.
2. Russell RB, Petrini JR, Damus K, et al. The changing epidemiology of multiple births in the United States. Obstet Gynecol 2003;101:129–35.
3. Evans MI, Yaron Y, Wapner RJ. CVS. In: Evans MI, Johnson MP, Yaron Y, et al, editors. Prenatal diagnosis: genetics, reproductive risks, testing, and management. New York: McGraw-Hill; 2006. p. 433–42.
4. Spencer K, Nicolaides KH. Screening for trisomy 21 in twins using first trimester ultrasound and maternal serum biochemistry in a one-stop clinic: a review of three years experience. BJOG 2003;110:276–80.
5. Luke B. Monozygotic twinning as a congenital defect and congenital defects in monozygotic twins. Fetal Diagn Ther 1990;5(2):61–9.
6. Holmes A, Jauniaux E. Prospective study of parental choice for aneuploidy screening in assisted conception versus spontaneously conceived twins. Reprod Biomed Online 2004;8(2):243–5.
7. Geipel A, Berg C, Katalinic A, et al. Different preferences for prenatal diagnosis in pregnancies following assisted reproduction versus spontaneous conception. Reprod Biomed Online 2004;8:119–24.
8. Brambati B, Tului L, Alberti E. Prenatal diagnosis by chorionic villus sampling. Eur J Obstet Gynecol Reprod Biol 1996;65:11–6.
9. Alfirevic Z, Sundberg K, Brigham S. Amniocentesis and chorionic villus sampling for prenatal diagnosis. Cochrane Database Syst Rev 2003;3:CD003252.
10. Alfirevic Z, Tabor A. Pregnancy loss rates after midtrimester amniocentesis. Obstet Gynecol 2007;109:1203–4.
11. Mujezinovic F, Alfirevic Z. Procedure related complications of amniocentesis and chorionic villus sampling. Obstet Gynecol 2007;110:687–94.
12. Yaron Y, Bryant-Greenwood PK, Dave N, et al. Multifetal pregnancy reductions of triplets to twins: comparison with nonreduced triplets and twins. Am J Obstet Gynecol 1999;180:1268–71.
13. Sepulveda W, Sebire NJ, Hughes K, et al. The lambda sign at 10–14 weeks of gestation as a predictor of chorionicity in twin pregnancies. Ultrasound Obstet Gynecol 1996;7:421–3.
14. Vayssiere CF, Heim N, Camus EP, et al. Determination of chorionicity in twin gestations by high-frequency abdominal ultrasonography: counting the layers of the dividing membrane. Am J Obstet Gynecol 1996;175:1529–33.
15. Evans MI, Galen RS, Drugan A. Biochemical screening. In: Evans MI, Johnson MP, Yaron Y, et al, editors. Prenatal diagnosis: genetics, reproductive risks, testing, and management. New York: McGraw-Hill; 2006. p. 277–88.
16. Wald NJ, Rish S, Hackshaw AK. Combining nuchal translucency and maternal serum markers in prenatal screening for Down Syndrome in twin pregnancies. Prenat Diagn 2000;23:588–92.
17. Sebire NJ, Snijders RJM, Hughes K, et al. Screening for Trisomy 21 in twin pregnancies by maternal age and fetal nuchal translucency thickness at 10–14 weeks of gestation. Br J Obstet Gynaecol 1996;103:999–1003.

18. Obrien JE, Dvorin E, Yaron Y, et al. Differential increases in AFP, hCG, and uE3 in twin pregnancies: impact on attempts to quantify Down Syndrome screening calculations. Am J Med Genet 1997;73:109–12.
19. Cleary-Goldman J, Berkowitz RL. First trimester screening for Down Syndrome in multiple pregnancy. Semin Perinatol 2005;29:395–400.
20. Henry GP, Britt DW, Evans MI. Screening advances and diagnostic choice: the problem of residual risk. Fetal Diagn Ther 2008;23:308–15.
21. Wald NJ, Rodeck C, Hackshaw AK, et al. SURUSS in perspective. Br J Obstet Gynaecol 2004;111:521–31.
22. Gonce A, Borrell A, Fortuny A, et al. First trimester screening for trisomy 21 in twin pregnancy: does the addition of biochemistry make an improvement? Prenat Diagn 2005;25:1156–61.
23. Evans MI, Van Decruyes H, Nicolaides KH. Nuchal translucency (NT) measurements for 1st trimester screening: the "price" of inaccuracy. Fetal Diagn Ther 2007;22:401–4.
24. Bang J, Nielsen H, Philip J. Prenatal karyotyping of twins by ultrasonically guided amniocentesis. Am J Obstet Gynecol 1975;123:695–6.
25. Nicolini U, Monni G. Intestinal obstruction in babies exposed in utero to methylene blue. Lancet 1990;336:1258–9.
26. Cragan JD, Martin ML, Khoury MJ, et al. Dye use during amniocentesis and birth defects. Lancet 1993;341:1352.
27. Jeanty P, Shah D, Roussis P. Single-needle insertion in twin amniocentesis. J Ultrasound Med 1990;9:511–7.
28. Machin GA. Some causes of genotypic and phenotypic discordance in monozygotic twin pairs. Am J Med Genet 1996;61:216–28.
29. Evans MI, Rodeck CH, Johnson MP, et al. Selective termination in Evans MI. In: Johnson MP, Yaron Y, Drugan A, editors. Prenatal diagnosis: genetics, reproductive risks, testing, and management. New York: McGraw-Hill; 2006. p. 571–8.
30. Nieuwint A, Zalen-Sprock R, Hummel P, et al. 'Identical' twins with discordant karyotypes. Prenat Diagn 1999;19:72–6.
31. Evans MI, Wapner RJ. Invasive prenatal diagnostic procedures 2005. In: Reddy U, Mennuti MT, editors. Seminars in perinatology, 29. Elsevier; 2005. p. 215–8.
32. Eddleman KA, Malone FD, Sullivan L, et al. Pregnancy loss rates after midtrimester amniocentesis. Obstet Gynecol 2006;108(5):1067–72.
33. Wapner RJ, Evans MI, Platt LD. Pregnancy loss rates after midtrimester amniocentesis. Obstet Gynecol 2007;109:780.
34. Tabor A, Philip J, Madsen M, et al. Randomised controlled trial of genetic amniocentesis in 4606 low-risk women. Lancet 1986;1:1287–93.
35. De Catte L, Foulon W. Obstetric outcome after fetal reduction to singleton pregnancies. Prenat Diagn 2002;22:206–10.
36. Evans MI, Kaufman M, Urban AJ, et al. Fetal reduction from twins to a singleton: a reasonable consideration. Obstet Gynecol 2004;104:102–9.
37. Wapner RJ, Johnson A, Davis G, et al. Prenatal diagnosis in twin gestations: a comparison between second-trimester amniocentesis and first-trimester chorionic villus sampling. Obstet Gynecol 1993;82:49–56.
38. Rhoads GG, Jackson LG, Schlesselman SE, et al. The safety and efficacy of chorionic villus sampling for early prenatal diagnosis of cytogenetic abnormalities. N Engl J Med 1989;320:609–17.
39. Brambati B, Tului L, Guercilena S, et al. Outcome of first-trimester chorionic villus sampling for genetic investigation in multiple pregnancy. Ultrasound Obstet Gynecol 2001;17:209–16.

40. Caughey AB, Hopkins LM, Norton ME. Chorionic villus sampling compared with amniocentesis and the difference in the rate of pregnancy loss. Obstet Gynecol 2006;108:612–6.
41. Brambati B, Tului L, Baldi M, et al. Genetic analysis prior to selective fetal reduction in multiple pregnancy: technical aspects and clinical outcome. Humanit Rep 1995;10:818–25.
42. Jenkins TM, Wapner RJ. The challenge of prenatal diagnosis in twin pregnancies. Curr Opin Obstet Gynecol 2000;12:87–92.
43. Britt DW, Evans MI. Sometimes doing the right thing sucks: frame combinations and multifetal pregnancy reduction decision difficulty. Soc Sci Med 2007;65: 2342–56.

Noninvasive Prenatal Diagnosis: 2010

Mark I. Evans, MD[a,b,c,]*, Michael Kilpatrick, PhD[d]

KEYWORDS

- Noninvasive prenatal diagnosis • Cell-free fetal DNA/RNA
- Fetal cells

For more than 40 years, definitive prenatal diagnosis of chromosome and mendelian disorders has been possible and widely available, but it has been done only by obtaining fetal cells through invasive diagnostic procedures.[1,2] Because such procedures carry associated risks for miscarriage, are expensive, and require labor intensive care and sophisticated technology, they cannot be realistically offered to all patients.[3] For more than 20 years, a maternal age of 35 years at delivery has been the medicolegal standard in the United States for offering invasive tests. Screening tests, such as maternal serum screening and ultrasound, can alter odds but are not diagnostic.[3] The authors Bahado-Singh and Argoti describe these issues extensively in another chapter,[4] and they are not be repeated here.

Looking for fetal cells and now nucleic acids has been the holy grail of prenatal diagnosis for more than a century.[5] The first approach that has occupied much of the past 30 years has centered on the search for fetal cells in the maternal circulation.[6–8] Over the past decade a second front has been added to the attack and has focused first on free-fetal DNA and then free-fetal RNA in the mother's circulation.[9,10] The cell-free approaches have made considerable progress. However, the recent fiasco with data irregularities and the unprofessional marketing attempts by Sequenom to push the technology before there were any refereed publications using their data has probably set back the field considerably. The alleged fraud has brought taint to the genuine investigators in the field, and there will be continuing damage that will occur as the jurisprudence from the Securities and Exchange Commission and possibly other legal authorities will be headline news across the globe.

The use of noninvasive diagnostics has potential far beyond aneuploidy; in fact its use for Rhesus disease is already commonplace in Europe.[11] Its use allows for women who are Rh negative to assess whether their fetus is Rh negative and potentially avoid

[a] Fetal Medicine Foundation of America, New York, NY, USA
[b] Comprehensive Genetics, 131 East 65th Street, New York, NY 10065, USA
[c] Department of Obstetrics and Gynecology, Mount Sinai School of Medicine, 131 East 65th Street, New York, NY 10065, USA
[d] Ikonisys Inc, 5 Science Park, New Haven, CT 06511, USA
* Corresponding author. Comprehensive Genetics, 131 East 65th Street, New York, NY 10065.
E-mail address: evans@compregen.com

Clin Lab Med 30 (2010) 655–665
doi:10.1016/j.cll.2010.04.011
0272-2712/10/$ – see front matter © 2010 Elsevier Inc. All rights reserved.

the use of RhoGAM to avoid sensitization. For sensitized women, a decision could also be made about continuation of the pregnancy in situations when prior bad outcomes would predispose to a high likelihood of hemolytic anemia.

FETAL CELLS

The presence of fetal cells in maternal circulation was initially described more than a century ago, but attempts to use fetal cells as a diagnostic or screening test to date have been very frustrating.[5,8] The number of fetal cells found in maternal blood is extremely low, speculated at perhaps 1 part per 10 million.[6] In 20 mL of maternal blood there may be no more than 20 fetal cells so that isolation, purification, and enhancement methods need to be nearly perfect to find and reliably analyze these cells. Even slight handling losses can render the technique nearly or completely useless, and conversely imperfections in techniques can produce high proportions of false-positive cases by reading maternal cells as fetal. It is well appreciated in the screening literature that in situations in which rare-event detection is required, even a great screening test will have a high proportion of false positive cases.[12]

The considerable difficulty in separating signal to noise of fetal cells from maternal ones has been a function of many factors, including ignorance of the total number and type of fetal cells, the timing of their appearance, the possibility of detecting them in all pregnancies, and the best approach for their enrichment and analysis.[8] For example, the 2002 National Institute of Child Health and Human Development (NICHD)-sponsored NIH Fetal Cell Study (NIFTY) trial was only able to detect the correct fetal gender or aneuploidy in less than 50% of cases.[5] There were many important contributions from NIFTY and many lessons were learned that will be important to the ultimate success of the concept. However, the overall conclusion from NIFTY was that the technology was not yet ready for a clinical trial. There were far too many variables that needed to be standardized within and across the centers involved before a real clinical trial could have been feasible. Furthermore, it appeared as if the available fluorescence in situ hybridization (FISH) probes could not easily penetrate and stain the fetal cells that were isolated.[13]

Since the end of the NIFTY trial, the NICHD has taken a step back and encouraged the private sector to develop the technology. Several companies have jumped into the fray. There have been several recent publications with the differing groups focusing on slightly different areas of expertise. The rarity of the cells being sought would appear to lend itself to an automated approach to sample analysis.[14] One such approach, automated fluorescence microscopy, has been taken to improve the detection and analysis of fetal cells based on immunohistochemical and molecular markers (**Fig. 1**). Using this system, Seppo and colleagues[15] showed rapid and reliable detection of apparently fetal cells on slides of maternal blood. Huang used a microfluidic filtration device to separate erythrocytes from other nucleated cells in maternal blood samples (**Fig. 2**).[16] The next step still needs to be optimized (ie, the definitive identification of fetal cells). There have been suggestions that laser capture microdissection methodologies might be useful, but there are too few data to reach any conclusions.[17]

ENDOCERVICAL FETAL TROPHOBLASTS

Although most approaches to noninvasive prenatal diagnosis have centered on maternal peripheral blood as a source of fetal material, other potential sources of cells have been suggested. An attractive alternative to peripheral blood is isolation and analysis of transcervical trophoblasts. Unlike maternal blood in which the fetal cells consist of multiple circulating fetal-cell types, fetal cells in the cervix are

Fig. 1. Automated scanning of slides to find candidate cells.

all of placental origin and probably overwhelmingly trophoblasts. Thus, fetal-cell recovery has the potential to be more amenable to unique markers that distinguish fetal from surrounding maternal cells. Noninvasive recovery of endocervical fetal trophoblasts during early pregnancy could permit definitive prenatal genetic testing (**Fig. 3**). Several studies support the potential of this approach.[18,19] Although the optimal endocervical sampling procedure may have yet to be determined, fetal-cell detection rates from 60% to more than 80% of cases have been reported.[20,21] Millions of pregnant women have undergone some type of cervical sampling while pregnant and several studies have shown no increase in adverse pregnancy events following endocervical sampling.[21–24] Fetal cells obtained by such an approach are amenable to analysis by immunohistochemical and molecular techniques, making the approach suitable for the various analytical methods described in this review. The fetal-cell story is not dead.

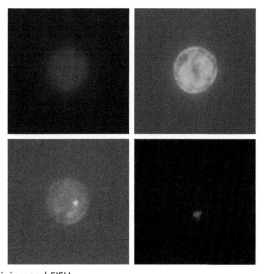

Fig. 2. Immunostaining and FISH.

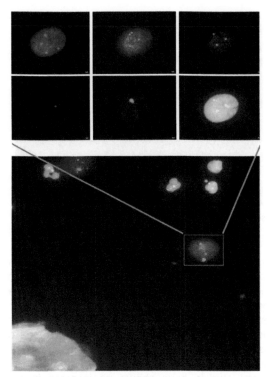

Fig. 3. Fetal cell recovery from endocervical canal.

FREE-FETAL DNA AND RNA

In 1997 Lo and colleagues[25] published and patented the concept that, instead of looking for intact fetal cells that leaked through to the maternal circulation, break down free-fetal DNA and other nucleotides that might be a better source of fetal material to study. They suggested that the concentration of cell-free fetal DNA (cff DNA) was perhaps a 100-fold to 1000-fold higher and have suggested that the proportion might be between 3% and 6%.[9] Nevertheless, the amount of cff DNA is still a small percentage of the circulating DNA, and proper identification is crucial.

Most investigators have focused on the fact that fetal fragments tend to be of shorter length than maternal fragments, averaging only about 300 versus more than 500 base pairs for maternal fragments.[26,27] The difference has been attributed to differential mechanisms of apoptosis between syncytiotrophoblasts and maternal physiology. Unfortunately, there is no current laboratory methodology for the efficient detection of these size differences.

Epigenetic mechanisms have also been proposed to differentiate between fetal and maternal cff DNA.[28] Following basic work, Chim and colleagues[29] investigated markers on Chromosome 21 that might be amenable to epigenetic differences and found 19 markers that are differentially methylated between maternal and fetal tissues. Unfortunately, it is unlikely that epigenetic methods will be useful because the chemical steps needed to use them are traumatic and can destroy much of the materials being interrogated.

RNA–SINGLE-NUCLEOTIDE POLYMORPHISM ALLELIC RATIOS

In an effort to overcome the similarity between fetal and maternal DNA and the minor increases in concentration of DNA in maternal plasma from the fetus, the strategy of searching for RNA from placental specific alleles emerged. Thus, instead of perhaps a 3% to 6% increase in DNA, there should be a 2:1 ratio of any gene on a trisomic chromosome 21 in comparison to a euploid control, such as chromosome 12 (**Fig. 4**). Tsui and colleagues developed a systematic microarray approach for identification of placental mRNA in maternal plasma. In 2007, the placenta specific 4 (PLAC 4) gene was identified forming the basis for the thought that noninvasive diagnosis using RNA might be practical.[10]

Data presented at investor meetings (as opposed to peer-reviewed scientific literature) by senior scientists at Sequenom, Inc. generated enormous interest among physicians and investors. Some of these investor meetings were held concurrently with major scientific meetings, such as the International Society for Prenatal Diagnosis and Society for Maternal Fetal Medicine, but had no affiliation with the actual scientific meeting. Press releases and coverage failed to make the distinction and, likely as a direct consequence, the stock price of Sequenom skyrocketed more than 1000%.

In January 2009, the company announced plans to launch the technology commercially in 6 months before any of the clinical trials they were discussing would be

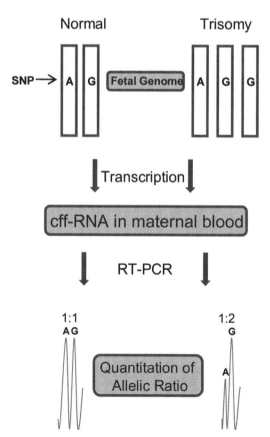

Fig. 4. RNA ratio can be 2:1.

anywhere near completion or any substantive data actually published in the medical literature. At public professional forums and meetings, such as the Society for Maternal Fetal Medicine and American College of Medical Genetics, several well-informed critics argued that the stability of RNA was such that a national transport system of specimens to 1 or 2 laboratories was likely to be impractical and that launching a clinical fee for service test was very premature. The leaders of the company declined to show actual data to support claims that their system worked satisfactorily. To process specimens on a commercial basis, the specimens need an intermediary fixation step within hours of blood collection such that even routine overnight shipment to a centralized laboratory becomes problematic.

It was the attempted use of the RNA method by Sequenom that lead to serious concerns about the science and the marketing. Papers by Lo suggested a 90% sensitivity for a 96.5% specificity.[10,30] If those numbers held up on large series of subjects, the technique would be competitive against existing screening methodologies.[4] However, the claims by the company of a 100% sensitivity for a 99% specificity were unbelievable to many observers. Multiple warning flags were raised when the company did not have any significant refereed publications and was rushing to the market place before appropriate trials were even initiated let alone finished.

Ultimately, it appears that there was malfeasance in the process, which was first acknowledged by the company in April 2009. The Securities and Exchange Commission has initiated action against Sequenom and there are multiple class action lawsuits already filed and criminal indictments initiated.[31] There is now a completely new leadership for Sequenom that is trying to rebuild the image and assets of the company.

DIGITAL POLYMERASE CHAIN REACTION

The development of microfluidic chambers, with literally thousands of reaction chambers, has made the technique of digital polymerase chain reaction (PCR) one of intense investigation.[30,32–34] The technique is appealing for its ability to discern small differences in concentrations at low levels of targets. For aneuploidy, it is dependent upon the absolute differences in overall DNA concentrations between the normal and abnormal chromosomes and what percentage of the analyzed material is the target material (fetal) versus the background of maternal. For example, if one assumes that the cff DNA represents 5% of the overall concentration of DNA in the maternal circulation, then the technique requires the ability to differentiate a 5% difference in normal pregnancy and a 10% difference in a trisomic pregnancy (**Fig. 5**). Clinical issues, such as mosaicism, coefficient of variation of the measured findings, and other confounders, are yet to be determined.

MULTIPLE PARALLEL GENOMIC SEQUENCING

Multiple parallel genomic sequencing, otherwise called shot-gun sequencing, is a method developed by Solexa that was later bought by Illumina in which short tags across the genome are amplified and sequenced.[35] Fan and colleagues[36] demonstrated more than 10 million 25 base-pair sequences with about 65,000 tags for chromosome 21. They then subjected these to digital PCR for identification with a high sensitivity on a limited number of cases. The method has major theoretical advantages over others in that multiple chromosomes can be assayed simultaneously, and the technology appears to be robust. However, the technique is currently not practical because the machinery costs approximately $700,000, the reagents are approximately $700 per case, and throughput is approximately 10 cases per week. However,

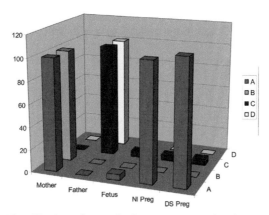

Fig. 5. Digital PCR identification of aneuploidy. Assume 100 of each parental allele: Mother A and B, Father B and C. Assume fetus contributes 5 of its alleles in maternal circulation: Fetus is A and C. Maternal levels in normal pregnancy: A, 105; B, 100; C, 5; D, 0. Down syndrome pregnancy with second meiotic division nondisjunction: A, 110; B, 100; C, 5; D, 0.

it is likely that methodological improvements may make such sequencing part of the armamentarium.[37]

RH DISEASE AND OTHER MENDELIAN DISORDERS

The one clinical use of cff DNA already in widespread use in much of Europe is the identification of fetal Rh status in women who are Rh negative.[11] As such, the use of RhoGAM can be avoided in a large number of women. The methods for the Rh gene determination have varied tremendously around the globe.[38] The available technology in the United States until recently had a 14% inconclusive rate, which is far too high of a false-negative rate rendering it unusable.[11] More recently, a reverse transcriptase PCR has become available with the suggestion of much greater accuracy. A meta-analysis in 2006 suggested 97% accuracy, which is still too low for reliability but moving in the correct direction.[39] It seems likely that an accurate assessment of Rh status will replace routine use of RhoGAM and amniocentesis to determine actual fetal Rh status in high-risk situations.

Logic dictates that the identification of single gene disorders, if anything, should be easier than aneuploidy. Extensive experience with preimplantation diagnosis has shown the same principle (ie, that single genes are more reliable than chromosomes, but that all these methodologies have a nonzero error rate). It is far too early to speculate on which disorders are likely to go on line first other than that single mutation, single genes (eg, sickle cell) are far more likely to be successful than disorders with multiple mutations (eg, cystic fibrosis) or with nontraditional inheritance (eg, fragile X).[40,41]

FETAL GENDER DETERMINATION

The identification of fetal gender from either fetal cells or cff DNA or RNA is straight forward.[42] In some cultures, in which there is still a profound difference in the perceived value of female versus male offspring, a market exists for gender determination early in pregnancy. Some of these companies have come and gone and there have been lawsuits filed against claims of 100% accuracy that proved to be wrong. Recently appropriately rigorous publications have begun to emerge. Scheffer and colleagues[42] in 2010 used real-time PCR to study the SRY gene and multicopy DYS14 marker sequence and required to be considered a test-positive male. Females were diagnosed by 24 biallelic insertion/deletion polymorphisms or paternally inherited blood group antigens confirming fetal DNA. They reported on 201 women with a median gestational age of 9 weeks for whom a test result was determined in 94%. Of those subjects for whom a test was completed and outcome available, the authors reported a 100% sensitivity and specificity. They concluded that this approach is a "clinical reality," and "there is no longer a need for invasive procedures to determine fetal sex."[42] They may be scientifically correct, but such a conclusion seems premature, however, given the single center and the unfortunate history of similar claims that were false . Societal problems will arise over this issue given the differential status of gender in certain parts of the world, the potential for misuse of the technology, and the potential for some couples to forego more extensive, true genetic analysis and missing serious disorders that would be diagnosable by more traditional methods.

SUMMARY

Accurate segregation of fetal cells from maternal cells or identification of cff DNA or RNA is critical to the development of fetal cells as a screening or diagnostic prenatal technique. The large number of approaches that have been used is testimony to the fact that none of them have been particularly successful.

The search for fetal cells in maternal blood has been the object of unrelenting investigation during the past decades of prenatal diagnosis. Everyone knows they are there. Although there is general agreement that fetal cells are present in the maternal circulation, proving such and getting them to be useful and reliable for prenatal diagnosis has been frustrating.[5,35] In contrast, far more progress has been made for invasive procedures, such as chorionic villus sampling, amniocentesis, and fetal blood and tissue sampling.[2] However, all carry some associated procedural risks and are expensive. Therefore, such services, even those that have been available for more than 30 years, have never been used by more than 5% to 10% of the population. Furthermore, there have been considerable differences in use around the country and world because of differences in religions and ethnic groups, and with how much difficulty the pregnancy was achieved.[43] For most patients, there is a question of balance that needs resolution between the degree of risk for an underlying problem, their motivation not to have a child with serious medical issues, and the risks they are willing to take to get an answer. Ultrasound has improved by orders of magnitude and can be useful for the diagnosis of structural abnormalities.[44] Ultrasound can be a screen for aneuploidy but its sensitivity and specificity have varied enormously from study to study.[45–47] Ultrasound is, however, not a substitute for karyotype or molecular answers in most cases. Several papers have reported on the limitations of just looking.[47]

The psychosocial arm of the NIFTY trial showed that if a noninvasive, accurate screen for aneuploidy were available, it would be highly desired and used.[48] Ideally, such a test would be noninvasive (ie, have no risk, have perfect sensitivity and specificity, and be inexpensive). Such a test does not exist, and likely will not exist anytime soon, if ever. Fetal cells, even when isolated, cannot be reliably cultured and karyotyped. Therefore, fetal cells can only be a screening test and not completely replace the karyotype.[48] Today, the data from fetal cells are either PCR-based or FISH-based molecular tests for aneuploidy or mendelian disorders. Until molecular karyotypes or effective culture techniques are developed, fetal-cell technology can only be a screening test. Just how close to perfect the parameters can get will determine the role for fetal-cell and DNA technology.

REFERENCES

1. Evans MI, Johnson MP, Yaron Y, et al, editors. Prenatal diagnosis: genetics, reproductive risks, testing, and management. New York: McGraw Hill Publishing Co; 2006.
2. Evans MI, Wapner RJ. Invasive prenatal diagnostic procedures 2005. Semin Perinatol 2005;29(4):215–8.
3. Evans MI, Krivchenia EL, Wapner RJ, et al. Principles of screening. In: Evans MI, editor. Clinical obstetrics and gynecology – new genetics for the clinician. Philadelphia: Lippincott, Williams & Wilkins; 2002. p. 657–60.
4. Evans MI, Andriole S. Screening and testing in multiples. In: Odibo A, Krantz DA, editors. Prenatal screening and diagnosis clinics in laboratory medicine. Philadelphia: Elsevier Saunders Publishing C, in press.
5. Bianchi DW, Simpson JL, Jackson LG, et al. Fetal gender and aneuploidy detection using fetal cells in maternal blood: analysis of NIFTY I Data. Prenat Diagn 2002;22:609–15.
6. Herzenberg LA, Bianchi DW, Schroeder J, et al. Fetal cells in the blood of pregnant women: detection and enrichment by fluorescence-activated cell sorting. Proc Natl Acad Sci U S A 1979;76:1453–5.
7. Hahn S, Holzgreve W, editors. Fetal cells and fetal DNA in maternal blood: new developments for a new millennium. Basel (Switzerland): Karger Publishing Co; 2001.
8. Holzgreve W, Zhong XY, Troeger C, et al. Fetal cells in maternal blood: an overview of the basel experience. In: Hahn S, Holzgreve W, editors. Fetal cells and fetal DNA in maternal blood: new developments for a new millennium. Basel (Switzerland): Karger Publishing Co; 2001. p. 28–36.
9. Lo YMD, Tein MS, Lau TK, et al. Quantitative analysis of fetal DNA in maternal plasma and serum: implications for noninvasive prenatal diagnosis. Am J Hum Genet 1999;64:218–24.
10. Lo YMD, Tsui NBY, Leung TY, et al. Development of extraction protocols to improve the yield for fetal RNA in maternal plasma. Nat Med 2007;13:218–23.
11. Moise KJ. Management of Rhesus alloimmunization in pregnancy. Obstet Gynecol 2008;112:164–76.
12. Evans MI, Hyett J, Nicolaides KH. Genetic screening and clinical testing. In: Funai E, Evans MI, Lockwood J, editors. High risk obstetrics in the requisites in obstetrics and gynecology. Philadelphia: Elsevier Science; 2008. p. 33–60.
13. Bischoff F, Hahn S, Johnson K, et al. Intact fetal cells in maternal plasma: are they really there? Lancet 2003;361:139–40.
14. Kilpatrick MW, Tafas T, Evans MI, et al. Getting fetal cells in maternal blood to work: eliminating the false positive XY signals in XX pregnancies. Am J Obstet Gynecol 2004;190:1571–81.
15. Seppo A, Frisova V, Ichetovkin I, et al. Detection of circulating fetal cells utilizing automated microscopy: potential for noninvasive prenatal diagnosis of chromosomal aneuploidies. Prenat Diagn 2008;28(9):815–21.
16. Huang R, Barber TA, Schmidt MA, et al. A microfluidics approach for the solation of nucleated red blood cells (NRBCs) from peripheral blood of pregnant women. Prenat Diagn 2008;28:892–9.

17. Burgemeister R. New aspects of laser microdissection in research and routine. J Histochem Cytochem 2005;53:409–12.

18. Adinolfi M, Sherlock J. First trimester prenatal diagnosis using transcervical cells: an evaluation. Hum Reprod Update 1997;3:383–92.

19. Fejgin MD, Diukman R, Cotton Y, et al. Fetal cells in the uterine cervix: a source for early non-invasive prenatal diagnosis. Prenat Diagn 2001;21:619–21.

20. Bussani C, Cioni R, Scarselli B, et al. Strategies for the isolation and detection of fetal cells in transcervical samples. Prenat Diagn 2002;22:1098–101.

21. Cioni R, Bussani C, Scarselli B, et al. Comparison of two techniques for transcervical cell sampling performed in the same study population. Prenat Diagn 2005; 25:198–202.

22. Rodeck C, Tutschek B, Sherlock J, et al. Methods for the transcervical collection of fetal cells during the first trimester of pregnancy. Prenat Diagn 1995;15:933–42.

23. Massari A, Novelli G, Colosimo A, et al. Non-invasive early prenatal molecular diagnosis using retrieved transcervical trophoblast cells. Hum Genet 1996;97: 150–5.

24. Katz-Jaffe MG, Mantzaris D, Cram DS. DNA identification of fetal cells isolated from cervical mucus: potential for early non-invasive prenatal diagnosis. BJOG 2005;112:595–600.

25. Lo YMD, Corbetta N, Chamberlain PF, et al. Presence of fetal DNA in maternal plasma and serum. Lancet 1997;350:485–7.

26. Chan KCA, Zhang J, Jui AB, et al. Size distributions of maternal and fetal DNA in maternal plasma. Clin Chem 2004;50:88–92.

27. Li Y, DiNaro E, Vitucci A, et al. Detection of paternally inherited fetal point mutations for beta-thalassemia using size fractionated cell free DNA in maternal plasma. JAMA 2005;293:843–9.

28. Poon LLM, Leung TN, Lau TK, et al. Differential DNA methylation between fetus and mother as a strategy for detecting fetal DNA in maternal plasma. Clin Chem 2002;48:35–41.

29. Chim SSC, Tong YK, Chiu RWK, et al. Detection of the placental epigenetic signature of the maspin gene in maternal plasma. Clin Chem 2002;48:35–41.

30. Lo YMD. Non invasive prenatal detection of fetal chromosomal aneuploidies by maternal plasma nucleic acid analysis: a review of the current state of the art. Br J Obstet Gynaecol 2009;116:152–7.

31. Available at: http://finance.yahoo.com/news/Sequenom-Announces-Settlement-prnews-939367606.html?x=0&.v=1. Accessed June 1, 2010.

32. Lo YMD, Lun FMF, Chan KCA, et al. Digital PCR for the molecular detection of fetal chromosomal aneuploidy. Proc Natl Acad Sci U S A 2007;104:13116–21.

33. Fan HC, Blumenfeld YJ, El-Sayed YY, et al. Microfluidic digital PCR enables rapid prenatal diagnosis of fetal aneuploidy. Am J Obstet Gynecol 2009;200:543. e1–543.e7.

34. Vogelstein B, Kintzler KW. Digital PCR. Proc Natl Acad Sci U S A 1999;96: 9236–41.

35. Hahn S, Jackson LG, Kolla V, et al. Noninvasive prenatal diagnosis of fetal aneuploidies and Mendelian disorders: new innovative strategies. Expert Rev Mol Diagn 2009;9:613–21.

36. Fan HC, Blumenfeld YJ, Chirkara U, et al. Noninvasive diagnosis of fetal aneuploidy by shotgun sequencing DNA from maternal blood. Proc Natl Acad Sci U S A 2008;105:16266–71.

37. Chiu RW, Chan KC, Gao Y, et al. Noninvasive prenatal diagnosis of fetal chromosomal aneuploidy by massively parallel genomic sequencing of DNA in maternal plasma. Proc Natl Acad Sci U S A 2008;105:20458–63.
38. Geifman-Holtzman O, Grotegut CA, Gaughan JP. Diagnostic accuracy of noninvasive fetal Rh genotyping from maternal blood – a meta analysis. Am J Obstet Gynecol 2006;195:1163–73.
39. Brown S, Kellner LH, Munson M, et al. Non-invasive prenatal testing: technical strategies to achieve testing of cell free fetal DNA RhD genotype in a clinical lab. Am J Obstet Gynecol 2007;197:S173.
40. Chiu RWK, Lau TK, Leung TN, et al. Prenatal exclusion of beta thalassaemia major by examination of maternal plasma. Lancet 2002;360:998–1000.
41. Li Y, Page-Christiaens GC, Gille JJ, et al. Non-invasive prenatal detection of achondroplasia in size fractionated cell-free DNA by MALDI-TOF MS assay. Prenat Diagn 2007;27:11–7.
42. Scheffer PG, van der Schoot CE, Godelieve CML, et al. Reliability of fetal sex determination using maternal plasma. Obstet Gynecol 2010;115:117–26.
43. Baker C, Feldman B, Shalhoub AG, et al. Demographic factors for utilization of invasive genetic testing after multifetal pregnancy reduction (MFPR). Fetal Diagn Ther 2003;18:140–3.
44. Abuhamad A, Chaoui R. A practical guide to fetal echocardiography. 2nd edition. Philadelphia: Wolters Kluwer/Lippincott; 2010.
45. Malone FD, Canick JA, Ball RH, et al. First trimester or second trimester screening or both for Down's Syndrome. N Engl J Med 2005;353:2001–11.
46. Henry GP, Britt DW, Evans MI. Screening advances and diagnostic choice: the problem of residual risk. Fetal Diagn Ther 2008;23:308–15.
47. Evans MI, Pergament E. Impact of quality of nuchal translucency measurements on detection rates of Trisomies 13 and 18. Fetal Diagn Ther 2010;27:68–71.
48. Zamerowski ST, Lumley MA, Arreola RA, et al. Favorable attitudes toward testing for chromosomal abnormalities via analysis of fetal cells in maternal blood. Genet Med 2001;4:301–9.

The Role of Second-Trimester Serum Screening in the Post–First-Trimester Screening Era

Alireza A. Shamshirsaz, MD[a], Peter Benn, PhD, DSc[b,*], James F.X. Egan, MD[a]

KEYWORDS

• Prenatal • Screening • Diagnosis • Down syndrome
• Aneuploidy • Maternal serum • Ultrasound

Down syndrome (DS) is the most common clinically significant chromosomal abnormality, with a live birth rate of about 1 in 700.[1] The original prenatal screening criterion for DS was a maternal age of 35 years or older or a history of a previously affected infant.

In the 1970s, when prenatal diagnosis through amniocentesis first became possible, approximately 5% of the pregnant women in the United States were 35 years or older but only 28% of the cases of DS could have been detected prenatally using advanced maternal age alone.[2,3] This lack of efficacy of maternal age as a screening tool can be further illustrated by considering the implications if it had been used as the sole criterion for invasive testing in more recent years. For example, by 2005, 14.4% of children in the United States were born to women who were 35 years or older and the women would therefore have needed to be offered amniocentesis.[4,5] Although up to 52.6% of DS births might have been detected[5,6] using maternal age as a screening strategy, this also means that 47.4% of the cases in the total population would have been missed. In actuality, screening for DS using advanced maternal age alone has largely been replaced by far more efficacious screening methods.

Invasive diagnostic tests, such as amniocentesis and chorionic villous sampling, carry a small but real risk of procedure-related losses. This fueled the search for more efficacious screening methods. A broad range of second-trimester maternal

[a] Department of Obstetrics and Gynecology, Division of Maternal-Fetal Medicine, University of Connecticut Health Center, 263 Farmington Avenue, Farmington, CT 06030-2947, USA
[b] Department of Genetics and Developmental Biology, University of Connecticut Health Center, 263 Farmington Avenue, BB5, Farmington, CT 06030-6140, USA
* Corresponding author.
E-mail address: benn@nso1.uchc.edu

Clin Lab Med 30 (2010) 667–676
doi:10.1016/j.cll.2010.04.013   labmed.theclinics.com

serum and ultrasound markers have emerged, and this has facilitated the expansion of the screening to the obstetric population.[7] The current American College of Obstetrics and Gynecology guidelines recommend offering prenatal screening to all women, regardless of maternal age.[8]

Early screening and diagnosis was carried out through the introduction of fetal nuchal translucency (NT) measurement. This approach to DS screening became popular in Europe in the 1990s.[9] The first-trimester combined test includes NT and the serum markers of human chorionic gonadotropin (hCG), or free β-hCG, and pregnancy-associated plasma protein-A (PAPP-A). Two large studies, the Serum, Urine and Ultrasound Screening Study (SURUSS)[10] and First- and Second-Trimester Evaluation of Risk for Fetal Aneuploidy (FASTER)[11] trial, have documented the efficacy of first-trimester screening for DS in prospective studies of large populations.

Comparisons of the efficacies of first-trimester versus second-trimester screening protocols are confounded by the fact that some aneuploid fetuses are spontaneously lost during pregnancy. This means that the prevalence of DS decreases as the pregnancy progresses. Current screening modalities are benchmarked to a specific time in the pregnancy, usually 16 to 18 weeks, to standardize the results and compare the efficacies. First-trimester screening may also change the efficacy of second-trimester screening strategies because widespread use with pregnancy intervention may alter the prevalence of DS fetuses in the second trimester. The magnitude of the impact of first-trimester screening on DS prevalence in the second trimester is not known as there is no National Birth Defects Registry in the United States.

The purpose of this review is to summarize the expected performance of the currently available first- and second-trimester screening methods and to describe how to use both to calculate the best estimate of fetal DS risk.

SCREENING MARKERS

Although attention is focused on DS, it must be stressed that serum and ultrasound markers also help to identify women at risk for other aneuploidies, structural malformations, and obstetric complications. Of the more than 50 maternal blood, maternal urine, or ultrasound markers of DS, 7 are widely used in routine multimarker screening today. These are maternal serum α-fetoprotein (AFP), hCG, the free β-subunit of hCG, unconjugated estriol (uE_3), inhibin A (Inh-A), PAPP-A, and ultrasound NT. A subset of additional ultrasound markers are also used sometimes. The role of the "genetic sonogram" is only briefly mentioned because it is discussed in detail in the article by Timms and Campbell elsewhere in this issue.

Maternal serum AFP was the first serum marker associated with an increased risk of aneuploidy.[12,13] AFP already had an established role in screening for open neural tube defects and also identifies pregnancies at increased risk for ventral wall defects, other fetal anomalies, pregnancy complications, and fetal death.[14,15] In the absence of a second-trimester ultrasonography to rule out fetal anatomic abnormalities, the second-trimester maternal serum AFP test remains an important component of prenatal screening.

Maternal serum hCG[16] and free β-subunit of hCG[17] levels increase in DS pregnancies in the first and second trimesters, although the extent of increase is greater in the second trimester. Before 11 weeks, free β-hCG is discriminatory but hCG is not. Between 11 and 13 gestational weeks, free β-hCG is univariately a more discriminatory DS screening marker than hCG. When combined with maternal age, NT, and PAPP-A, free β-hCG performs better than hCG (2%–3% higher detection) at 11 weeks. At 13 weeks, hCG may perform slightly better than free β-hCG (1%–2% higher detection). hCG and free β-hCG levels are also markedly elevated in some triploid pregnancies, complete molar pregnancies, trisomy 16 mosaic pregnancies, and probably other conditions associated with an abnormal placenta.[18–22]

Maternal serum uE_3 is lower[23] in the second trimester in DS pregnancies. Undetectable levels of maternal serum uE_3 are found when the fetus has steroid sulfatase deficiency, deletion of genes contiguous with the steroid sulfatase gene, or other disorders of steroid metabolism or when there is fetal death.[24] Very low uE_3 level, in conjunction with low maternal serum AFP and low hCG levels, can be the basis of a protocol to screen for Smith-Lemli-Opitz syndrome.[25,26]

Inh-A levels are increased in DS pregnancies.[27,28] These increases are not as marked before 13 weeks of gestation as they are in the second trimester.

PAPP-A levels are reduced in first-trimester DS pregnancies,[29] but this reduction diminishes as the pregnancy progresses; there is little difference in maternal serum PAPP-A levels between DS and unaffected pregnancies in the second trimester. Low levels of PAPP-A are associated with fetal death, intrauterine growth retardation, and preeclampsia.

NT thickness usually increases in DS pregnancies.[30] This is measured between 11 0/7 weeks and 13 6/7 weeks (crown-rump length 45–85 mm) when subcutaneous edema can be identified in the fetal neck. NT is visualized in the sagittal section used for crown-rump length, and it is essential that a standardized technique be adopted for this measurement.[31] Increased NT is also seen with other aneuploidies, cardiac defects, and many other fetal disorders and syndromes.[32] There are several other first-trimester ultrasound markers that are sometimes used in DS screening. These include absence of a nasal bone (also useful in the second trimester), abnormal Doppler ductus venosus blood flow, and tricuspid regurgitation. In the second trimester, many fetal anomalies and markers associated with aneuploidy are seen on ultrasonography (see the article by Timms and Campbell elsewhere in this issue for further exploration of this topic).

SECOND-TRIMESTER SCREENING

Second-trimester screening is performed between 15 0/7 weeks and 21 6/7 weeks of gestation. The combination of maternal serum AFP, hCG, and uE_3 is commonly used as a "triple test." More recently, Inh-A was added to provide a "quadruple test," which further improved the screening performance. In 2007, 85.6% of second-trimester serum screenings in the United States used the quadruple test.[33]

The second-trimester genetic sonogram consists of a combination of structural abnormalities and soft markers, which are sometimes present in DS and other aneuploid fetuses, that are diagnosed by ultrasonography (see the article by Timms and Campbell elsewhere in this issue for further exploration of this topic). The genetic sonogram is often provided as a second step after second-trimester serum screening.[34]

The names and components of currently used screening tests are listed in **Table 1**.

In the era of first-trimester screening, there remains an important role for the second-trimester tests. If all women were to receive first-trimester screening, and all were to terminate affected pregnancies, the prevalence of DS in the second trimester would be markedly reduced (**Table 2**). However, even in this unlikely scenario, there would still remain many women whose individual risk will be relatively close to the screening cutoff and who could therefore benefit from the added efficacy that second-trimester tests can provide. In addition, many women will not receive prenatal care until after 13.9 weeks or may not receive the combined first-trimester screening

Table 1
Current screening protocols

Trimester	Name of Protocol	Tests	Comments
First	Combined	NT, PAPP-A, hCG	Completed in first trimester
Second	Triple	AFP, hCG, uE$_3$	
	Quadruple	AFP, hCG, uE$_3$, Inh-A	
	Genetic sonogram	Anatomic abnormalities and markers	Usually offered after triple or quadruple test
Both	Integrated	NT, PAPP-A, AFP, hCG, uE$_3$, Inh-A	Nondisclosure of results until all tests are completed
	Independent sequential	NT, PAPP-A, hCG; AFP, hCG, uE$_3$, Inh-A	Second-trimester test risks do not consider first-trimester results
	Stepwise sequential	NT, PAPP-A, hCG; AFP, hCG, uE$_3$, Inh-A	Results disclosed in first trimester; patients with very high risk are offered chorionic villous sampling or amniocentesis
	Contingent	NT, PAPP-A, hCG; AFP, hCG, uE$_3$, Inh-A	Results disclosed in first trimester; only patients with intermediate risks are offered second-trimester screening tests

hCG may include free β-hCG or intact hCG.

Table 2
Overall prevalence of DS in women who are screened negative by the first-trimester combined test (NT, PAPP-A, hCG)

Maternal Age (y)	Prevalence (1/n)
<20	3595
20–24	3442
25–29	2948
30–34	2039
35–39	1191
40–44	697
>44	447

Based on modeling for first-trimester screening for all women in the United States in 2006 using a second-trimester cutoff of 1:270 to define the high-risk group. This prevalence does not include any pregnancies (affected or unaffected) that were screened positive by first-trimester screening.

for other reasons (eg, availability, affordability). In the authors' region, where first-trimester screening is readily available, they estimate that 40% to 50% of women receive only the second-trimester tests. Some of the second-trimester markers are associated with other disorders not identifiable in the first trimester, and therefore, additional benefits are accrued when the markers are included in prenatal screening.

CURRENT CROSS-TRIMESTER MULTIMARKER SCREENING PROTOCOLS

Several large, prospective studies have compared first- and second-trimester risk assessments and various combinations of first- and second-trimester risk assessments. Given the number of potential markers with efficacies that vary by gestational age, numerous approaches for risk assessment are possible (see **Table 1**).

In this section, the combinations of cross-trimester tests that can be offered and the net effect in DS screening are considered.

The Integrated Test

The integrated test combines first-trimester NT measurement and serum PAPP-A levels with second-trimester AFP, β-hCG, uE_3, and Inh-A levels.[35,36] In the initial report, Wald and colleagues[35] estimated that the detection rate for the integrated test was 94% at a 5% false-positive rate. The high detection rate and low false-positive rate imply that fewer women will undergo invasive testing with the inherent risk of miscarriage after screening with the integrated test. Also, fewer women will become anxious about their pregnancy.[37] The integrated test presents an ethical challenge to the providers and the patient because the first-trimester results are withheld until the second trimester, thus denying the mother the potential advantages of early decision making regarding pregnancy termination. Another disadvantage is the high cost compared with contingency screening.

The Sequential Test

Sequential testing involves the performance of first- and second-trimester testing but with the immediate disclosure of first-trimester results for use in clinical management. There are 3 approaches to such sequential risk management: (1) independent, (2) stepwise, and (3) contingent.

1. Independent sequential testing involves the independent interpretation of first-trimester combined test and second-trimester serum test. The first-trimester result is given to the patient for clinical decision making. The second-trimester test is interpreted without taking into account the first-trimester results, that is, maternal age is used as the a priori risk for first- and second-trimester testing. Although the sensitivity is high, this is the least efficacious risk assessment strategy because the test's additive false-positive rate is unacceptably high.[11,38,39] Even more problematic is that the second-trimester risk presented can be misleading because it fails to take into account all available information (ie, the first-trimester findings). Consequently, independent sequential testing is not appropriate.[40]

2. Stepwise sequential testing offers an early invasive procedure if the first-trimester result is more than a specific cutoff. If the first-trimester risk assessment result is less than this cutoff, then the patient is offered second-trimester testing, with the final risk determined by combining all the markers. The advantage of this approach is that the sensitivity and the false-positive rate approached those obtained using integrated risk assessment, but with the option that the early results are available in the first trimester for the highest-risk patients.

3. Contingent sequential testing begins with the performance of first-trimester risk assessment. Based on these results, women are grouped into 1 of 3 risk categories: high risk, intermediate risk, and low risk. The cutoff points of the groups and their specific risks vary depending on how these groups are defined.[38] For contingent sequential risk assessment to be successful, careful determination of

Table 3
Expected performance of various combinations of first- and second-trimester screenings for DS

Screening Test	DR for 5% FPR	At a 1:270 Second-Trimester Cutoff	
		DR	FPR
First Trimester			
NT Alone	71–77	69–76	3.8–4.1
Combined	81–85	77–82	3.4–3.9
Second Trimester			
Double	56	62	7.6
Triple	60	63	6.8
Quad	67	73	5.9
First and Second Trimester			
Serum Integrated	73–78	74–75	4.5–5.2
Full Integrated	89–93	86–89	2.1–2.7
Independent	84	86	6.3–6.4
Stepwise Sequential	91–94	87–90	2.1–2.6
Contingent	88–90	85–87	1.8–2.3

Stepwise sequential, contingent, and independent tests use a 1 in 38 midtrimester high-risk cutoff, and the contingent test uses a 1 in 1200 midtrimester low-risk cutoff. Ranges reflect the variable performance of NT depending on gestational week.

Abbreviations: DR, detection rate; FPR, false-positive rate.

Data from Cuckle H, Benn PA. Multi-marker maternal serum screening for chromosome abnormalities. In: Milunsky A, Milunsky JA, editors. Genetic disorders and the fetus. 6th edition. Chichester: Wiley-Blackwell; 2010. p. 771–818.

Table 4
Detection rate corresponding to a 5% false-positive rate for various test protocols followed by using a genetic sonogram

Protocol	Before Genetic Sonogram	After Genetic Sonogram
Combined	81	90
Quad Screen	81	90
Integrated	93	98
Stepwise Sequential	97	98
Contingent Sequential	95	97

Data from Aagaard-Tillery KM, Malone F, Nyberg D, et al. Role of second-trimester genetic sonography after Down syndrome screening. Obstet Gynecol 2009;114:1189–96.

the risk cutoffs is required. The first-trimester cutoff must identify a significant proportion of DS pregnancies with only a small number of false positives.[41] Of all the potential sequential screening protocols, contingent sequential screening seems to have the most advantages with a high detection rate, a low false-positive rate, an early detection of many affected pregnancies, and the highest cost-effectiveness.[42] Most importantly, most women would have their screening completed in the first trimester, which will substantially reduce patient anxiety and increase test satisfaction. Patients would benefit from first- and second-trimester screenings, yet the obstetricians would not have to wait until the second trimester to disclose the test results. Thus, this protocol is highly likely to increase patient and provider satisfaction.

A comparison of the performance of the various screening tests described thus far is shown in **Table 3**.

Sequential First-Trimester Combined Screening and a Genetic Sonogram

Based on patients enrolled in the FASTER trial, who received the first-trimester combined test, the addition of a second-trimester genetic sonogram improves the overall detection and lowers the false-positive rate of DS screening.[43] However, the increase in detection rate is less than that achieved by offering these patients a quadruple serum test. The incremental increase in detection rate by providing the genetic sonogram to patients who have received one of the serum sequential protocols described earlier also seems to be small (**Table 4**).

The provision of the genetic sonogram to patients who have previously received complex combinations of other first- and second-trimester screening tests should be approached with caution.[34] The individual likelihood ratios used in the genetic sonogram are assumed to be independent of each other and also independent of each of the prior test results; there is some uncertainty about the accuracy of each of the likelihood ratios, and the final risks are subject to the compounding of the errors inherent in the multiple test measurements.

SUMMARY

Although first-trimester screening provides effective early screening for DS, many patients can still benefit from second-trimester screening tests that can further refine risks and identify several disorders that are not readily identifiable in the first trimester. Correct calculation of risk using sequential first- and second-trimester screening tests involves recognition of the possible correlation between test results.

In the future, with refinements in the use of existing first-trimester markers, or with the development of new ones, it may be possible to achieve efficacy comparable with those of the sequential protocols, without the need to wait for second-trimester tests.

REFERENCES

1. Korenberg JR, Chen XN, Schipper R, et al. Down syndrome phenotypes: the consequences of chromosomal imbalance. Proc Natl Acad Sci U S A 1994;91: 4997–5001.
2. Mathews TJ, Hamilton BE. Mean age of mother, 1970–2000. Natl Vital Stat Rep 2002;51:1–13.
3. Egan JF, Benn P, Borgida AF, et al. Efficacy of screening for fetal Down syndrome in the United States from 1974 to 1997. Obstet Gynecol 2000;96(6):979–85.
4. Martin JA, Hamilton BE, Sutton PD, et al. Births: final data for 2002. Natl Vital Stat Rep 2003;52:1–113.
5. National Vital Statistics Reports. Centers for Disease Control and Prevention, Atlanta, GA. Available at: http://www.cdc.gov/nchs/data/nvsr/nvsr56/nvsr56_06.pdf. Accessed May 30, 2010.
6. Odibo AO, Stamilio DM, Nelson DB, et al. A cost-effectiveness analysis of prenatal screening strategies for Down syndrome. Obstet Gynecol 2005;106:562–8.
7. Cuckle H, Benn PA. Multi-marker maternal serum screening for chromosome abnormalities. In: Milunsky A, Milunsky JA, editors. Genetic disorders and the fetus. 6th edition. Chichester: Wiley-Blackwell; 2010. p. 771–818.
8. ACOG Committee on Practice Bulletin. ACOG practice bulletin NO.77: screening for fetal chromosomal abnormalities. Obstet Gynecol 2007;109:217–27.
9. Snijders RJ, Noble P, Sebire N, et al. UK multicentre project on assessment of risk of trisomy 21 by maternal age and fetal nuchal-translucency thickness at 10–14 weeks of gestation. Fetal Medicine Foundation First Trimester Screening Group. Lancet 1998;352:343–6.
10. Wald NJ, Rodeck C, Hackshaw AK, et al. First and second trimester antenatal screening for Down's syndrome: the results of the Serum, Urine and Ultrasound Screening Study (SURUSS). Health Technol Assess 2003;7:1–77.
11. Malone FD, Canick JA, Ball RH, et al. First and Second Trimester Evaluation of Risk for Fetal Aneuploidy (FASTER): principal results of the NICHD multicenter Down syndrome screening study. N Engl J Med 2005;353:2001–11.
12. Merkatz IR, Nitowsky HM, Macri JN, et al. An association between low maternal serum alpha-fetoprotein and fetal chromosome abnormalities. Am J Obstet Gynecol 1984;148:886–94.
13. Cuckle HS, Wald NJ, Lindenbaum RH. Maternal serum alpha-fetoprotein measurement: a screening test for Down syndrome. Lancet 1984;1:926–9.
14. Milunsky A, Alpert E. Maternal serum AFP secreening. N Engl J Med 1978; 298(13):738–9.
15. Crandall BF, Robinson L, Grau P. Risks associated with an elevated maternal serum alpha-fetoprotein level. Am J Obstet Gynecol 1991;165(3):581–6.
16. Bogart MH, Pandian MR, Jones OW. Abnormal maternal serum chorionic gonadotropin levels in pregnancies with fetal chromosome abnormalities. Prenat Diagn 1987;7:623–30.
17. Macri JN, Kasturi RV, Krantz DA, et al. Maternal serum Down syndrome screening: free beta-protein is a more effective marker than human chorionic gonadotropin. Am J Obstet Gynecol 1990;163(4 Pt 1):1248–53.

18. Lambert-Messerlian G, Pinar H, Rubin LP, et al. Second-trimester maternal serum markers in twin pregnancies with complete mole, report of 2 cases. Pediatr Dev Pathol 2005;8:230–4.
19. Paradinas FJ, Sebire NJ, Fisher RA, et al. Pseudo-partial moles, placental stem vessel hydrops and the association with Beckwith-Wiedemann syndrome and complete moles. Histopathology 2001;39:447–54.
20. Benn PA, Gainey A, Ingardia CJ, et al. Second trimester maternal serum analytes in triploid pregnancies, correlation with phenotype and sex chromosome complement. Prenat Diagn 2001;21(8):680–6.
21. Saller DN Jr, Canick JA, Schwartz S, et al. Multiple-marker screening in pregnancies with hydropic and nonhydropic Turner syndrome. Am J Obstet Gynecol 1992;167(4 Pt 1):1021–4.
22. Lambert-Messerlian GM, Saller DN Jr, Tumber MB, et al. Second-trimester maternal serum inhibin A levels in fetal trisomy 18 and Turner syndrome with and without hydrops. Prenat Diagn 1998;18(10):1061–7.
23. Canick JA, Knight GJ, Palomaki GE, et al. Low second trimester maternal serum unconjugated oestriol in pregnancies with Down's syndrome. Br J Obstet Gynaecol 1988;95:330–3.
24. Kashork CD, Sutton VR, Fonda Allen JS, et al. Low or absent unconjugated estriol in pregnancy, an indicator for steroid sulfatase deficiency detectable by fluorescence in situ hybridization and biochemical analysis. Prenat Diagn 2002;22(11):1028–32.
25. Bradley LA, Palomaki GE, Knight GJ, et al. Levels of unconjugated estriol and other maternal serum markers in pregnancies with Smith-Lemli-Opitz (RSH) syndrome fetuses. Am J Med Genet 1999;82(4):355–8.
26. Craig WY, Haddow JE, Palomaki GE, et al. Major fetal abnormalities associated with positive screening test for Smith-Lemli-Opitz syndrome (SLOS). Prenat Diagn 2007;27:409–14.
27. Van Lith JM, Pratt JJ, Beekhuis JR, et al. Second-trimester maternal serum immunoreactive inhibin as a marker for fetal Down's syndrome. Prenat Diagn 1992; 12(10):801–6.
28. Wallace EM, Grant VE, Swanston IA, et al. Evaluation of maternal serum dimeric inhibin A as a first-trimester marker of Down's syndrome. Prenat Diagn 1995; 15(4):359–62.
29. Brambati B, Lanzani A, Tului L. Ultrasound and biochemical assessment of first trimester pregnancy. In: Chapman M, Grudzinskas G, Chard T, editors. The embryo: normal and abnormal development and growth. New York: Springer-Verlag; 1991. p. 181–94.
30. Nicolaides KH, Azar G, Byrne D, et al. Fetal nuchal translucency: ultrasound screening for chromosomal defects in first trimester of pregnancy. Br Med J 1992;304(6831):867–9.
31. Snijders RJ, Thom EA, Zachary JM, et al. First-trimester trisomy screening: nuchal translucency measurement training and quality assurance to correct and unify technique. Ultrasound Obstet Gynecol 2002;19(4):353–9.
32. Montenegro N, Matias A, Areias JC, et al. Increased fetal nuchal translucency, possible involvement of early cardiac failure. Ultrasound Obstet Gynecol 1997; 10(4):265–8.
33. Fang YMV, Benn P, Campbell W, et al. Down syndrome screening in the United States in 2001 and 2007: a survey of maternal-fetal medicine specialists. Am J Obstet Gynecol 2009;201:97 e1–5.
34. Benn PA, Egan JF. Second trimester prenatal ultrasound and screening for Down syndrome. Prenat Diagn 2007;27(9):884.

35. Wald NJ, Watt HC, Hackshaw AK. Integrated screening for Down's syndrome on the basis of tests performed during the first and second trimesters. N Engl J Med 1999;341:461–7.
36. Canick JA, MacRae AR. Second trimester serum markers. Semin Perinatol 2005; 29:203–8.
37. Marteau TM, Kidd J, Michie S, et al. Anxiety, knowledge and satisfaction in women receiving false positive results on routine prenatal screening: a randomized controlled trial. J Psychosom Obstet Gynaecol 1993;14:185–96.
38. Wapner R, Thom E, Simpson JL, et al. First-trimester screening for trisomies 21 and 18. N Engl J Med 2003;349:1405–13.
39. Cuckle H, Benn P, Wright D. Down syndrome screening in the first and/or second trimester: model predicted performance using meta-analysis parameters. Semin Perinatol 2005;29:252–7.
40. Benn P, Donnenfeld AE. Sequential Down syndrome screening: the importance of first and second trimester test correlations when calculating risk. J Genet Couns 2005;14(6):409–13.
41. Benn P, Wright D, Cuckle H. Practical strategies in contingent sequential screening for Down syndrome. Prenat Diagn 2005;25:645–52.
42. Gekas J, Gagné G, Bujold E, et al. Comparison of different strategies in prenatal screening for Down's syndrome: cost effectiveness analysis of computer simulation. BMJ 2009;338:b138.
43. Aagaard-Tillery KM, Malone F, Nyberg D, et al. Role of second-trimester genetic sonography after Down syndrome screening. Obstet Gynecol 2009;114:1189–96.

Modifying Risk for Aneuploidy with Second-Trimester Ultrasound After a Positive Serum Screen

Diane Timms, DO*, Winston A. Campbell, MD

KEYWORDS

- Genetic sonogram • Down syndrome • Aneuploidy screening
- Maternal serum markers • Risk reduction • Likelihood ratios

Prenatal diagnosis for aneuploidy (primarily Down syndrome) has evolved over the past 4 decades. It started as a screening process using advanced maternal age (AMA) of 35 years or older as a risk factor to offer pregnant mothers the option for prenatal diagnosis. The actual diagnosis involved undergoing an invasive procedure (amniocentesis) to obtain fetal cells for processing to determine fetal karyotype. This approach had several shortcomings: (1) it limited potential diagnosis to only a small portion of the pregnant population (AMA); (2) it would only detect 30% of cases of Down syndrome, and (3) it presented a 0.3%[1] to 1.0%[2] potential risk for miscarriage as a complication of the procedure.

The development of noninvasive prenatal screening to better identify pregnant patients at high risk for Down syndrome (second-trimester risk, ≥1:270) improved the ability to detect cases of aneuploidy and limit amniocentesis to only patients considered at high risk. This approach has a higher detection rate and a lower procedure-related rate of fetal loss than use of maternal age of 35 years or older alone. Abandoning the practice of offering invasive prenatal diagnosis (amniocentesis) to pregnant women without prior assessment by maternal serum analyte screening has been recommended.[3]

Division of Maternal-Fetal Medicine, Department of Obstetrics & Gynecology, University of Connecticut Health Center-School of Medicine-John Dempsey Hospital, 263 Farmington Avenue, Room CG 214, Farmington, CT 06030-2946, USA
* Corresponding author.
E-mail address: DTimms@resident.uchc.edu

Clin Lab Med 30 (2010) 677–692
doi:10.1016/j.cll.2010.04.016
0272-2712/10/$ – see front matter © 2010 Elsevier Inc. All rights reserved.

This article presents an overview of how prenatal diagnosis has evolved and then focuses on the current status of using ultrasound to evaluate patients considered to be screen positive for Down syndrome based on first-trimester screening (10–14 weeks) or second-trimester (15–22 weeks) maternal serum analyte screening.

EVOLUTION OF PRENATAL DIAGNOSIS

Several watershed events have facilitated the evolution of prenatal diagnosis. The first was the introduction of amniocentesis to obtain fetal cells from amniotic fluid, and culture of the cells to determine fetal karyotype, in 1967 and 1968.[1] This procedure allowed women who were considered at high risk for aneuploidy to be offered the opportunity to determine if their fetus had an abnormal karyotype. Although all trisomies increase with maternal age (**Table 1**), the initial focus of prenatal diagnosis was on the detection of Down syndrome (Trisomy 21). In the United States, a maternal age of 35 years was used as the risk level at which to start offering amniocentesis to pregnant women for prenatal diagnosis. This approach has a 30% detection rate with a 5% false-positive rate.

The second watershed event occurred with reports that a second-trimester maternal blood test (alpha-fetoprotein) was better able to identify pregnancies at risk for Down syndrome, with a detection rate of 40% and false-positive rate of 6.8%.[4,5] In the late 1980s, additional maternal serum analytes (elevated human chorionic gonadotropin [hCG][6] and low unconjugated estriol[7]) were reported as beneficial in identifying cases of Down syndrome. As reviewed by Cuckle,[8] 17 large prospective studies showed that second-trimester triple-marker screening (low alpha-fetoprotein, high hCG, and low unconjugated estriol) improved the detection rate for Down syndrome to 66%, with a 4.5% false-positive rate. The most recent analyte added

Table 1
Estimate of chromosomal abnormalities at mid-trimester and term according to maternal age[a]

| Maternal Age | Mid-Trimester | | Term | |
	Down Syndrome	All Chromosomal Abnormalities	Down Syndrome	All Chromosomal Abnormalities
33	416	185	625	285
34	322	153	500	238
35	250	132	384	204
36	192	105	303	167
37	149	83	227	130
38	115	65	175	103
39	89	53	137	81
40	69	40	106	63
41	53	31	81	50
42	41	25	64	39
43	31	19	50	30
44	25	15	38	24
45	19	12	30	19

[a] Expressed as 1/x.

Data from Hook EB, Cross PK, Schreinemachers DM. Chromosomal abnormality rates at amniocentesis and in live-born infants. JAMA 1983;249:2034–8.

to the second-trimester maternal serum screen was an elevated inhibin-A. With the addition of this last analyte the maternal serum quadruple-marker screen (low alpha-fetoprotein, high hCG, low unconjugated estriol, and high inhibin-A) has a reported detection rate of 70% with a false-positive rate of 5%.[9]

The third watershed event evolved when multiple-marker serum analyte screening was developing. This new procedure used a detailed ultrasound examination (genetic sonogram) to identify anatomic markers reported to be more frequent in Down syndrome fetuses.[10,11] The genetic sonogram has been used in women considered at high risk based on (1) maternal age–related risk alone, (2) maternal serum marker screening (regardless of maternal age), and (3) maternal age–related risk that was not reduced despite maternal serum analyte screen adjustment. An eight-center study on the use of the genetic sonogram reported detection rates of 71.6% (range, 63.6%–80%).[12]

Another watershed event is discussed in article by Shamshirsaz and colleagues elsewhere in this issue. This development is first-trimester screening using a combination of an ultrasound evaluation (nuchal translucency measurement) and serum analyte markers (pregnancy-associated plasma protein-A [PAPP-A], and free β-hCG). Reports from Europe[13] and the United States[14] have shown that this is a viable approach to prenatal screening in early gestation (10–14 weeks), with detection rates of approximately 80% to 90% using a fixed false-positive rate of 5%. First-trimester screening was recently endorsed as a national guideline for prenatal care in the United States.[15]

The evolution of screening for aneuploidy has allowed more flexibility and options for clinical management. Although the genetic sonogram alone has detection rates similar to maternal serum analyte screening, it does have a limitation. The genetic sonogram was only evaluated in women who were identified as being at high risk for aneuploidy. Its use in a low-risk population has not been evaluated. Therefore, its detection and false-positive rates might differ from those reported in high-risk patients. In contrast, maternal serum analyte screening can be offered to all women because it will adjust their underlying age-related risk (see **Table 1**), and thus identify patients who need additional evaluation if desired. This additional evaluation could be either an invasive procedure (amniocentesis) or a genetic sonogram, with amniocentesis reserved for pregnancies still found to be at high risk after the genetic sonogram.

THE GENETIC SONOGRAM

Use of ultrasound was one of the watershed events in the evolution of prenatal diagnosis. Fetal ultrasound was not considered a tool in prenatal diagnosis unless an obvious abnormality that had been described as a pediatric finding of Down syndrome could be seen on an ultrasound examination (eg, endocardial cushion defect, duodenal atresia). The use of ultrasound to determine other specific features associated with Down syndrome was first described by Benacerraf and colleagues[16,17] in 1985, who noted that affected fetuses tended to have an increased nuchal thickness. Subsequently, other investigators reported sonographic markers observed in fetuses confirmed to have Down syndrome (**Box 1**). These sonographic signs, also known as *soft markers*, do not impact fetal outcome and have varying sensitivity for detecting aneuploidy.[18] An ultrasound examination to assess for the presence or absence of these markers in women at high risk for Down syndrome is known as a *genetic sonogram*. The development of this approach and its use in modifying risk derived from the second-trimester maternal serum analyte screen are discussed in this section.

Box 1
Second trimester structural anomalies and sonographic markers of Down syndrome

Structural anomalies

Cardiac anomalies

Duodenal atresia

Brachycephaly

Hydrocephalus

Cystic hygroma

Hydrops

Sonographic soft markers

Increased nuchal thickness

Short femur

Short humerus

Renal pyelectasis

Echogenic bowel

Intracardiac echogenic focus

Absent or hypoplastic nasal bone

Clinodactyly

Decreased ear length

Two-vessel umbilical cord

Sandal-gap deformity

The major, or structural, anomalies associated with Down syndrome include cardiac defects, duodenal atresia, ventriculomegaly, and cystic hygroma.[18] However, these structural malformations may be seen in only 25% of fetuses with Down syndrome.[19] In affected fetuses, the rate of cardiac defects, including ventricular septal defect, is approximately 50%.[20,21] However, many of these may be missed on a second-trimester ultrasound.[19] The use of nonstructural, or soft, markers became possible with advancements in ultrasound technology. Since the identification of increased nuchal thickness as a marker for Down syndrome, numerous other markers have been evaluated, not only for Down syndrome (Trisomy 21) but also for Trisomies 18 and 13. The specific pattern of markers may suggest the particular diagnosis.

The genetic sonogram identifies as many as 50% to 75% of fetuses with Down syndrome, with a screen-positive rate of 4% to 15%.[22] Each ultrasonographic marker studied has its own sensitivity and false-positive rate. Likelihood ratios (LR) for each marker are calculated by dividing the sensitivity of a particular marker by its false-positive rate.[23] An LR of greater than 1 increases the probability of the condition to be present, with values of 2 to 5, 5 to 10, and greater than 10 showing small, moderate, and large probabilities, respectively, for the condition.[24] LRs calculated for several commonly used ultrasonographic markers for Down syndrome in several studies can be seen in **Table 2**.

The strongest soft marker for Down syndrome is an increased nuchal fold thickness (**Fig. 1**). It must be measured in the transcerebellar scanning plane of the fetal head. This view plane is angled posteriorly to include the key landmarks: frontal horns of

Table 2
Likelihood ratios for Down syndrome using isolated ultrasound markers

Marker	Nyberg & Souter[18]	Smith-Bindman et al[29]	Smith-Bindman et al[25]	Aagaard-Tillery et al[40]
Thickened nuchal fold	11	12.9	17	49
Short femur	1.5	1.1	2.7	4.6
Short humerus	5	1.6	7.5	5.0
Intracardiac echogenic focus	1.8	1.43	2.8	6.3
Renal pyelectasis	1.5	1.6	1.9	5.5
Echogenic bowel	6.7	2.5	6.1	24
No markers	0.4	0.55	NA	0.41

lateral ventricles, cavum septum pellucidum, thalami, cerebellum, cisterna magna, and occipital bone.[19] The nuchal thickness is measured from the external surface of the occipital bone to the outer surface of the fetal scalp. A value of 6 mm or greater is considered abnormal. This marker has a sensitivity of 11.8%, with a false-positive rate of 0.9%, for detecting Down syndrome.[25] This result yields an LR of 12.9, significantly increasing the risk for Down syndrome even in the absence of a major structural anomaly.

Other ultrasonographic markers may be useful in detecting Down syndrome. Both the humerus and the femur tend to be shortened in affected fetuses compared with normal fetuses. A shortened femur or humerus length may be used to detect Down syndrome through calculating a ratio of the actual measured bone length to an expected bone length, with expected femur length of $-9.3105 + 0.9028 \times$ biparietal diameter (BPD).[26] A femur length ratio of less than 0.91 has a sensitivity of 40% to 50%, with a false-positive rate of 2.2% to 6.5%.[19] A humerus ratio of less than 0.90 using expected humerus length of $-7.9404 + 0.8492 \times$ BPD has a sensitivity of up to 50% for detecting fetuses with Down syndrome.[27] Additionally, a (femur + humerus) / foot length ratio of less than 1.75 has a reported sensitivity of 51%, with

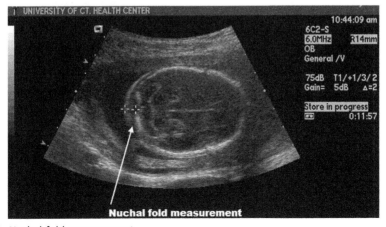

Fig. 1. Nuchal fold measurement.

a false-positive rate of 7% for detecting Down syndrome.[28] These markers may be less reliable because of natural variations in bone length at different gestational ages, and based on the ethnic group and gender of the fetus.[18]

Renal pyelectasis is defined as an anterior–posterior measurement of the renal pelves of 4 mm or greater on a cross-sectional view (**Fig. 2**). Although pyelectasis has been associated with Down syndrome, it is also a common finding in normal fetuses. A meta-analysis performed by Smith-Bindman and colleagues[29] in 2001 showed pyelectasis had a sensitivity of only 2% but a low false-positive rate of 0.06% to 2.9%, with an LR of 1.9.

Another finding that is considered a marker for Down syndrome is hyperechoic (echogenic) bowel (**Fig. 3**). Although echogenic bowel can be a variant of normal, the differential diagnosis is broad and includes chromosomal abnormalities (especially Down syndrome), in utero infection (especially cytomegalovirus), meconium ileus, intra-amniotic bleeding, and cystic fibrosis.[30] The finding can be graded by comparing bowel with liver echogenicity. In grade 0, the bowel and liver are isoechoic, whereas the bowel is mildly echogenic in grade 1, moderately echogenic in grade 2, and markedly echogenic and nearly as bright as bone in grade 3 (used as a marker by most centers).[30] In addition, the finding tends to be focal.[18] This marker has a sensitivity of 17% and a false-positive rate of 0.5% for detecting Down syndrome, giving it an LR of 6.7.[18]

An intracardiac echogenic focus (**Fig. 4**) may also increase suspicion for Down syndrome, with a sensitivity of 0.11 and an LR of 2.8 when seen as an isolated abnormality.[29] Bromley and colleagues[31] found in their patient population that 18% of fetuses with Down syndrome had an intracardiac echogenic focus, whereas 4.7% of normal fetuses had this finding. It is most commonly noted in the left ventricle, but may be a more suspicious finding when an echogenic focus is present in both ventricles.

Absence or hypoplasia of the nasal bone has also been used as a soft marker (**Fig. 5**). The nasal bone should be measured with the ultrasound beam at an angle of 45° to 60°

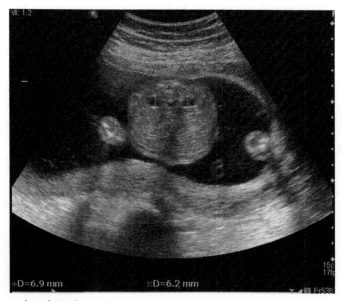

Fig. 2. Bilateral pyelectasis.

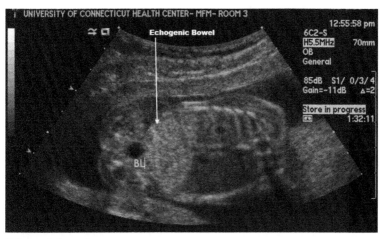

Fig. 3. Echogenic bowel.

to the mid-sagittal fetal profile and 60° to 90° with the fetal nose. In the second trimester, Viora and colleagues,[32] found an absent nasal bone in 0.47% of 418 normal fetuses but in 55% of 18 fetuses with Down syndrome, and nasal bone hypoplasia was present in 25% of fetuses with Down syndrome.[32] Nasal bone hypoplasia can be quantified using the ratio of BPD to nasal bone length, with a value greater than 9 suggesting hypoplasia,[33] or using a nasal bone measurement of less than 2.5 mm.[34]

Other more subtle ultrasound findings have been suggested for use as markers for Down syndrome, including clenched hands and clinodactyly, a curvature of the 5th finger toward the 4th finger caused by hypoplasia of the middle phalanx (**Fig. 6**). These findings are rarely seen in the absence of other anomalies.[25] Fetal ear length has also been proposed as a marker for aneuploidy. The maximal distance between the superior and inferior borders of the external ear is measured in a coronal view (**Fig. 7**). Letierri and colleagues[35] developed a nomogram for fetal ear length and reported

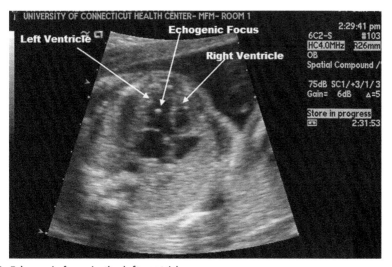

Fig. 4. Echogenic focus in the left ventricle.

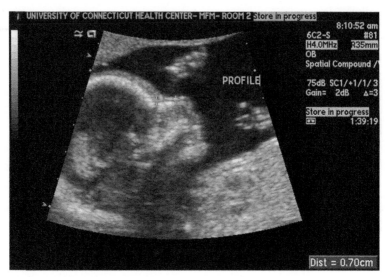

Fig. 5. Fetal nasal bone measurement.

that an ear length measurement in less than the 10th percentile had a 71% sensitivity with a 8% false-positive rate (LR, 8.8) for detecting Down syndrome. The benefit of fetal ear length has been confirmed in larger studies.[36]

A two-vessel umbilical cord (**Fig. 8**) also has been used as a marker for Down syndrome, but sensitivity of this marker is only 0.41% despite a low false-positive rate of 0.31%. This finding yields an LR of 1.3, making a single umbilical artery a weak marker for Down syndrome.[25] A widely separated great toe has been noted in children with Down syndrome, commonly known as the *sandal-gap deformity* (**Fig. 9**). This finding also may be seen on ultrasound.[37] However, the sensitivity for Down syndrome is only 3%.[12]

The predictive value of soft markers is improved when a major structural anomaly is also present.[25] In addition, the presence of multiple markers increases the risk. Nyberg

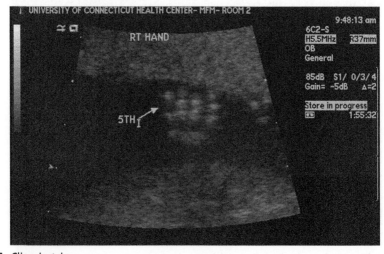

Fig. 6. Clinodactyly.

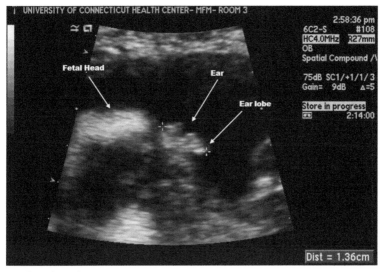

Fig. 7. Fetal ear length measurement.

and Souter[18] reported that when two markers are present, the LR is 9.6, and increases to 115 for three or more markers. In addition, other markers that may not predict an increased risk for Down syndrome may be more frequently identified in fetuses with other chromosomal anomalies. The presence of choroid plexus cysts (**Fig. 10**), for example, is associated with Trisomy 18 but does not significantly impact the risk for Trisomy 21.[18,38]

MODIFYING ANEUPLOIDY RISK WITH THE GENETIC SONOGRAM

LRs have been calculated for most of the commonly used ultrasonographic markers reported to be associated with Down syndrome. When a marker is identified on the

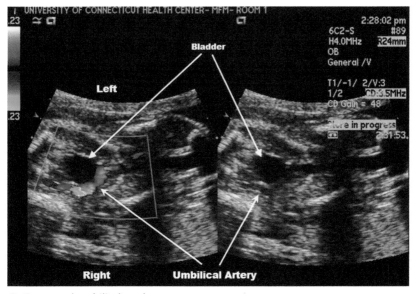

Fig. 8. Two vessel umbilical cord.

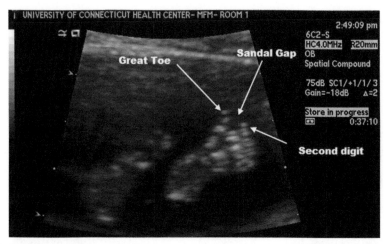

Fig. 9. Sandal-gap toes.

genetic sonogram, multiplying the Down syndrome risk by the marker's LR yields the adjusted risk. If multiple markers are seen, various approaches to adjust risk have been suggested. The individual LRs may be multiplied to determine an overall likelihood ratio,[39] or likelihood ratios based on number of markers observed may be used.[40] Other methods of determining risk when multiple markers are present include a scoring system assigning points for each marker seen.[19] At the authors' center, when multiple markers are identified, the marker with the highest LR is used to adjust the risk. The total LR can then be multiplied by the maternal age–related risk to calculate the specific risk for Down syndrome. Application of this principle to risks derived from either first-trimester, second-trimester, or integrated screening approaches have been examined.

In the case of second-trimester serum screening, statistical analysis has allowed for the creation of risk-estimate tables that can be used to modify triple screen–derived risk (**Table 3**).[41] This improved risk estimate can then be used when counseling

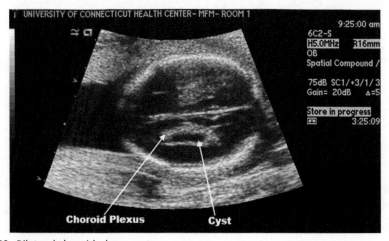

Fig. 10. Bilateral choroid plexus cysts.

Table 3
Mid-trimester risk for Trisomy 21 based on triple screen result as modified by genetic sonogram[a]

Triple Screen Risk	Normal Genetic Sonogram	Short Femur	Short Humerus	Pyelectasis	Increased Nuchal Fold	Echogenic Bowel
15,000	160,000	5631	3661	2359	347	1100
12,000	128,000	4505	2929	1888	277	880
9,000	96,000	3379	2197	1416	208	660
6,000	64,000	2253	1465	944	139	440
3,000	32,000	1127	733	473	70	221
1000	10,667	376	245	158	24	74
500	5333	188	123	80	13	38

[a] Risks expressed as 1/x.
Data from Vintzileos A, Egan J. Adjusting the risk of trisomy 21 on the basis of second-trimester ultrasonography. Am J Obstet Gynecol 1995;172:837–44.

patients regarding invasive testing and may decrease procedure-related fetal loss. Even in women identified as high-risk by age or second-trimester serum screening, the absence of ultrasonographic markers may be able to decrease risk estimates by 55% to 91%.[18,41,42] Using this approach, the rate of amniocentesis in women at high risk for aneuploidy based on age alone may be decreased to 20% without missing any cases of Trisomy 21.[41] However, because the genetic sonogram reduced risk in high-risk patients, the potential for missing a case still existed.

The use of the genetic sonogram to modify aneuploidy risk after a first-trimester combined screen alone has been evaluated in several studies. The concept of using an integrated screen for detecting Down syndrome was first introduced by Wald.[43] Data from published studies were used to calculate a Down syndrome risk from first-trimester screening, and then this value was combined with the risk derived from a second-trimester triple or quadruple screen to produce an integrated risk. The approach was prospectively evaluated by the First and Second-Trimester Evaluation of Risk (FASTER) research consortium.[44] Subsequently, several different screening approaches have been developed that modify risk either according to serum markers or a genetic sonogram (**Table 4**).

In an integrated approach, first-trimester screening results are withheld until the genetic sonogram is completed and a final risk assessment can be calculated. Stepwise sequential screening may have fewer ethical implications because first-trimester results are shared with the patient, who then can opt either to undergo invasive testing if aneuploidy risk exceeds a predetermined threshold level, or to continue on to the next level of screening, in this case the genetic sonogram. In contingent screening, patients at low risk based on first-trimester screening results are not offered further testing, whereas those at high risk are offered immediate invasive testing. Patients with an intermediate risk proceed to the next stage of screening, which is the genetic sonogram.[22]

In a statistical model using the genetic sonogram after normal first-trimester screening results as an integrated test, the detection rate for Down syndrome increased from 88.5% to 94.6%, with an increase in the screen-positive rate from 4.2% to 5.4%.[45] When the genetic sonogram was used in a contingent approach to further screen only women with an intermediate risk for Down syndrome (1:300–1:2500 on first-trimester screening), the detection rate improved to 93.3%, with a screen positive rate of 4.9%.[45] However, these results were challenged by Wax and colleagues[46] when applied to a high-risk population of women at advanced maternal age. First-trimester screening failed to identify only one fetus with Down syndrome, which was detected using the genetic sonogram, yielding a detection rate of 100%. Unfortunately, the screen-positive rate jumped to greater than 20%, regardless of whether the genetic sonogram was used as part of an integrated approach to screening or in a stepwise sequential manner.

An early study evaluating use of the genetic sonogram after integrated first- and second-trimester screening tests found that when a screen-positive cutoff of 1:150 was used, the false-positive rate decreased from 2.5% to 1.8%, but the detection rate also decreased from 83% to 75%.[47] The investigators concluded that the absence of ultrasonographic markers should not prevent the offering of invasive testing to women with high-risk screening results, and conversely that women with low-risk screening results and one soft marker should not be offered invasive testing.[47]

Most recently, data from the FASTER trial were used to prospectively examine the use of the genetic sonogram to improve the detection rate of Down syndrome with and without different screening methods.[40] The detection rate for the genetic sonogram

Table 4
Approaches to Down syndrome screening

Screening Test	Evaluation	Results	Advantage	Disadvantage
First-trimester NT	NT measurement using ultrasound	Short-interval turnaround[b]	Potential for early diagnosis	Lower detection rate compared with first trimester combined
First trimester serum analyte	PAPP-A, free β-hCG	Short-interval turnaround[b]	Potential for early diagnosis	Lower detection rate compared with first trimester combined
First trimester combined	Fetal NT by ultrasound + serum PAPP-A/free β-hCG	Short-interval result turnaround[b]	Potential for early diagnosis	Higher detection rate when combined with second-trimester testing
Second-trimester quadruple screen	Serum hCG (free β or total), estriol, AFP, inhibin-A	Short-interval result turnaround[b]	No specialized ultrasound examination needed	Diagnosis delayed until second trimester
Genetic sonogram	Ultrasound at 18–20 wk	Immediate	Allows for evaluation of multiple fetal anomalies	Lower sensitivity when used alone, diagnosis delayed until second trimester
Integrated	First trimester combined + quadruple screen[a]	Withheld after first-trimester screen, given after second-trimester screen complete	Lowest false-positive rate, highest sensitivity	Patient kept unaware of first-trimester screening result, diagnosis delayed
Sequential	First trimester combined + quadruple screen[a]	Short interval after first-trimester screen, second-trimester testing modifies risk	Intervention possible after first-trimester screening; risk modification with second-trimester testing	Marginally increased false-positive rate Decreased sensitivity versus integrated Diagnosis delayed
Contingent	First trimester combined ± quadruple screen[a]	Short interval after first trimester screening, only intermediate-risk patients offered second-trimester screen or genetic sonogram	Lowest cost, allows for first-trimester intervention	Marginally increased false-positive rate Decreased sensitivity versus integrated Diagnosis delayed

Abbreviations: AFP, alpha-fetoprotein; hCG, human chorionic gonadotropin; NT, nuchal translucency; PAPP-A, pregnancy-associated plasma protein-A.
[a] The genetic sonogram may be substituted for second-trimester serum screening.
[b] Short-interval turnaround is usually less than a week but can vary depending on the reference laboratory performing the testing.

alone (without prior screening) was 83%, with a false-positive rate of 12% using a risk cutoff of 1:270. When used after previous screening with a false-positive rate set at 5%, the detection rate for Down syndrome was increased by the genetic sonogram, regardless of the type of screening used. The detection rate using integrated screening alone was 93% and increased to 98% when genetic sonogram was added. Used in conjunction with sequential or contingent screening, the detection rate increased only marginally because the screening tests were so effective (97% and 95% detection, respectively). When the genetic sonogram was used along with first-trimester screening (without second-trimester serum screening) in a sequential or contingent strategy, the detection rate was 90%.[40] The LR in the absence of any markers was 0.41, suggesting again that use of the genetic sonogram to decrease risk assigned by screening tests could lead to a corresponding decrease in the need for invasive testing for false-positive screening.

SUMMARY

Prenatal diagnosis for aneuploidy has moved away from the limited option of invasive diagnostic testing with its associated risk of fetal loss. The development of noninvasive first- and second-trimester maternal serum screening allows clinicians to better identify patients, of any maternal age, who would be considered at high risk for aneuploidy. Identification of ultrasonographic markers to aid in recognition of fetuses with Down syndrome has improved detection of aneuploidy. The genetic sonogram is proving to be a useful adjunct to adjust risk results from screening tests to detect Down syndrome, and significantly increases the detection rate regardless of the screening modality used. A normal genetic sonogram can also decrease age-related or screening test–derived Down syndrome risk, preventing unnecessary invasive procedures.

REFERENCES

1. NICHD National Registry for Amniocentesis Study Group Midtrimester amniocentesis for prenatal diagnosis: safety and accuracy. JAMA 1976;236:1471–6.
2. Tabor A, Madsen M, Obel EB, et al. Randomized controlled trial of genetic amniocentesis in 4606 low-risk women. Lancet 1986;1:1287–93.
3. Egan JFX, Benn P, Borgida AF, et al. Efficacy of screening for fetal Down syndrome in the United States from 1974–1997. Obstet Gynecol 2000;96:979–85.
4. Merkatz IR, Nitowsky HM, Macri JN, et al. An association between low maternal serum alpha-fetoprotein and fetal chromosomal abnormalities. Am J Obstet Gynecol 1984;148:886–94.
5. Cuckle HS, Wald NJ, Lindenbaum RH. Maternal serum alpha-fetoprotein measurement: a screening test for Down's syndrome. Lancet 1984;323:926–9.
6. Bogart MH, Pandian MR, Jones OW. Abnormal maternal serum chorionic gonadotropin levels in pregnancies with fetal chromosome abnormalities. Prenat Diagn 1987;7(9):623–30.
7. Canick JA, Knight GJ, Palomaki GE, et al. Low second-trimester serum unconjugated oestriol in pregnancies with Down's syndrome. Br J Obstet Gynaecol 1988; 95(4):330–3.
8. Cuckle H. Established markers in second-trimester serum. Early Hum Dev 1996; 47(Suppl):S27–9.
9. Wald NJ, Densem J, George L, et al. Prenatal screening for Down's syndrome using inhibin-A as a serum marker. Prenat Diagn 1996;16:143–53.

10. Benacerraf BR, Neuberg B, Bromley B, et al. Sonographic scoring index for prenatal detection of chromosomal abnormalities. J Ultrasound Med 1992;9:449–58.
11. Vintzileos AM, Campbell WA, Rodis JF, et al. The use of second-trimester genetic sonogram in guiding clinical management of patients at increased risk for fetal trisomy 21. Obstet Gynecol 1996;87:948–52.
12. Hobbins JC, Lezotte DC, Persutte WH, et al. An 8-center study to evaluate the utility of mid-term genetic sonograms among high-risk pregnancies. J Ultrasound Med 2003;22(1):33–8.
13. Spencer K, Souter V, Tul N, et al. A screening program for trisomy 21 at 10-14 weeks using fetal nuchal translucency, maternal serum free ß-human chorionic gonadotropin and pregnancy-associated plasma protein-A. Ultrasound Obstet Gynecol 1999;13:231–7.
14. Wapner R, Thom E, Simpson JL, et al. First-trimester screening for trisomies 21 and 18. First-trimester Maternal Serum Biochemistry and Fetal Nuchal Translucency Screening (BUN) Study Group. N Engl J Med 2003;349:1405–13.
15. ACOG Practice Bulletin No. 77. Screening for fetal chromosomal abnormalities. Obstet Gynecol 2007;109:217–27.
16. Benacerraf BR, Barss VA, Laboda LA. A sonographic sign for the detection in the second-trimester of the fetus with Down's syndrome. Am J Obstet Gynecol 1985; 151:1078–9.
17. Benacerraf BR, Frigoletto FD, Laboda LA. Sonographic diagnosis of Down syndrome in the second-trimester. Am J Obstet Gynecol 1985;153:49–52.
18. Nyberg DA, Souter VL. Sonographic markers for fetal trisomies: second trimester. J Ultrasound Med 2001;20:655–74.
19. Benacerraf BR. The role of the second-trimester genetic sonogram in screening for fetal Down syndrome. Semin Perinatol 2005;29:386–94.
20. Paladini D, Tartaglione A, Agangia A, et al. The association between congenital heart disease and Down syndrome in prenatal life. Ultrasound Obstet Gynecol 2000;15:104–8.
21. Respondek-Liberska M, Nowicki G, Krason A, et al. Can we suspect fetal down syndrome by heart evaluation during the second half of pregnancy? Fetal Diagn Ther 1999;14:143–8.
22. Driscoll DA, Gross S. Prenatal screening for aneuploidy. N Engl J Med 2009;360: 2556–62.
23. McGee S. Simplifying likelihood ratios. J Gen Intern Med 2002;17(8):646–9.
24. Jaeschke R, Guyatt GH, Sackett DL. Users' guides to the medical literature. III. How to use an article about a diagnostic test. B. What are the results and will they help me in caring for my patients? The Evidence-Based Medicine Working Group. JAMA 1994;271(9):703–7.
25. Smith-Bindman R, Chu P, Goldberg JD. Second-trimester prenatal ultrasound for the detection of pregnancies at increased risk of Down' syndrome. Prenat Diagn 2007;27:535–44.
26. Benacerraf BR, Gelman R, Frigoletto F. Sonographic identification of second-trimester fetuses with Down's syndrome. N Engl J Med 1987;317:1371–6.
27. Benacerraf BR, Neuberg D, Frigoletto F. Humeral shortening in second-trimester fetuses with Down syndrome. Obstet Gynecol 1991;77:223–7.
28. Johnson MP, Michaelson JE, Barr M, et al. Combining humerus and femur length for improved ultrasonographic identification of pregnancies at increased risk for trisomy 21. Am J Obstet Gynecol 1995;172:1229–35.
29. Smith-Bindman R, Hosmer W, Feldstein V. Second-trimester ultrasound to detect fetuses with Down syndrome: a meta-analysis. JAMA 2001;285:1044–55.

30. Nyberg D, Dubinsky T, Resta R, et al. Echogenic fetal bowel during the second-trimester: clinical importance. Radiology 1993;188:527–31.
31. Bromley B, Lieberman E, Laboda L, et al. Echogenic intracardiac focus: a sonographic sign for fetal Down's syndrome. Obstet Gynecol 1995;86:998–1001.
32. Viora E, Errante G, Sciarrone A, et al. Fetal nasal bone and trisomy 21 in the second-trimester. Prenat Diagn 2005;25:511–5.
33. Bromley B, Lieberman E, Shipp TD, et al. Fetal nasal bone length. A marker for Down syndrome in the second-trimester. J Ultrasound Med 2002;21:1387–94.
34. Cicero S, Sonek JD, Mckenna DS, et al. Nasal bone hypoplasia in trisomy 21 at 15-22 weeks' gestation. Ultrasound Obstet Gynecol 2003;21:15–8.
35. Letierri L, Rodis JF, Vintzileos, et al. Ear length in second-trimester aneuploid fetuses. Obstet Gynecol 1993;81(1):57–60.
36. Chitkara U, Lee L, Oehlert JL, et al. Fetal ear length measurement: a useful predictor of aneuploidy? Ultrasound Obstet Gynecol 2002;19(2):131–5.
37. Wilkins I. Separation of the great toe in fetuses with Down syndrome. J Ultrasound Med 1994;13:229–31.
38. Bottalico J, Chen X, Tartaglia M, et al. Second-trimester genetic sonogram for detection of fetal chromosomal abnormalities in a community-based antenatal testing unit. Ultrasound Obstet Gynecol 2009;33:161–8.
39. Nyberg DA, Luthy DA, Resta BC, et al. Age-adjusted ultrasound risk assessment for fetal Down's syndrome during the second-trimester: description of the method and analysis of 142 cases. Ultrasound Obstet Gynecol 1998;12:8–14.
40. Aagaard-Tillery KM, Malone FD, Nyberg DA, et al. Role of second-trimester genetic sonography after Down's syndrome screening. Obstet Gynecol 2009;114:1189–96.
41. Vintzileos A, Egan J. Adjusting the risk of trisomy 21 on the basis of second-trimester ultrasonography. Am J Obstet Gynecol 1995;172:837–44.
42. Benn PA, Egan JF. Expected performance of second-trimester maternal serum testing followed by a 'genetic sonogram' in screening of fetal Down syndrome. Prenat Diagn 2008;28:230–5.
43. Wald NJ, Watt HC, Hackshaw AK. Integrated screening for Down's syndrome based on tests performed during the first and second trimesters. N Engl J Med 1999;341:461–7.
44. Malone FD, Canick JA, Ball RH, et al. First-trimester or second-trimester screening, or both for Down's syndrome. N Engl J Med 2005;353:2001–11.
45. Krantz DA, Hallahan TW, Macro VJ, et al. Genetic sonography after first-trimester Down syndrome screening. Ultrasound Obstet Gynecol 1993;168:534–8.
46. Wax JR, Pinnette MG, Cartin A, et al. Second-trimester genetic sonography after first-trimester combined screening for trisomy 21. J Ultrasound Med 2009;28:321–5.
47. Weisz B, Pandya PP, David AL, et al. Ultrasound findings after screening for Down's syndrome using the integrated test. Obstet Gynecol 2007;109:1046–52.

Biophysical and Biochemical Screening for the Risk of Preterm Labor

Joseph R. Wax, MD*, Angelina Cartin, Michael G. Pinette, MD

KEYWORDS

- Cervical cerclage • Cervical length • Fetal fibronectin
- Preterm birth • Progesterone • Ultrasound

Preterm birth, defined as delivery at less than 37 weeks' gestation, is the leading cause of perinatal morbidity and mortality in developed nations. Twelve to thirteen percent of births in the United States are preterm, representing more than 500,000 births annually. In 2007, the preterm birth rate decreased to 12.7%, the first drop in more than 2 decades (**Fig. 1**).[1] Medical costs for preterm newborns are more than 10 times those of term infants, and the average length of hospitalization is more than 6 times that of term infants.

Preterm deliveries, including births following preterm labor and/or preterm membrane rupture, may be categorized as spontaneous or due to maternal or fetal complications. This article addresses only spontaneous preterm birth. Risk factors for spontaneous preterm birth are listed in **Box 1**. This lengthy catalog of heterogeneous associations of spontaneous preterm births suggests causal heterogeneity as well. Although mechanisms of labor initiation are unknown, broad categories for these associations include inflammation, decidual hemorrhage, uterine overdistension, and early initiation of normal parturition.[2] Not surprisingly, long-standing goals identifying women destined to preterm delivery and offering effective preventive measures remain only partially fulfilled.

Proposed techniques for detecting at-risk pregnancies include risk factor–based scoring systems, home uterine activity monitoring, maternal serum chemistries, salivary estriol, cervicovaginal chemistries, and amniotic fluid analytes (**Box 2**). These modalities are characterized by inadequate screening efficiencies, invasiveness, expense, or lack of commercial availability. Moreover, their use does not

Division of Maternal-Fetal Medicine, Department of Obstetrics and Gynecology, Maine Medical Center, Portland, ME, USA
* Corresponding author. Maine Medical Partners Women's Health, 887 Congress Street, Suite 200, Portland, ME 04102.
E-mail address: waxj@mmc.org

Clin Lab Med 30 (2010) 693–707
doi:10.1016/j.cll.2010.04.006
0272-2712/10/$ – see front matter © 2010 Elsevier Inc. All rights reserved.

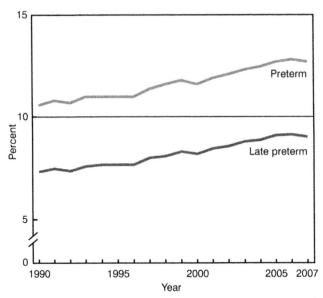

NOTE: Preterm is less than 37 completed weeks of gestation. Late preterm is 34–36 completed weeks of gestation.
SOURCE: CDC/NCHS, National Vital Statistics System.

Fig. 1. Preterm birth rates in the United States: final 1990 to 2006 and preliminary 2007.

demonstrate reduced spontaneous preterm birth rates. The remainder of this article discusses the respective biophysical and biochemical tests of sonographic cervical length measurement and cervicovaginal fetal fibronectin (FFN) that are widely evaluated and incorporated into the clinical care of patients at risk for spontaneous preterm birth.

CERVICAL LENGTH ASSESSMENT
Rationale

Labor is defined as regular uterine contractions resulting in progressive dilation and effacement of the cervix. Thus, the cervix provides the definitive window to diagnosing labor. Traditionally the cervix has been viewed in dichotomous terms, either as capable of maintaining pregnancy until term (competent) or not (incompetent). More recently, this paradigm has been challenged, with cervical function now viewed along a continuum. Landmark research in the mid-1990s compared cervical lengths measured by transvaginal ultrasound (TVUS) in women with prior preterm births with cervical lengths in control subjects without previous preterm births. The investigators found that gestational age at delivery of the prior pregnancy correlated significantly with the cervical length at 20 to 30 weeks in the subsequent gestation.[3]

These findings were expanded later in a multicenter study of 2915 women undergoing TVUS at 24 weeks' gestation. The investigators observed that cervical lengths were normally distributed (**Fig. 2**) and that the risk of spontaneous preterm birth in the current pregnancy increased with decreasing cervical length (see **Fig. 2; Fig. 3**). A cervical length of 25 mm (10th percentile) seemed to be a clinically appropriate

Box 1
Risk factors for spontaneous preterm birth
Demographic
Age less than 18 years and more than 40 years
Lower socioeconomic status
Unmarried
Poor nutritional status
Psychosocial stressors
Inadequate prenatal care
Black race
Underweight
Smoker
Anemia
Interpregnancy interval less than 6 months
Drug abuse
Prior preterm birth
Obstetric/Gynecologic
Uterus/Cervix
Fibroids
Mullerian anomaly
Conization or loop electrosurgical excision procedure
Laceration
Diethylstilbestrol exposure
Overdistension
Multiple gestations
Polyhydramnios
Obstetric bleeding
Abruption
Threatened miscarriage
Inflammation
Bacterial vaginosis
Cystitis
Systemic infection

threshold for identifying preterm delivery risk, offering 37.3% sensitivity, 92.2% specificity, and a negative predictive value of 97.4%.[4] Occasionally, echogenic material is noted within the amniotic fluid at the level of the cervix (**Fig. 4**). Initially thought to represent blood clot, this debris is an inflammatory exudate consisting of fibrous tissue, white blood cells, and bacteria.[5] Presence of this material, known as "sludge," incurs a risk of preterm birth significantly more than that incurred by the cervical length noted earlier (**Fig. 5**).[6]

Box 2
Proposed biomarkers of preterm birth

Amniotic Fluid

    Interleukin (IL)-6

    Glucose

    Monocyte chemotactic protein-1

    Culture

    Whole blood cell count

    Gram stain

    C-reactive protein (CRP)

    Pregnancy-associated placental protein A

Maternal Serum

    IL-6

    IL-8

    Tumor necrosis factor α (TNF-α)

    Ferritin

    CRP

    Maternal serum α-fetoprotein

    Unconjugated estriol uE$_3$ (saliva)

    Corticotropin-releasing hormone

    Human chorionic gonadotropin (hCG)

Maternal Genital Tract

    pH

    FFN

    IL-6

    IL-8

    TNF-α

    Bacterial vaginosis

Technique

A proper technique is critical for accurate and reproducible cervical length measurements. The patient should be examined with an empty bladder to avoid dynamic cervical changes. The TVUS probe is introduced into the anterior vaginal fornix under real-time visualization. Use of TVUS limits measurement variation to 5% to 10%, a marked improvement over digital examination or transabdominal US. A midsagittal view of the cervix is obtained. The probe is then withdrawn just enough to allow the image to blur and then advanced just until the image comes back into focus. This sequence avoids excessive probe pressure on the cervix, which can result in falsely lengthened cervical measurements.

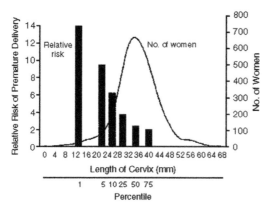

Fig. 2. Distribution of subjects among percentiles for cervical length measured by transvaginal ultrasonography at 24 weeks of gestation (*solid line*) and relative risk of spontaneous preterm delivery before 35 weeks of gestation according to percentiles for cervical length (*bars*). The risks among women with values at or below the 1st, 5th, 10th, 25th, 50th, and 75th percentiles for cervical length are compared with the risks among women with values above the 75th percentile. (*Reproduced from* Iams JD, Goldenberg RL, Meis PJ, et al. The length of the cervix and the risk of spontaneous premature delivery. N Engl J Med 1996;334:569; copyright 1996, Massachusetts Medical Society. All rights reserved; with permission.)

The on-screen electronic calipers are placed at the notches representing the internal os and external cervical os, thereby identifying the bounds of the cervical length measurement (**Fig. 6**). Three such measurements are taken, and the shortest of the 3 is reported as the cervical length, because the initially determined length is often longer than the others.

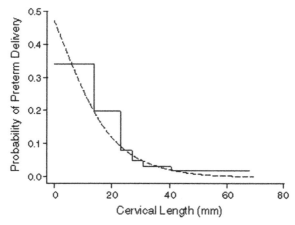

Fig. 3. Estimated probability of spontaneous preterm delivery before 35 weeks of gestation from a logistic regression analysis (*dashed line*) and observed frequency of spontaneous preterm delivery (*solid line*) according to cervical length measured by transvaginal ultrasonography at 24 weeks' gestation. (*Reproduced from* Iams JD, Goldenberg RL, Meis PJ, et al. The length of the cervix and the risk of spontaneous premature delivery. N Engl J Med 1996;334:569, copyright 1996, Massachusetts Medical Society. All rights reserved; with permission.)

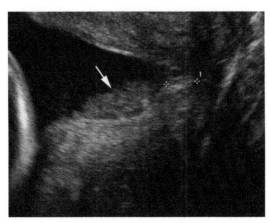

Fig. 4. Echogenic debris (*arrow*), known as "sludge," at level of internal cervical os.

Despite these safeguards for ensuring proper cervical length assessments, several pitfalls may still affect this measurement. At less than 20 weeks' gestation the lower uterine segment is not particularly well developed, making it difficult to reliably determine the location of the internal os (**Fig. 7**). Commonly observed focal myometrial contractions of the lower uterine segment may give a false impression of either increased cervical length or dilation of the internal cervical os (**Fig. 8**). Cervical dynamicism, that is, spontaneous cervical lengthening or shortening, may occur during the examination, precluding an accurate evaluation.[7]

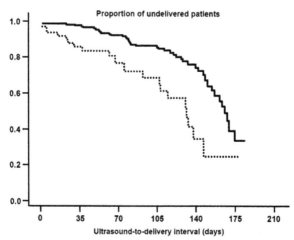

Fig. 5. Kaplan-Meier survival analysis of the ultrasound-to-delivery interval (in days) according to the presence or absence of amniotic fluid (AF) sludge in asymptomatic high-risk patients for preterm delivery. Patients with sludge (*dotted line*) had a shorter ultrasound-to-delivery interval than those without AF sludge (*solid line*) (median of 127 days [95% confidence interval (CI), 120–134] for those positive for AF sludge versus median of 161 days [95% CI, 153–169] for those negative for AF sludge; $P<.001$; log-rank test). (*Reproduced from* Kusanovic JP, Espinoza J, Romero R, et al. Clinical significance of the presence of amniotic fluid 'sludge' in asymptomatic patients at high risk for spontaneous preterm delivery. Ultrasound Obstet Gynecol 2007;30:710; with permission from John Wiley & Sons, Inc.)

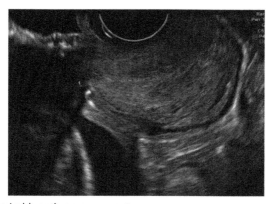

Fig. 6. Normal cervical length measurement.

FETAL FIBRONECTIN
Rationale

FFN, a glycoprotein, is a component of the amniochorionic extracellular matrix. It is believed to act as a "glue," aiding in membrane adherence to the decidua. FFN may normally be detected in cervicovaginal secretions at less than 20 weeks' gestation and more than or equal to 37 weeks' gestation (**Fig. 9**).[8] Between these gestational ages, cervicovaginal FFN is associated with an increased risk of spontaneous preterm birth, suggesting inappropriate release and leakage of FFN in response to inflammation or uterine activity. A recent meta-analysis of FFN testing among women symptomatic for preterm labor calculated a spontaneous preterm birth detection rate of 76.1% (95% confidence interval [CI], 69.1%–81.9%), positive predictive value of 25.9%, and negative predictive value of 97.6% for delivery within 7 days of testing.[9] Among asymptomatic, generally low-risk patients, FFN testing at 24 to 30 weeks' gestation demonstrated test-positive rates of 3.1% to 3.5%, detection rates of 17% to 19%, and positive predictive values of 13% to 24%, with 97% specificity.[10] Although intended for use in singleton pregnancies, a recent study evaluated FFN testing in symptomatic women carrying twins. The results demonstrated somewhat

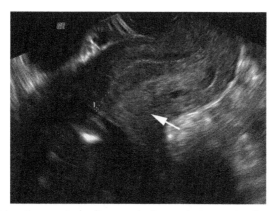

Fig. 7. Second trimester cervical ultrasound demonstrates undeveloped lower uterine segment (*arrow*).

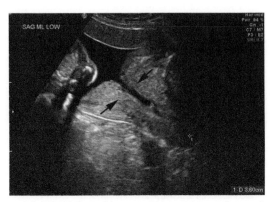

Fig. 8. Focal myometrial contraction of lower uterine segment (*arrows*).

diminished sensitivity for delivery within 14 days of testing for these women versus that for singletons (71% vs 82%) but similar negative predictive values (97% vs 99%).[11]

Technique

A specimen for FFN testing is obtained from the patient during a vaginal speculum examination. The test is intended for women symptomatic for preterm labor with minimal (<3 cm) cervical dilation at 24 0/7 to 34 0/7 weeks' gestation or asymptomatic women from 22 0/7 to 30 6/7 weeks' gestation to provide additional information regarding preterm delivery risk. The manufacturer-provided polyester swab is rotated across the posterior vaginal fornix for 10 seconds to absorb secretions and then placed in the provided tube of buffer. The specimen is labeled and transported to the laboratory for analysis. Validity of the test requires no antecedent cervical manipulation such as sexual intercourse, digital examination, vaginal US, culturing, or

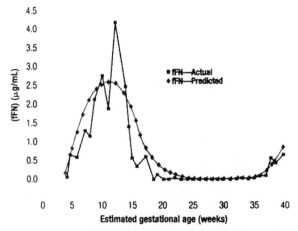

Fig. 9. FFN may normally be detected in cervicovaginal secretions at less than 20 weeks' gestation and more than or equal to 37 weeks' gestation. (*Reproduced from* Ascarelli MH, Morrison JC. Use of fetal fibronectin in clinical practice. Obstet Gynecol Surv 1997; 52:1S–12S; with permission from Lippincott Williams & Wilkins, Inc.)

Papanicolaou smear. Likewise, contamination of the collection swab with lubricants, soaps, or disinfectants may interfere with the test, invalidating results.

To improve patient acceptance and permit nonphysician personnel to obtain samples for FFN testing, investigators have evaluated "blind" collection techniques without a speculum examination. FFN test results after collection by speculum and blind methods were in agreement more than 95% of the time, indicating excellent agreement as measured by the κ statistic (κ = 0.90).[12] Another study found that blind collection offered similar detection rates and negative predictive values in patients observed with the recommended speculum examination.[13]

FFN may be distinguished from other fibronectins by FDC-6 monoclonal antibodies directed against the unique III-CS region of FFN, forming the basis for the available laboratory test. The assay is a solid-phase enzyme-linked immunosorbent assay. Specimen processing via an autoanalyzer requires approximately 20 minutes. If spectrophotometric evaluation at a wavelength of 550 nm notes a sample signal intensity greater than or equal to the calibrated value corresponding to the FFN concentration of 0.050 µg/mL, the result is reported as positive. If the signal intensity is less than the calibrated value, the test result is negative. Internal controls are run with every sample and if unmet, they lead to an invalid test result.

GESTATIONAL AGE- AND RISK-SPECIFIC APPROACH TO USING CERVICAL LENGTH AND FFN IN CLINICAL EVALUATION AND MANAGEMENT

From a clinical perspective, integrating cervical length and FFN into preterm birth risk assessment algorithms is best done in the context of gestational age at evaluation (<24 weeks, ≥24 weeks), history of previous spontaneous preterm birth (yes = high risk, no = low risk), and presence or absence of preterm labor symptoms. Thus, the following discussion is framed in the context of these variables. In general, routine screening of low-risk asymptomatic patients using TVUS or FFN is not recommended because of (1) false-positive test results with low positive predictive values and (2) lack of evidence-based consensus on how to respond to positive test results in these women. Most importantly, the importance of cervical lengths and FFN lies in their extremely high negative predictive values.[14] FFN testing among symptomatic women in particular is associated with fewer hospital admissions for preterm labor, shorter lengths of stay, fewer medical interventions, and lower costs.[15–19]

Earlier than 24 Weeks' Gestation
Cervical length and cerclage
FFN is usually not performed at less than 24 weeks' gestation, as noted earlier. A shortened (<25 mm) cervix in high-risk patients at this gestational age raises the question of cervical insufficiency, classically referred to as "incompetent cervix." No objective diagnostic criteria exist for this condition, and there is no definition uniformly agreed on. However, a reasonable description is "a clinical diagnosis characterized by recurrent painless dilation and spontaneous midtrimester birth, generally in the absence of predisposing conditions, such as spontaneous membrane rupture, bleeding, and infection, characteristics that shift the presumed underlying cause away from cervical incompetence and support other components of the preterm birth syndrome."[20]

At 20 to 24 weeks' gestation, the clinician should rule out uterine contractions, ruptured membranes, acute chorioamnionitis, and fetal death. If present, these conditions are managed according to existing guidelines.[14,21,22] If absent, cervical cerclage may be considered. If the patient is less than 20 weeks pregnant, one may first consider repeating the cervical length after 3 to 7 days of restricted physical activity to ensure accuracy, because performing cervical length sonography at less than 20 weeks' gestation is technically difficult.[23] A recent meta-analysis of randomized trials of cerclage for preterm birth prevention in singleton high-risk pregnancies with a short cervix suggested that cerclage was associated with a significantly lower risk of delivery at less than 35 weeks' gestation, giving a relative risk (RR) of 0.61 (95% CI, 0.40–0.92). Among singletons with a shortened cervix and prior midtrimester loss, cerclage was also associated with a reduced likelihood of delivery at less than 35 weeks' gestation (39% vs 23.4%, number needed to treat = 8; RR = 0.57; 95% CI, 0.33–0.99).[24] Similar findings were noted in a recent randomized trial of cerclage versus no cerclage in women with a history of spontaneous preterm birth.[25]

Current evidence does not support cerclage for the incidental finding of a shortened cervix in women without a prior spontaneous preterm birth or midtrimester pregnancy loss.[26] Other groups known to be at increased risk for spontaneous preterm birth include women carrying twins and women who have undergone prior cervical cone biopsy or loop electrosurgical excision procedures.[26–32] In the former group, cerclage for a short cervix is associated with an increased rate of preterm birth at less than 35 weeks' gestation, with an RR of 2.15 (95% CI, 1.15–4.01).[24] In the latter group, efficacy of cerclage for a shortened cervix has not been evaluated, leaving management speculative.[23]

Additional investigations evaluated the presence or absence of various biomarkers to improve identification of candidates for cerclage on the basis of midtrimester cervical sonography. Sakai and colleagues[33] performed cervical US on 16,508 women in a general obstetric population at 20 to 24 weeks' gestation. Clinicians made the decision to offer cerclage for those with a cervix less than 25 mm in length without knowing cervical interleukin (IL)-8 levels, a marker of inflammation. Women undergoing cerclage with normal IL-8 levels were less likely to deliver at less than 37 weeks' gestation than similar patients not receiving a cerclage (33% vs 54.5%, P = .01). In contrast, subjects undergoing cerclage with elevated IL-8 levels were more likely to deliver preterm than similar subjects not receiving a cerclage (78% vs 54.1%, P = .03). Thus, IL-8 levels, although not commercially available for this purpose, may deserve further evaluation for identifying patients who may experience benefit or even harm from a cerclage.

In another study, Keeler and colleagues[34] stratified outcomes of delivery using results of FFN testing obtained from 18 to 24 weeks' gestation at the time of TVUS. Subjects with cervical lengths less than 25 mm were randomized to cerclage or no cerclage without clinician knowledge of the FFN result. Spontaneous preterm birth at less than 35 weeks' gestation occurred with similar frequency among women who tested positive in FFN with (44.1%) or without (55.2%) cerclage (P = .45), as well as subjects who tested negative in FFN with (17.8%) or without (17%) cerclage (P = .99). The investigators concluded that although FFN does not aid cerclage candidate selection, it may aid in counseling on pregnancy outcome.

Cervical length and progesterone

Supplemental progesterone administered to women with a singleton pregnancy after a previous spontaneous preterm birth significantly reduces the risk of recurrent spontaneous preterm birth.[35] It is remarkable that the effect is most pronounced in patients having deliveries that are very preterm (<32 weeks' gestation). Unfortunately, no such protective effect is observed in twin and triplet gestations.[36–38] The mechanism by which progesterone acts is unclear, but may involve suppressing the fetal inflammatory response and inhibiting cervical ripening.[39–41] Regardless, not all women benefit from progesterone, and among those who do, the benefits may vary. Several studies have therefore evaluated midtrimester cervical length to identify women potentially benefiting from progesterone therapy.

O'Brien and colleagues[42] randomized 659 women with a history of spontaneous preterm birth to receive daily treatment with either 90 mg vaginal progesterone gel or placebo from 16 to 22 6/7 weeks' gestation until 37 weeks' gestation, or until early delivery occurred. There was no difference between groups in the primary outcome of delivery at less than or equal to 32 weeks' gestation: 10% and 11.3%, respectively. A secondary analysis reevaluated the original results by cervical length at study enrollment. Outcomes of subjects with cervical lengths less than or equal to 28 mm were compared by assignment to progesterone or placebo. Among women with a shortened cervix, progesterone therapy was associated with significantly less frequent delivery at less than or equal to 32 weeks' gestation, neonatal intensive care admissions, and shorter neonatal intensive care length of stay.[43]

Another multicenter trial evaluated cervical lengths measured by TVUS at 20 to 25 weeks' gestation in a general obstetric population of singletons and twins. Women with cervical lengths less than or equal to 15 mm were offered randomization to daily oral progesterone, 200 mg or placebo from 24 to 33 6/7 weeks' gestation. The frequency of spontaneous preterm birth at less than 34 weeks' gestation was significantly lower in the group taking progesterone (19.2% vs 34.4%). Although no differences were observed in perinatal morbidity or mortality, the study was not powered to evaluate these outcomes.[44] At present, the American College of Obstetricians and Gynecologists notes that the ideal formulation of progesterone for preterm birth prevention is unknown and that its use should be restricted to women with a documented history of spontaneous preterm birth at less than 37 weeks' gestation.[45]

24 to 34 Weeks' Gestation

The period of 24 to 34 weeks' gestation in pregnancy is beyond the window of classical cervical insufficiency and also marks the early phase of ex utero fetal viability. Thus, clinicians are now concerned with the prevention, diagnosis, and treatment of preterm labor. Unfortunately, the ability to predict and prevent preterm birth remains limited. Therefore, efforts have concentrated on the accurate diagnosis of preterm labor to allow selective and timely obstetric interventions for optimizing neonatal outcomes of fetuses destined for early delivery. Such measures include maternal administration of antibiotics for prophylaxis against invasive group B streptococcal infections, glucocorticoid administration to accelerate fetal lung maturity, and tocolysis to abate uterine contractions and permit transport to a facility capable of providing specialized care of preterm infants. Equally important is the ability to reliably rule out preterm labor among symptomatic women to avoid the potential morbidity, expense, and inconvenience of such treatment.

At less than 37 weeks' gestation, clinical symptoms of at least 6 contractions per hour accompanied by cervical dilation by digital examination of at least 3 cm and 80% effacement, particularly in the presence of ruptured membranes or vaginal bleeding, comfortably allows the diagnosis of preterm labor. Contractions without these associated findings are less clear, leaving the diagnosis uncertain. Therefore, in the authors' practice, a guideline that incorporates TVUS and FFN testing is adopted for evaluating patients presenting with suspected preterm labor.[2]

During the initial assessment, the patient undergoes a vaginal speculum examination. If the membranes are unruptured, a vaginal swab for FFN testing is obtained and held aside. A group B streptococcal culture is obtained as well. If a digital cervical examination and contraction frequency establish a diagnosis of preterm labor, treatment proceeds as outlined. If the diagnosis remains unclear, TVUS is performed. A cervical length more than 30 mm effectively rules out preterm labor; the FFN swab does not need to be sent, and the patient can be managed expectantly. A cervical length less than 20 mm effectively confirms the diagnosis of preterm labor, allowing treatment to proceed. Again, the FFN swab may be discarded. Diagnosis is considered inconclusive for a cervical length of 20 to 30 mm. The FFN swab is sent to the laboratory for processing. A positive FFN result leads to the presumptive diagnosis of preterm labor, whereas a negative result permits expectant care.

The authors recommend screening women presenting with preterm labor symptoms for asymptomatic bacteriuria. Identification and treatment of this condition significantly reduces the risk of preterm delivery (RR = 0.56; 95% CI, 0.43–0.73).[46] Likewise, diagnosis and treatment of bacterial vaginosis in symptomatic women with a prior spontaneous preterm birth can also reduce recurrent preterm delivery risk (RR = 0.42; 95% CI, 0.27–0.67).[47]

It is understandable that not all obstetric care providers always have resources available for TVUS. In such cases, the authors believe that FFN offers sufficiently high sensitivity and negative predictive value to assist in guiding initial clinical decision making. Similarly, not all facilities offer FFN testing. Moreover, cervical manipulation may have occurred before deciding on FFN testing. In these cases, where available, incorporating TVUS with other available clinical information may assist clinical decision making.

SUMMARY

Etiologic and physiologic heterogeneity confound the clinical prediction and prevention of spontaneous preterm birth. Research over the past 15 years demonstrates the remarkable progress made in these areas. Results of these labors include TVUS, cervicovaginal FFN, progesterone therapy, and more selective use of cervical cerclage. Future research is likely to evaluate other markers of preterm birth, maternal abdominal surface uterine electromyography, and proteomic evaluation of maternal and amniotic fluids.[48–51] Imaging and clinical and research laboratories will play central roles in the unfolding story of preterm birth prediction and prevention.

REFERENCES

1. Hamilton BE, Martin JA, Ventura SJ. Births: preliminary data for 2007. National vital statistics reports, March 18, 2009. Available at: http://www.cdc.gov/nchs/data/nvsr/nvsr57/nvsr57_12.pdf. Accessed April 28, 2010.
2. Iams JD. Prediction and early detection of preterm labor. Obstet Gynecol 2003; 101:402–12.
3. Iams JD, Johnson FF, Sonek J, et al. Cervical competence as a continuum: a study of ultrasonographic cervical length and obstetric performance. Am J Obstet Gynecol 1995;172(4 Pt 1):1097–106.
4. Iams JD, Goldenberg RL, Meis PJ, et al. The length of the cervix and the risk of spontaneous premature delivery. National Institute of Child Health and Human Development Maternal Fetal Medicine Unit Network. N Engl J Med 1996; 334(9):567–72.
5. Romero R, Kusanovic JP, Espinoza J, et al. What is amniotic fluid 'sludge'? Ultrasound Obstet Gynecol 2007;30(5):793–8.
6. Kusanovic JP, Espinoza J, Romero R, et al. Clinical significance of the presence of amniotic fluid 'sludge' in asymptomatic patients at high risk for spontaneous preterm delivery. Ultrasound Obstet Gynecol 2007;30(5):706–14.

7. Yost NP, Bloom SL, Twickler DM, et al. Pitfalls in ultrasonic cervical length measurement for predicting preterm birth. Obstet Gynecol 1999;93(4):510–6.

8. Ascarelli MH, Morrison JC. Use of fetal fibronectin in clinical practice. Obstet Gynecol Surv 1997;52(Suppl 4):S1–12.

9. Sanchez-Ramos L, Delke I, Zamora J, et al. Fetal fibronectin as a short-term predictor of preterm birth in symptomatic patients: a meta-analysis. Obstet Gynecol 2009;114(3):631–40.

10. Goldenberg RL, Mercer BM, Meis PJ, et al. The preterm prediction study: fetal fibronectin testing and spontaneous preterm birth. NICHD Maternal Fetal Medicine Units Network. Obstet Gynecol 1996;87(5 Pt 1):643–8.

11. Singer E, Pilpel S, Bsat F, et al. Accuracy of fetal fibronectin to predict preterm birth in twin gestations with symptoms of labor. Obstet Gynecol 2007;109(5):1083–7.

12. Stafford IP, Garite TJ, Dildly GA, et al. A comparison of speculum and nonspeculum collection of cervicovaginal specimens for fetal fibronectin testing. Am J Obstet Gynecol 2008;199(2):131, e1–4.

13. Roman AS, Koklanaris N, Paidas MJ, et al. "Blind" vaginal fetal fibronectin as a predictor of spontaneous preterm delivery. Obstet Gynecol 2005;105(2):285–9.

14. ACOG Practice Bulletin No. 43. Management of preterm labor Obstet Gynecol 2003;101(5 Pt 1):1039–47

15. Joffe GM, Jacques D, Bemis-Heys R, et al. Impact of the fetal fibronectin assay on admissions for preterm labor. Am J Obstet Gynecol 1999;180(3 Pt 1):581–6.

16. Incerti M, Ghidini A, Korker V, et al. Performance of cervicovaginal fetal fibronectin in a community hospital setting. Arch Gynecol Obstet 2007;275(5):347–51.

17. Abenhaim HA, Morin L, Benjamin A. Does availability of fetal fibronectin testing in the management of threatened preterm labor affect the utilization of hospital resources? J Obstet Gynaecol Can 2005;27(7):689–94.

18. Mozurkewich EL, Naglie G, Krahn MD, et al. Predicting preterm birth: a cost-effectiveness analysis. Am J Obstet Gynecol 2000;182(6):1589–98.

19. Lowe MP, Zimmerman B, Hansen W. Prospective randomized controlled trial of fetal fibronectin on preterm labor management in a tertiary care center. Am J Obstet Gynecol 2004;190(2):358–62.

20. Owen J, Iams JD, Hauth JC. Vaginal sonography and cervical incompetence. Am J Obstet Gynecol 2003;188(2):586–96.

21. ACOG Practice Bulletin No. 80. Premature rupture of membranes. Obstet Gynecol 2007;109(4):1007–19.

22. ACOG Practice Bulletin No. 102. Management of stillbirth. Obstet Gynecol 2009;113(3):748–61.

23. Harger JH. Cerclage and cervical insufficiency: an evidence-based analysis. Obstet Gynecol 2003;100(6):1313–27.

24. Berghella V, Odibo AO, To MS, et al. Cerclage for short cervix on ultrasonography: meta-analysis of trials using individual patient-level data. Obstet Gynecol 2005;106(1):181–9.

25. Owen J, Hankins G, Iams JD, et al. Multicenter randomized trial of cerclage for preterm birth prevention in high-risk women with shortened mid-trimester cervical length. Am J Obstet Gynecol 2009;201:375, e1–8.

26. ACOG Practice Bulletin No. 48. Cervical insufficiency Obstet Gynecol 2003;102(5 Pt 1):1091–9.

27. Sjoborg KD, Vistad I, Myhr SS, et al. Pregnancy outcome after cervical cone excision: a case-control study. Acta Obstet Gynecol Scand 2007;86(4):423–8.

28. Berghella V, Pereira L, Gariepy A, et al. Prior cone biopsy: prediction of preterm birth by cervical ultrasound. Am J Obstet Gynecol 2004;191(4):1393–7.

29. Crane JM. Pregnancy outcome after loop electrosurgical excision procedure: a systematic review. Obstet Gynecol 2003;102(5 Pt 1):1058–62.

30. Samson SA, Bentley JR, Fahey TJ, et al. The effect of loop electrosurgical excision procedure on future pregnancy outcome. Obstet Gynecol 2005;105(2):325–32.

31. Noehr B, Jensen A, Fredericksen K, et al. Loop electrosurgical excision of the cervix and risk for spontaneous preterm delivery in twin pregnancies. Obstet Gynecol 2009;114(3):511–5.

32. Jakobsson M, Gissler M, Paavonen J, et al. Loop electrosurgical excision procedure and the risk for preterm birth. Obstet Gynecol 2009;114(3):504–10.

33. Sakai M, Shiozaki A, Tabata M, et al. Evaluation of effectiveness of prophylactic cerclage of a short cervix according to interleukin-8 in cervical mucus. Am J Obstet Gynecol 2006;194(1):14–9.

34. Keeler SM, Roman AS, Coletta JM, et al. Fetal fibronectin testing in patients with short cervix in the midtrimester: can it identify optimal candidates for ultrasound-indicated cerclage? Am J Obstet Gynecol 2009;200(2):158, e1–6.

35. Meis PJ, Klebanoff M, Thom E, et al. Prevention of recurrent preterm birth by 17 alpha-hydroxyprogesterone caproate. N Engl J Med 2003;348(24):2379–85.

36. Norman JE, Mackenzie F, Owen P, et al. Progesterone for the prevention of preterm birth in twin pregnancy (STOPPIT): a randomized, double-blind, placebo controlled study and meta-analysis. Lancet 2009;373(9680):2034–40.

37. Rouse DJ, Caritis SN, Peaceman AM. A trial of 17 alpha-hydroxyprogesterone caproate to prevent prematurity in twins. N Engl J Med 2007;357(5):454–6.

38. Caritis SN, Rouse DJ, Peaceman AM, et al. Prevention of preterm birth in triplets using 17 alpha-hydroxyprogesterone caproate—a randomized controlled trial. Obstet Gynecol 2009;113(2 Pt 1):285–92.

39. Peltier MR, Berlin Y, Tee SC, et al. Does progesterone inhibit bacteria-stimulated interleukin-8 production by lower genital tract epithelial cells? J Perinat Med 2009;37(4):328–33.

40. Yellon SM, Ebner CA, Elovitz MA. Medroxyprogesterone acetate modulates remodeling, immune cell census, and nerve fibers in the cervix of a mouse model for inflammation-induced preterm birth. Reprod Sci 2009;16(3):257–64.

41. Schwartz N, Xue X, Elovitz MA, et al. Progesterone suppresses the fetal inflammatory response ex vivo. Am J Obstet Gynecol 2009;201(2):211, e1–9.

42. O'Brien JM, Adair CD, Lewis DF, et al. Progesterone vaginal gel for the reduction of recurrent preterm birth: primary results from a randomized, double-blind, placebo-controlled trial. Ultrasound Obstet Gynecol 2007;30(5):687–96.

43. DeFranco EA, O'Brien JM, Adair CD, et al. Vaginal progesterone is associated with a decrease in risk for early preterm birth and improved neonatal outcome in women with a short cervix: a secondary analysis from a randomized, double-blind, placebo-controlled trial. Ultrasound Obstet Gynecol 2007;30(5):697–705.

44. Fonseca EB, Celik E, Parra M, et al. Progesterone and the risk of preterm birth among women with a short cervix. N Engl J Med 2007;357(5):462–9.

45. ACOG Committee Opinion No. 419. Use of progesterone to reduce preterm birth Obstet Gynecol 2008;112(4):963–5

46. Romero R, Oyarzun E, Mazor M, et al. Meta-analysis of the relationship between asymptomatic bacteriuria and preterm delivery/low birth weight. Obstet Gynecol 1989;73(4):576–82.

47. Leitich H, Brunbauer M, Bodnar-Aderl B, et al. Antibiotic treatment of bacterial vaginosis in pregnancy: a meta-analysis. Am J Obstet Gynecol 2003;188(3): 752–8.
48. Verdenik I, Pajntar M, Leskosek B. Uterine electrical activity as predictor of preterm birth in women with preterm contractions. Eur J Obstet Gynecol Reprod Biol 2001;95(2):149–53.
49. Grgic O, Matijevic R. Uterine electrical activity and cervical shortening in the mid-trimester of pregnancy. Int J Gynaecol Obstet 2008;102(3):246–8.
50. Garfield RE, Maner WL, Maul H, et al. Use of uterine EMG and cervical LIF in monitoring pregnant patient. BJOG 2005;112(Suppl 1):103–8.
51. Marque CK, Terrien J, Rihana S, et al. Preterm labour detection by use of a biophysical marker: the uterine electrical activity. BMC Pregnancy Childbirth 2007;7(Suppl 1):S1–5.

Toxoplasmosis, Parvovirus, and Cytomegalovirus in Pregnancy

Deborah M. Feldman, MD[a], Diane Timms, DO[b],
Adam F. Borgida, MD[a],*

KEYWORDS

- Toxoplasmosis • Parvovirus • Cytomegalovirus
- Diagnosis • Management

TOXOPLASMOSIS

Toxoplasmosis is caused by the *Toxoplasma gondii* protozoan, an obligate intracellular parasite. The organism can infect any warm-blooded animal or may be found in soil, but its definitive host is the cat family. The organism completes its sexual cycle in feline intestinal epithelial cells and oocysts are shed in the feces for several weeks after the reproductive cycle is completed.[1] Three routes of infection have been identified. Oocysts may be ingested from contaminated cat feces, water, or fruits and vegetables as well as gardening in contaminated soil. Tissue cysts are ingested in infected raw or undercooked meat. In a study of 148 patients including 76 pregnant women with recently acquired infection, age 50 years or more, male sex, Midwest region, working with meat, having 3 or more kittens, eating locally produced cured, dried, or smoked meat, rare lamb, raw ground beef, and unpasteurized goat's milk were found to be associated with infection.[2] A third route of infection is via vertical transmission. Vertical transmission from a pregnant woman to her fetus can cause congenital toxoplasmosis, with consequences including stillbirth, chorioretinitis, deafness, microcephaly, and developmental delay.[3,4]

The true prevalence of toxoplasmosis is unknown because it is not a reportable disease in the United States; however, it was estimated by the fourth National Health

---

[a] Prenatal Testing Center, Division of Maternal Fetal Medicine, Department of Obstetrics and Gynecology, University of Connecticut School of Medicine, Hartford Hospital, 85 Jefferson Street, #625, Hartford, CT 06102, USA
[b] Maternal Fetal Medicine, UConn Health Center, Department of Obstetrics and Gynecology, University of Connecticut School of Medicine, 263 Farmington Avenue, Farmington, CT 06030, USA
* Corresponding author.
E-mail address: aborgid@harthosp.org

Clin Lab Med 30 (2010) 709–720
doi:10.1016/j.cll.2010.04.009
0272-2712/10/$ – see front matter © 2010 Elsevier Inc. All rights reserved.

labmed.theclinics.com

and Nutrition Examination Survey (NHANES) performed from 1999 to 2000.[1] Of 4234 people tested for immunoglobulin (Ig) G antibodies to *Toxoplasma*, 15.8% were positive. Of 2221 women aged 12 49 years, 14.9% were seropositive, leaving 85% of women of child-bearing age susceptible to infection. The rate of congenital toxoplasmosis has been reported to be as high as 10 per 10,000. In a more recent study of 635,000 infants in the New England Regional Newborn Screening Program, it was found to be 1 per 10,000 live births.[3] With approximately 4 million live births in the United States annually, it can be estimated that between 400 and 4000 infants will be born with congenital toxoplasmosis.

Vertical transmission of infection to the fetus is most likely to occur with a primary infection during the pregnancy. However, immunocompromised women with chronic infection may also transmit the disease.[5] More than 90% of pregnant women who acquire a primary infection are asymptomatic, as are 85% of neonates born with congenital toxoplasmosis.[6] Transmission is rare in early pregnancy and increases with duration of pregnancy. Transmission frequency in the first trimester is approximately 15%, 30% in the second trimester, and 60% in the third trimester.[6] Exposure to infection acquired in the first trimester causes more severe congenital toxoplasmosis, with fetuses exposed in the third trimester most likely to be asymptomatic. These infants require treatment to prevent manifestations later in life. Transmission can be decreased by antenatal treatment, and appropriate therapy should be initiated for suspected fetal infection.

Diagnosis

Diagnosis can be made by testing maternal serum for antibodies. Initial testing should measure IgG and IgM antibodies. If both are negative, infection has not occurred. A negative IgM result with a positive IgG during the first or second trimester often indicates an infection that predated the pregnancy; this is also likely in the third trimester but the infection could have occurred early in pregnancy with the IgM level decreased to undetectable levels.[7] A positive IgM result with or without IgG to *Toxoplasma* requires further testing to determine the status of the infection. IgM antibodies may represent false-positive results or chronic or past infection, as they can persist for 1 year or more.[8]

Up to 60% of patients positive for IgM in the community have results inconsistent with recent infection on confirmatory testing at the reference laboratory.[9] Therefore, confirmation is important before consideration of elective termination of pregnancy. In 1 study, confirmatory testing decreased the rate of abortion from 17.2% to 0.4%.[9]

Confirmatory testing consists of the *Toxoplasma* serologic profile (TSP), performed at reference laboratories such as the Toxoplasma Serology Laboratory of the Palo Alto Medical Foundation. The panel of tests available includes the Sabin-Feldman test, the differential agglutination (AC/HS) test, IgG avidity, and enzyme-linked immunosorbent assay (ELISA) for IgM, IgE, and IgA.

ELISA is used to qualitatively determine the presence or absence of antibodies by adding serum to a well containing *T gondii* antigen bound to an enzyme. A fluorescent substrate is then added that will fluoresce if antigen-antibody linking has occurred.[10] The presence of IgA and IgE on ELISA implies recent infection.

The IgG avidity test measures the strength of antigen-antibody binding, which increases with duration of infection. Avidity is determined by diluting the substrates in an immunoassay with urea and comparing the ratio of antibody titer in an untreated well with that of the urea-treated well.[11] High avidity requires at least 3 months to develop, and so helps to rule out acute infection.

Ultrasound can be used to detect certain fetal manifestations of infection. Findings suggestive of congenital toxoplasmosis include unilateral or bilateral ventriculomegaly, ascites, intracranial or intrahepatic calcifications, hepatomegaly, and splenomegaly.[7] In the absence of abnormalities, monthly ultrasonographic monitoring should continue throughout the pregnancy.

Amniocentesis can be offered for polymerase chain reaction (PCR) testing of the amniotic fluid. The procedure should be performed after 18 weeks's gestation and 4 or more weeks after the estimated date of infection. Amplification of the B1 gene of the parasite is used to assess for the presence of infection. In a study performed at 3 centers in France, overall sensitivity was 64% with a negative predictive value of 98.8%. There were no false-positives, yielding a specificity of 100%, as well as a positive predictive value of 100%.[12] The sensitivity of PCR diagnosis was highest when maternal infection occurred between 17 and 21 weeks. Although other studies have suggested a higher sensitivity,[13,14] a negative PCR result does not rule out congenital disease and adequate treatment and follow-up are still indicated for these patients.

Treatment

Vertical transmission of newly acquired infection during early pregnancy at 18 weeks or more can be prevented by administration of oral spiramycin, 1 g every 8 hours. This macrolide antibiotic does not cross the placenta, so is not appropriate for fetal treatment. In the absence of signs of fetal infection, spiramycin should be continued until delivery. The drug is not commercially available in the United States, but can be obtained at no cost from the Food and Drug Administration or the reference laboratories that perform confirmatory testing.[6] Spiramycin does not seem to have any fetal effects, however a small percentage of women may develop gastrointestinal side effects.[6,15]

If seroconversion occurs after 18 weeks or fetal infection is confirmed by PCR or ultrasound findings, treatment should be initiated. Pyrimethamine 50 mg twice daily for 2 days followed by 50 mg per day, sulfadiazine 75 mg/kg per day in 2 divided doses for 2 days followed by 50 mg/kg twice daily, and folinic acid 10 to 20 mg per day, may prevent congenital infection at later gestational ages and also treat the fetus.[6] Pyrimethamine is a folic acid anatagonist that is teratogenic early in pregnancy, therefore its use in the first trimester should be avoided. It is not associated with hyperbilirubinemia, but may cause bone marrow depression.[16] Folinic acid may help prevent hematologic toxicity.

Immunocompromised women with chronic infection may rarely transmit the parasite to the fetus, resulting in congenital infection. This includes women with AIDS as well as those on immunosuppressive treatment. Vertical transmission may occur in up to 4% of cases, particularly when the CD4 count is less than 100/mm^3.[17] The risk of transmission is low when the CD4 count is greater than 200/mm^3. Consideration should be given to screening all immunosuppressed women for evidence of a history of infection to establish an early diagnosis of reactivation. Seropositive women with low CD4 counts should receive trimethoprim-sulfamethoxazole to prevent reactivation of *Toxoplasma*. Because of reports of congenital toxoplasmosis in mild or moderately immunosuppressed women, it is recommended that women infected with human immunodeficiency virus with CD4 counts less than 200/mm^3 or immunocompromised women not infected with HIV be treated with spiramycin for the duration of pregnancy.[6]

Prevention

In a recent survey of pregnant women in the United States, only 48% of respondents had heard of toxoplasmosis but 60% were aware that *Toxoplasma* is shed in the feces of cats and can be contracted by changing cat litter. Only 30% knew of the association with raw or undercooked meat.[18] A 2009 survey of obstetricians practicing in the United States showed that 87.7% counsel patients about how to prevent toxoplasmosis and why, with 78% of counseling occurring only at the first prenatal visit.[19] The rate of primary infection may be decreased by as much as 63% to 92% by counseling pregnant woman on how to avoid infection.[20]

Secondary prevention strategies to prevent fetal infection in women who contract the disease are in place in many countries with a higher incidence of toxoplasmosis than the United States, including France and Austria. In these countries, all women are screened for antibodies to *Toxoplasma* on initiation of prenatal care. Seronegative women are rechecked monthly to allow for intervention if a new infection is detected. In the United States, several states have instituted newborn serologic screening for *Toxoplasma* IgM. However, this does not allow for prenatal intervention, and may miss neonates infected early in gestation or late in the third trimester.[5]

PARVOVIRUS

Parvovirus B19 is a small, single-stranded DNA virus that infects only humans. It most commonly presents as erythema infectiosum, or fifth disease, a common viral exanthem in children. Typically the disease is characterized by fever and an erythematous rash on the cheeks. It is self-limited and symptoms resolve within 7 to 10 days. Immunity after the disease is life-long, and at least 50% of adults are immune from exposure to the virus during childhood. Clinical manifestations for those adults who are susceptible to the virus include malaise, a reticular rash, and joint pain/swelling that may last from days to months. Approximately 20% to 30% of patients have no symptoms at all.[21]

Transmission of parvovirus B19 occurs most commonly through spread of respiratory droplets. The incubation period is 5 to 10 days after exposure and before any symptoms. By the time a rash is present, respiratory secretions and serum are usually free of the virus and the patient is no longer contagious.[22]

Because parvovirus B19 preferentially infects rapidly dividing cells and is cytotoxic for erythroid progenitor cells, there is concern about the effect of fetal transmission from an infected mother. Among the first reported association between parvovirus B19 and fetal nonimmune hydrops was a case series published in the mid to late 1980s after an outbreak of the virus in a Connecticut community in 1986.[23] Since then, several hundred publications have reported the potential risks and outcomes, and management plans for parvovirus in pregnancy have been outlined.

Diagnosis of Maternal Infection

Maternal serology using ELISA, Western blot, or radioimmunoassay is the most common method of detecting the presence of IgG and IgM immunoglobulins, which are both produced in response to infection with parvovirus B19. The sensitivity of these assays to detect IgG and IgM is generally around 70% to 80%.[24] The IgM-specific antibody is usually present by the third to fifth day after symptoms present, and may persist for several weeks to months. Positive IgM antibody indicates acute infection. The presence of IgG antibodies is noted approximately 7 days after the onset of symptoms and lasts indefinitely. In the absence of IgM antibodies, a positive IgG indicates an old infection and therefore immunity. Cases of recurrent or persistent parvovirus are extremely rare. The prevalence of IgG antibodies to the virus increases with age, with 2% to 10% rates of seropositivity in preschool-age children to 60% in adolescents and adults.[25]

Diagnosis of Fetal Infection

Ultrasound is the primary tool for diagnosing congenital parvovirus B19 infection. Because of the affinity of the virus for erythroid stem cells, infected fetuses may become profoundly anemic. In addition, the virus can attack the myocardium, causing a cardiomyopathy, as well as direct hepatic injury that may impair protein synthesis and lower colloid oncotic pressure. All of these effects may lead to hydrops fetalis, which is readily diagnosed with ultrasound (**Fig. 1**). Hydrops occurs in up to 10% of pregnancies in which parvovirus infection is documented before 20 weeks. The risk for hydrops lowers significantly if infection occurs in the late second or third trimester. Infection early in the first trimester is associated with a higher risk for spontaneous abortion than in uninfected pregnancies.[26] Fetal parvovirus B19 infection can also be diagnosed using PCR of amniotic fluid or in fetal/placental tissue after a fetal demise.[26,27]

Management of Parvovirus B19 Infection During Pregnancy

Following exposure to parvovirus B19, the pregnant patient should be tested for the presence of IgG and IgM antibodies. If immunity is documented by the presence of IgG and the absence of IgM antibodies, the patient can be reassured that her fetus is not at risk for prenatal infection. If IgG and IgM antibodies are undetectable, this indicates that the patient is susceptible to infection and titers should be repeated in 3 to 4 weeks. If they remain negative, the patient remains susceptible to the disease without evidence of infection. Continued hand-washing and avoidance of possible sources of infection are recommended. There is no vaccine or known medical treatment of the virus, so routine screening and avoidance of work among school teachers or daycare providers is recommended.

Should the patient have evidence of seroconversion with positive titers of IgG and IgM antibodies, ultrasound surveillance of the fetus should be initiated. Attention should be focused on the presence of ascites, pleural or pericardial effusions, or scalp edema. In addition, more recent evidence supports the use of middle cerebral artery (MCA) Doppler to evaluate for fetal anemia (**Fig. 2**), as this may be detected before fetal hydrops.[28,29] The incubation period for congenital infection may be longer than in adults, and reports of fetal hydrops have been made as long as 8 to 10 weeks after exposure. Therefore, we recommend weekly ultrasounds for approximately 10 weeks after exposure to the virus. If no hydrops or evidence of anemia has been

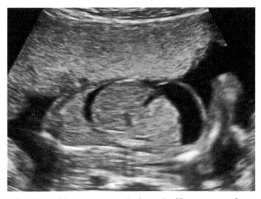

Fig. 1. Fetal hydrops diagnosed by ascites and pleural effusions in a fetus with known parvovirus B19 infection.

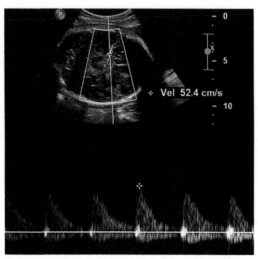

Fig. 2. MCA-peak systolic velocity to screen for fetal anemia after acute parvovirus B19 infection.

demonstrated by then, the likelihood of its development is small.[30] Few cases of fetal death in the absence of hydrops have been attributed to parvovirus B19.

If there is evidence of fetal hydrops or anemia by an increased peak systolic velocity through the MCA, a cordocentesis should be performed when technically possible. Although the disease is often self-limited and there have been cases of spontaneous resolution of hydrops reported,[10] an in utero blood transfusion is indicated in cases of severe anemia. This is best performed intravascularly through the umbilical vein using ultrasound guidance.[31,32]

Neonatal Outcomes after Parvovirus Infection

There have been few data published on the long-term outcomes of fetuses requiring in utero blood transfusion because of parvovirus B19 infection. Barring any complications related to the procedure itself, most fetuses do well after intravascular transfusion even if they are profoundly anemic before the procedure. Results regarding the neurodevelopment of these infants after birth are slightly conflicting. Most studies suggest normal neurologic outcomes after appropriate therapy. One small retrospective study reported a higher rate of delayed psychomotor development in children aged 6 to 8 years who had undergone intrauterine transfusion for parvovirus B19 infection, suggesting a potential effect of the virus on the central nervous system.[33] A larger controlled study suggested a similar rate of developmental delay among infants born to mothers with acute parvovirus infection during pregnancy compared with controls.[34]

CYTOMEGALOVIRUS

Human cytomegalovirus (CMV) is an enveloped DNA herpes virus. It has numerous characteristics of a herpes virus including the ability to cause congenital infection. The seroprevalence of CMV is approximately 50% in adults in industrialized countries. Approximately 0.6% to 0.7% of infants born in the United States are congenitally infected making it the most common cause of infection-related congenital handicaps.[35] Vertical transmission of CMV depends on numerous factors including type and timing of infection. Treatment of congenital CMV infection is an active area of research, and the Institute of Medicine has rated the development of a CMV vaccine a high priority.[36]

CMV infection is typically asymptomatic in immunocompetent adults. Less than 5% of pregnant women with a primary CMV infection are symptomatic, making the diagnosis of infection in pregnancy difficult.[37] CMV infection is known to cause neurologic sequelae in newborns; however, prediction of vertical transmission can be difficult. Neurologic handicap is possible after either primary or recurrent infection. However, after primary infections with CMV, about one-third of newborns acquire a CMV infection but only approximately 1% to 2% of newborns acquire CMV after a recurrent infection.[35,38] Up to 90% of infants who are symptomatic at birth will have serious long-term handicaps including hearing loss, visual impairment, mental retardation, and/or mild cognitive impairment.[39] In contrast, asymptomatic newborns are at much less risk for serious long-term impairment, in the range of 5% to 15%.[38,40] The timing in gestation has also been described as an important risk factor for vertical transmission. Third trimester infection seems to have a higher rate of vertical transmission, but the incidence of symptomatic newborns with these late infections is much less than first trimester vertical transmission.[41] In contrast, the rate of vertical transmission after maternal infection early in pregnancy is low, but in cases of congenital infection, the rate of severe disease is much higher.[42,43]

Maternal Infection

Acute maternal infection to CMV can be considered if a woman has seroconversion of CMV IgG during her pregnancy. In this situation, her nonimmune status would have to have been previously established. Another possible indicator of acute maternal infection is CMV IgG and/or IgM antibodies. However, CMV IgM antibodies can persist for more than 6 months making it difficult to determine the precise timing of infection.[44] In addition, there has been concern about the accuracy of commercially available CMV antibody test kits.[45] CMV IgM may also be present with reinfection and false-positive results have been reported from other viral infections.[45,46]

When there is a question of acute maternal CMV infection, IgG avidity testing may be the most reliable way to confirm the diagnosis. Low avidity IgG antibodies are present in acute or recent primary CMV infections.[47] If testing is performed at 16 to 18 weeks's gestation, anti-CMV IgG avidity testing has been reported to have a 100% sensitivity for newborn infection.[48] If high avidity CMV IgG is detected by 16 weeks, a recent infection can be ruled out.

Fetal Infection

If acute maternal infection is suspected in pregnancy, fetal infection can then be investigated. Historically, fetal blood sampling was performed by cordocentesis to determine fetal immune status. Because the fetus may not be immunocompetent in early gestation, fetal immune status may not be helpful until late in pregnancy. There is also concern about the safety and availability of cordocentesis.[49] Amniocentesis, which is much safer than cordocentesis, can obtain amniotic fluid for detection of CMV by PCR. PCR of amniotic fluid has a reported sensitivity and specificity of more than 90% for vertical transmission of CMV.[50,51] Viral culture or CMV early antigen testing has also been performed to confirm vertical transmission, but the speed and accuracy of PCR have made it the standard diagnostic test for fetal infection of CMV.

As mentioned earlier, fetal infection may be suspected during pregnancy from ultrasound findings suspicious for CMV infection. These findings include early onset intrauterine growth restriction, microcephaly, ventriculomegaly, liver calcifications, echogenic bowel, and fetal hydrops (**Fig. 3**). Unfortunately, only about 5% to 25% of infected newborns have ultrasound evidence of congenital infection.[52] However, if fetal anomalies are detected, it would infer a more severely affected newborn.[53] Any ultrasound findings suspicious for congenital CMV infection should prompt a serologic and/or invasive diagnostic evaluation to determine if an acute infection is present. Amniocentesis with CMV PCR has been reported to be most accurate for diagnosing fetal infection when performed after 20 weeks's gestation making this the ideal time for the procedure.[54,55]

Treatment

Once fetal CMV infection has been confirmed, no standard therapy for in utero treatment has been established. A recent nonrandomized trial of CMV hyperimmune globulin was promising for treatment of acute fetal CMV infection. Women who received CMV hyperimmune globulin during pregnancy had only a 3% incidence of a symptomatic newborn at birth and 2 years of age, whereas untreated women had a 50% incidence.[56] There are no specific antiviral regimens for fetal treatment of CMV infection but postnatal treatment of severely affected newborns has been reported with ganciclovir and valganciclovir with varying degrees of efficacy.[47,57] Pregnancy termination remains an option for pregnancies with CMV infection, but this should be reserved for cases with documented acute fetal infection after a thorough diagnostic evaluation and extensive counseling.

Routine screening for CMV infection in pregnancy is controversial and will remain so until an efficacious treatment of acute fetal infection is established. A recent study evaluated 3 screening strategies and showed that universal screening could be cost effective if treatment of CMV in pregnancy could achieve at least a 47% reduction in disease.[58] Until then, education on prevention with good hygiene makes most sense for women known to be at risk for primary CMV infection.

SUMMARY

There are many infections that may be asymptomatic or cause only mild clinical symptoms in an immunocompetent adult, but cause much more significant consequences in a developing fetus. Depending on the gestational age of infection, there is wide variation in the pregnancy outcomes of women who acquire toxoplasmosis, parvovirus, or CMV during pregnancy. Most fetal outcomes are favorable even for those with

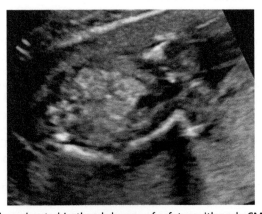

Fig. 3. Echogenic bowel noted in the abdomen of a fetus with early CMV infection.

documented infection during pregnancy. However, there remains much anxiety among patients who develop these infections. With proper screening, maternal and fetal testing, and treatment where appropriate, these patients can be provided with the best possible pregnancy outcome.

REFERENCES

1. Jones J, Kruszon-Moran D, Wilson M. *Toxoplasma gondii* infection in the United States, 1999–2000 [serial online] [2009 September]. Emerg Infect Dis 2003. Available at: http://www.cdc.gov/ncidod/EID/vol9no11/03-0098.htm. Accessed October 22, 2009.
2. Jones J, Dargelas V, Roberts J, et al. Risk factors for *Toxoplasma gondii* infection in the United States. Clin Infect Dis 2009;49:878–84.
3. Guerina NG, Hsu H-W, Meissner H, et al. Neonatal serologic screening and early treatment for congenital *Toxoplasma gondii* infection. N Engl J Med 1994;330: 1858–63.
4. McClure E, Goldenberg R. Infection and stillbirth. Semin Fetal Neonatal Med 2009;14:182–9.
5. Centers for Disease Control and Prevention. Preventing congenital toxoplasmosis. MMWR Recomm Rep 2000;49:57–75.
6. Montoya J, Remington J. Management of *Toxoplasma gondii* infection during pregnancy. Clin Infect Dis 2008;47:554–66.
7. Montoya J, Rosso F. Diagnosis and management of toxoplasmosis. Clin Perinatol 2005;32:705–26.
8. Del Bono V, Canessa A, Bruzzi P, et al. Significance of specific immunoglobulin M in the chronological diagnosis of 38 cases of toxoplasmic lymphadenopathy. J Clin Microbiol 1989;27:2133–5.
9. Liesenfeld O, Montoya J, Tathineni N, et al. Confirmatory serologic testing for acute toxoplasmosis and the rate of induced abortions among women reported to have positive *Toxoplasma* immunoglobulin M antibody titers. Am J Obstet Gynecol 2001;184:140–5.
10. Lequin RM. Enzyme immunoassay (EIA)/enzyme-linked immunosorbent assay (ELISA). Clin Chem 2005;51:2415–8.
11. Lefevre-Pettrazzoni M, Le Cam S, Wallon M. Delayed maturation of immunoglobulin G avidity: implication for the diagnosis of toxoplasmosis in pregnant women. Eur J Clin Microbiol Infect Dis 2006;25:687–93.
12. Romand S, Wallon M, Franck F, et al. Prenatal diagnosis using polymerase chain reaction on amniotic fluid for congenital toxoplasmosis. Obstet Gynecol 2001;97: 296–300.
13. Foulon W, Pinon J, Stray-Pederson B, et al. Prenatal diagnosis of congenital toxoplasmosis: a multicenter evaluation of different diagnostic parameters. Am J Obstet Gynecol 1999;181:843–7.
14. Bessieres M, Berrebi A, Cassaing S, et al. Diagnosis of congenital toxoplasmosis: prenatal and neonatal evaluation of methods used in Toulouse University Hospital and incidence of congenital toxoplasmosis. Mem Inst Oswaldo Cruz 2009;104: 389–92. [Online].
15. Cook G. Use of antiprotozoan and anthelmintic drugs during pregnancy: side-effects and contra-indications. J Infect 1992;25:1–9.
16. Peters PJ, Thigpen MC, Parise ME, et al. Safety and toxicity of sulfadoxine/pyrimethamine: implications for malaria prevention in pregnancy using intermittent preventive treatment. Drug Saf 2007;30:481–501.

17. Bachmeyer C, Mouchnino G, Thulliez P, et al. Congenital toxoplasmosis from an HIV-infected woman as a result of reactivation. J Infect 2006;52:e55–7.

18. Jones J, Ogunmodede G, Scheftel J, et al. Toxoplasmosis-related knowledge and practices among pregnant women in the United States. Infect Dis Obstet Gynecol 2003;11:139–45.

19. Ross D, Rasmussen S, Cannon M, et al. Obstetrician/gynecologists' knowledge, attitudes, and practices regarding prevention of infections in pregnancy. J Womens Health 2009;18:1187–93.

20. Breugelmans M, Naessens A, Foulon W. Prevention of toxoplasmosis during pregnancy–an epidemiologic survey over 22 consecutive years. J Perinat Med 2004;32:211–4.

21. Chorba T, Coccia P, Holman RC, et al. The role of parvovirus B19 in anaplastic crisis and erythema infectiosum (fifth disease). J Infect Dis 1986;154:383–93.

22. Thurn J. Human parvovirus B19: historical and clinical review. Rev Infect Dis 1988;10:1005–11.

23. Rodis JF, Hodick TJ, Quinn DL, et al. Human parvovirus in pregnancy. Obstet Gynecol 1988;72(5):733–8.

24. Anderson LJ, Tsou C, Parker RA, et al. Detection antibodies and antigens of human parvovirus B19 by enzyme-linked immunosorbent assay. J Clin Microbiol 1986;24:522–6.

25. Hall SM, Cohen BJ, Mortimer PP, et al. Prospective study of human parvovirus (B19) infection in pregnancy. Public Health Laboratory Service Working Party on Fifth Disease. BMJ 1990;300(6733):1166–70.

26. Riipinen A, Vaisanen E, Nuutila M, et al. Parvovirus B19 infection in fetal deaths. Clin Infect Dis 2008;47(12):1519–25.

27. Kovacs BW, Carlson DE, Shahbahrami B, et al. Prenatal diagnosis of human parvovirus B19 in nonimmune hydrops fetalis by polymerase chain reaction. Am J Obstet Gynecol 1992;167:461–6.

28. Moise KJ Jr. The usefulness of middle cerebral artery Doppler assessment in the treatment of the fetus at risk for anemia. Am J Obstet Gynecol 2008;198(2):161 e1–4.

29. Borna S, Mirzaie F, Hanthoush-Zadeh S, et al. Middle cerebral artery peak systolic velocity and ductus venosus velocity in the investigation of non-immune hydrops. J Clin Ultrasound 2009;37(7):385–8.

30. Rodis JF, Borgida AF, Wilson M, et al. Management of parvovirus infection in pregnancy and outcomes of hydrops: a survey of members of the Society of Perinatal Obstetricians. Am J Obstet Gynecol 1998;79(4):985–8.

31. Schild RL, Bald R, Plath H, et al. Intrauterine management of fetal parvovirus B19 infection. Ultrasound Obstet Gynecol 1999;13(3):161–6.

32. Odibo AO, Campbell WA, Feldman DM, et al. Resolution of human parvovirus B19-induced nonimmune hydrops after intrauterine transfusion. J Ultrasound Med 1998;17(9):547–50.

33. Nagel HT, de Haan TR, Vandenbussche FP, et al. Long-term outcome after fetal transfusion for hydrops associated with parvovirus B19 infection. Obstet Gynecol 2007;109(1):42–7.

34. Rodis JF, Rodner C, Hansen AA, et al. Long-term outcome of children following maternal human parvovirus B19 infection. Obstet Gynecol 1998;91(1):125–8.

35. Kenneson A, Cannon MJ. Review and meta-analysis of the epidemiology of congenital cytomegalovirus (CMV) infection. Rev Med Virol 2007;17:253–76.

36. Institute of Medicine Committee to Study Priorities for Vaccine Development. Vaccines for the 21st Century: a tool for decision making. In: Stratton KR, Durch JS, Lawrence RS, editors. Washington, DC: National Academy Press; 2000. p. 460.

37. Pass RF. Cytomegalovirus. In: Jeffries DJ, Hudson CN, editors. Viral infections in obstetrics and gynecology. New York: Arnold; 1999. p. 35–6.

38. Fowler FB, Stagno S, Pass RF, et al. The outcome of congenital cytomegalovirus in relation to maternal antibody status. N Engl J Med 1992;326:663–7.

39. Boppana SB, Pass RF, Britt WJ, et al. Symptomatic congenital cytomegalovirus infection: neonatal morbidity and mortality. Pediatr Infect Dis J 1992;11:93–9.

40. Fowler KB, Dahle AJ, Boppana SB, et al. Newborn hearing screening: will children with hearing loss caused by congenital cytomegalovirus infection be missed? J Pediatr 1999;135:60–4.

41. Gindes L, Teperberg-Oikawa M, Sherman D, et al. Congenital cytomegalovirus infection following primary maternal infection in the third trimester. BJOG 2008; 115:830–5.

42. Daiminger GJ, Bader U, Enders G. Pre- and periconceptional primary cytomegalovirus infection: risk of vertical transmission and congenital disease. Br J Obstet Gynaecol 2005;112:166–72.

43. Leisnard C, Donner C, Brancart F, et al. Prenatal diagnosis of congenital cytomegalovirus infection: prospective study of 237 pregnancies at risk. Obstet Gynecol 2000;95:881–8.

44. Stagno S, Pass RF, Cloud G, et al. Primary cytomegalovirus infection in pregnancy: incidence, transmission to fetus and clinical outcome. JAMA 1986;256: 1904–8.

45. Lazzarotto T, Brojanac S, Maine GT, et al. Search for cytomegalovirus-specific immunoglobulin M: comparison between a new western blot, conventional western blot and nine commercially available assays. Clin Diagn Lab Immunol 1997;4:483–6.

46. Lazzarotto T, Gabrielli L, Lanari M, et al. Congenital cytomegalovirus infection: recent advances in the diagnosis of maternal infection. Hum Immunol 2004;65: 410–5.

47. Lazzarotto T, Spezzacatena P, Pradelli P, et al. Avidity of immunoglobulin G directed against human cytomegalovirus during primary and secondary infections in immunocompetent and immunocompromised subjects. Clin Diagn Lab Immunol 1997;4:469–73.

48. Lazzarotto T, Varani S, Spezzacatena P, et al. Maternal IgG avidity and IgM detected by blot as diagnostic tools to identify pregnancy women at risk of transmitting cytomegalovirus. Viral Immunol 2000;13:137–41.

49. Weiner CP. Cordocentesis. Obstet Gynecol Clin North Am 1988;15:283–301.

50. Lipitz S, Yagel S, Shalev E, et al. Prenatal diagnosis of fetal primary cytomegalovirus infection. Obstet Gynecol 1997;89:763–7.

51. Guerra B, Lazzarotto T, Quarta S, et al. Prenatal diagnosis of symptomatic congenital cytomegalovirus infection. Am J Obstet Gynecol 2000;183:476–82.

52. Ville Y. The megalovirus. Ultrasound Obstet Gynecol 1998;12:151–3.

53. Guerra B, Simonazzi G, Puccetti C, et al. Ultrasound prediction of symptomatic congenital cytomegalovirus infection. Am J Obstet Gynecol 2008;198:380, e1–7.

54. Pass RF, Fowler KB, Boppana SB, et al. Congenital cytomegalovirus infection following first trimester maternal infection: symptoms at birth and outcome. J Clin Virol 2006;35:216–20.

55. Reullan-Eugene G, Barjot P, Campet M, et al. Evaluation of virologic procedures to detect fetal human cytomegalovirus infection: avidity of IgG antibodies, virus detection in amniotic fluid and maternal serum. J Med Virol 1996;50:9–15.
56. Nigro G, Adler SP, La Torre R, et al. Passive immunization during pregnancy for congenital cytomegalovirus infection. N Engl J Med 2005;353:1350–62.
57. Muller A, Eis-Hubinger AM, Brandhorts G, et al. Oral valganciclovir for symptomatic congenital cytomegalovirus infection in an extremely low birth weight infant. J Perinatol 2008;25:74–6.
58. Cahill AG, Odibo AO, Stamillo DM, et al. Screening and treating for primary cytomegalovirus infection in pregnancy: where do we stand? A decision-analytic and economic analysis. Am J Obstet Gynecol 2009;201:466, e1–7.

Screening for Open Neural Tube Defects

David A. Krantz, MA*, Terrence W. Hallahan, PhD,
John E. Sherwin, PhD

KEYWORDS

- Alpha-fetoprotein • Open neural tube defect
- Screening • Pregnancy

Maternal serum screening for fetal congenital anomalies began in the early 1970s with the advent of alpha-fetoprotein (AFP) screening for neural tube defects.[1,2] It was from this screening protocol that the initial observation that AFP is low in Down syndrome–affected pregnancies was made.[3] Today, screening for Down syndrome is highly complex with protocols that include various combinations of serum and ultrasound markers across the first and second trimesters of pregnancy. However, since its inception, maternal serum screening for open neural tube defects (open spina bifida and anencephaly) has remained quite simple and straightforward by relying on a single AFP test during the second trimester of pregnancy.

Maternal serum AFP (MSAFP) screening is conducted between 15 and 21 weeks of gestation. Blood specimens may be collected as liquid whole blood or dried blood spots.[4] Median MSAFP levels increase steadily by about 15% per week from a concentration of approximately 25 IU/mL at 15 weeks of gestation to a level of approximately 60 IU/mL at 21 weeks of gestation. To account for this upward trend in normal levels throughout pregnancy, values of AFP are converted into multiples of the gestational age–specific median (MoMs) by dividing the patient's analytical AFP concentration by the median concentration for that gestation. The MoM values are then typically corrected for demographic factors such as maternal weight, ethnicity, and diabetic status.

Patients with higher maternal weight have lower MSAFP levels than those with lower maternal weight.[5] As a result, the MoM values for patients with higher maternal weight are adjusted downward, whereas patients with lower maternal weight are adjusted upward (**Fig. 1**).

MSAFP levels have been demonstrated to vary by ethnicity. The most significant shift is observed in African American patients who tend to have MoM values that are on average 16% greater than in White patients after weight adjustment.

Biostatistics Department, NTD Labs/PerkinElmer, 80 Ruland Road, Melville, NY 11747, USA
* Corresponding author.
E-mail address: david.krantz@perkinelmer.com

Clin Lab Med 30 (2010) 721–725
doi:10.1016/j.cll.2010.04.010
0272-2712/10/$ – see front matter © 2010 Elsevier Inc. All rights reserved.

labmed.theclinics.com

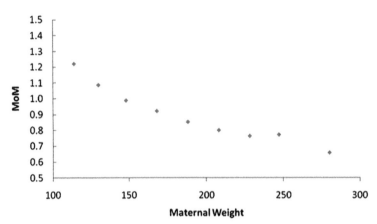

Fig. 1. Median AFP MoM versus median weight in 21,972 White patients.

Insulin-dependent diabetes mellitus (IDDM) affects open neural tube defect screening in 2 ways. First, the incidence of open neural tube defects is three- to four-fold higher in diabetic patients who are insulin dependent.[6] Second, MSAFP levels are approximately 20% lower in patients with IDDM compared with the general population.[7] However, recent publications have suggested that this adjustment factor may no longer be necessary.[8]

In cases of open spina bifida and anencephaly, openings in the spine or skull result in leakage of AFP into the amniotic fluid, which then diffuses into the maternal blood causing significant increases in MSAFP levels. The median MoM value in open spina bifida at 16 weeks of gestation is 3.8 MoM, whereas the median MoM value for anencephaly is 6.5 MoM.[9] The typical cutoff for MSAFP screening is 2.0 to 2.5 MoM. Using a cutoff of 2 MoM can increase detection of open spina bifida by approximately 10%. The detection rate for open spina bifida using a 2-MoM cutoff is 90%, whereas virtually all cases of anencephaly can now be detected unless there is a significantly incorrect gestational age.[10]

Twin pregnancies can be evaluated for open neural tube defects; however, the discrimination between the distribution of AFP levels in neural tube defect and unaffected pregnancy is much less than in singleton pregnancy. In an affected twin pregnancy, the median MoM is 4.4 in open spina bifida and 7.5 in anencephaly.[11] Compared with the unaffected twin median (1.9 MoM), this represents a 2.3- and 3.9-fold increase in affected cases for open spina bifida and anencephaly, respectively, compared with a 3.8- and 6.5-fold increase in a singleton pregnancy. The reason for the smaller discrimination is that the AFP level in affected twin pregnancy represents a mixture of AFP levels from both the unaffected and affected fetus. Thus, whereas the median MoM in unaffected twin pregnancy is approximately double that of a singleton pregnancy, the median MoM in an affected twin pregnancy is not twice as great as that in an affected singleton pregnancy.

Using a cutoff of 4 multiples of the singleton median, the detection rate in twins is 93% for anencephaly and 58% for open spina bifida with a 7.8% false positive rate. Using a 5-MoM cutoff, the detection rate is 83.0% for anencephaly and 39.0% for open spina bifida with a 3.3% false positive rate.[11] Laboratories may report the results in twins based on the singleton median, in which case the cutoff will be 4 or 5 MoM, or they may adjust the MoM for twins, in which case the cutoff will be identical to the cutoff used in singleton pregnancy (2.0–2.5 MoM).

Laboratories usually provide a patient-specific risk for open spina bifida, anencephaly, and ventral wall defect on patient reports. Risks are determined by factoring in the distribution of AFP MoM values and the prior incidence of these disorders. The incidence of open neural tube defects is approximately 1 to 2 per 1000 in the United States; however, these incidence rates vary from region to region. Incidence rates are highest in the southeastern United States and are lowest in the northwest. In addition, incidence rates vary by ethnic group with African Americans having a lower incidence than Whites.[12] In addition, the incidence of neural tube defects is increased in patients who previously have had a child with open neural tube defect and to a lesser extent if there is family history of open neural tube defect.[13] There is a 1% occurrence risk of open spina bifida in patients taking valproic acid or carbamazepine medication.[14,15] Today, however, it is difficult to accurately assess these risks because multiple factors make it difficult to ascertain the actual incidence of neural tube defects.

Since the early 1990s, the American College of Obstetricians and Gynecologists have recommended that pregnant women ingest 400 μg of folic acid daily to prevent neural tube defects, thus lowering the incidence of open neural tube defects.[16] In addition, because a large number of affected pregnancies are terminated, incidence rates at birth are no longer accurate. As a result, it is difficult to quantify the incidence rates compared with historically observed data. Thus risk figures provided by laboratories that rely on historical incidence rates may not be as precise as they were in the past. Furthermore, it is now possible to detect anencephaly during the nuchal translucency examination that is undertaken as part of first trimester Down syndrome screening.[17] Therefore, the risk of anencephaly quantitated based on MSAFP levels may no longer be relevant.

Specimens with results between 2.0 and 2.5 MoM may be considered to be borderline elevated. In such cases, a repeat maternal serum blood specimen can better differentiate between false positives and affected pregnancies. A second blood test result will tend to have "regression to the mean." In the case of open neural tube defects, the "regression to the mean" phenomenon has a significant advantage because the MSAFP levels in open spina bifida and anencephaly are significantly greater than 2.5 MoM. As a result, a second maternal serum blood specimen will tend to regress toward these higher MoM values, whereas a second maternal serum blood specimen from an unaffected pregnancy will tend to regress toward 1.0 MoM. Therefore, in open spina bifida and anencephaly pregnancies, a second blood specimen will tend to be higher, whereas in unaffected pregnancy, a second blood specimen will tend to be lower, thus improving screening performance.

For patients with MSAFP results above 2.5 MoM or those with 2 results over 2.0 MoM, follow-up testing should be offered. Biochemically, elevated amniotic fluid AFP with confirmation by acetylcholinesterase is an effective diagnostic test for neural tube defects. However, follow-up assessment with ultrasound to visualize the defect should be performed before any decision is made regarding continuation of the pregnancy. In recent years, it has been argued that it may be preferable to perform the detailed ultrasound before amniocentesis and offer amniocentesis only to confirm neural tube defects visualized on ultrasound.

In normal pregnancy, amniotic fluid AFP decreases by approximately 20% per week from a level of 15 μg/mL at 15 weeks of gestation to 4.4 μg/mL at 21 weeks of gestation. As mentioned previously, in cases of neural tube defect, AFP leaks into the amniotic fluid through openings in either the skull or spine, causing an increase in measured amniotic fluid AFP. Elevated amniotic fluid AFP may be associated with conditions other than neural tube defects and can also occur when there is fetal blood contamination of the amniotic fluid. As a result, confirmation should be performed using

Table 1
Incidence of adverse outcomes associated with elevated maternal serum AFP

Outcome	Relative Risk
Major nonchromosomal congenital defect	4.7
Fetal death	8.1
Neonatal death	4.7
Low birth weight	4.0
Newborn complications	3.6
Oligohydramnios	3.4
Abruption	3.0
Preeclampsia	2.3

Data from Milunsky A, Jick SS, Bruell CL, et al. Predictive values, relative risks, and overall benefits of high and low maternal serum alphafetoprotein screening in singleton pregnancies: new epidemiologic data. Am J Obstet Gynecol 1989;161:291–7.

acetylcholinesterase and fetal hemoglobin assays. Positive acetylcholinesterase results are an indication that an open neural tube defect may be suspected, whereas positive fetal hemoglobin results may explain elevated AFP results in the presence of negative acetylcholinesterase.

In cases where open neural tube defect has been ruled out, elevated MSAFP still imparts increased risk of adverse pregnancy outcome. Approximately 25% of patients with elevated MSAFP will have an adverse pregnancy outcome.[4,10] **Table 1** shows the increase in risk attributable to elevated MSAFP for specific disorders as provided by Milunsky and colleagues.[10]

REFERENCES

1. Brock DJ, Bolton AE, Monaghan JM. Prenatal diagnosis of anencephaly through maternal serum-alphafetoprotein measurement. Lancet. 1973;2(7835):923–4.
2. Macri JN, Weiss RR, Schell NB, et al. Progress in screening for neural tube defects. JAMA. 1977;237:2187.
3. Merkatz IR, Nitowsky HM, Macri JN, et al. An association between low maternal serum alpha-fetoprotein and fetal chromosomal abnormalities. Am J Obstet Gynecol. 1984;148:886–94.
4. Macri JN, Anderson RW, Krantz DA, et al. Prenatal maternal dried blood screening with alpha-fetoprotein and free beta-human chorionic gonadotropin for open neural tube defect and Down syndrome. Am J Obstet Gynecol. 1996; 174:566–72.
5. Wald N, Cuckle H, Boreham J, et al. The effect of maternal weight on maternal serum alpha-fetoprotein levels. Br J Obstet Gynaecol. 1981;88:1094–6.
6. Mills JL, Knopp RH, Simpson JL, et al. Lack of relation of increased malformation rates in infants of diabetic mothers to glycemic control during organogenesis. N Engl J Med 1988;318:671–6.
7. Henriques CU, Damm P, Tabor A, et al. Decreased alpha-fetoprotein in amniotic fluid and maternal serum in diabetic pregnancy. Obstet Gynecol. 1993;82:960–4.
8. Sancken U, Bartels I. Biochemical screening for chromosomal disorders and neural tube defects (NTD): is adjustment of maternal alpha-fetoprotein (AFP) still appropriate in insulin-dependent diabetes mellitus (IDDM)? Prenat Diagn. 2001; 21:383–6.

9. Fourth report of the UK collaborative study on alpha-fetoprotein in relation to neural tube defects. Estimating an individual's risk of having a fetus with open Spina Bifida and the value of repeat alpha-fetoprotein testing. J Epidemiol Community Health. 1982;36(2):87–95.
10. Milunsky A, Jick SS, Bruell CL, et al. Predictive values, relative risks, and overall benefits of high and low maternal serum alpha-fetoprotein screening in singleton pregnancies: new epidemiologic data. Am J Obstet Gynecol 1989;161:291–7.
11. Cuckle H, Wald N, Stevenson JD, et al. Maternal serum alpha-fetoprotein screening for open neural tube defects in twin pregnancies. Prenat Diagn 1990;10(2):71–7.
12. Greenberg F, James LM, Oakley GP Jr. Estimates of birth prevalence rates of spina bifida in the United States from computer-generated maps. Am J Obstet Gynecol. 1983;145:570–3.
13. Main DM, Mennuti MT. Neural tube defects: issues in prenatal diagnosis and counseling. Obstet Gynecol 1986;1:67.
14. Robert E, Guibaud P. Maternal valproic acid and congenital neural tube defects. Lancet 1982;320:937.
15. Rosa FW. Spina bifida in infants of women treated with carbamazepine during pregnancy. N Engl J Med 1991;324:675–7.
16. Centers for Disease Control (CDC). Use of folic acid for prevention of spina bifida and other neural tube defects—1983–1991. MMWR Morb Mortal Wkly Rep 1991; 40:513–6.
17. Johnson SP, Sebire NJ, Snijders RJ, et al. Ultrasound screening for anencephaly at 10–14 weeks of gestation. Ultrasound Obstet Gynecol 1997;9:14–6.

First- and Second-Trimester Screening for Preeclampsia and Intrauterine Growth Restriction

Methodius G. Tuuli, MD, MPH*, Anthony O. Odibo MD, MSCE

KEYWORDS

• Preeclampsia • Intrauterine growth restriction • Screening

Preeclampsia and intrauterine growth restriction (IUGR) are major contributors to perinatal mortality and morbidity.[1] Although there is increasing understanding of the pathophysiology of these conditions, their prevention remains a considerable challenge in obstetrics. It is now well understood that although the symptoms of preeclampsia and IUGR generally manifest in the second to third trimester of pregnancy, their underlying development largely takes place in the first trimester.[2] This finding has sparked great interest in the search for tests to predicting preeclampsia and IUGR early in pregnancy before these complications occur.

Regardless of the lack of effective prophylactic or therapeutic interventions, the ability to predict preeclampsia has several advantages. First, it would identify those women who require more intensive monitoring. Second, it would possibly permit earlier recognition and intervention. Third, it would further clarify the pathophysiology of these conditions and permit more mechanism-specific interventions. In addition, accurate prediction permits targeting of potential preventive measures to those at risk and allows the interventions to be timed early, before the underlying condition is established.

Several individual clinical factors, Doppler ultrasound parameters, and serum analytes have been evaluated for prediction of preeclampsia and/or IUGR. On their own these tests generally have poor predictive value. This finding may reflect the multifactorial nature of the preeclampsia syndrome. However, a combination of selected

Funding support: none.
Division of Maternal-Fetal Medicine and Ultrasound, Department of Obstetrics and Gynecology, Washington University School of Medicine, Campus Box 8064, 4566 Scott Avenue, St Louis, MO 63110, USA
* Corresponding author.
E-mail address: tuulim@wudosis.wustl.edu

parameters and results of recent novel measures seem promising. This article reviews first- and second-trimester screening tests for preeclampsia and IUGR. It begins with a brief overview of the pathophysiology of these conditions, followed by a discussion of the general principles underlying screening tests. The individual screening tests are then reviewed. Because there is considerable overlap between the underlying pathophysiology of preeclampsia and IUGR, the overlaps are not stratified separately but are highlighted when there are possible differences.

PATHOPHYSIOLOGY

Although the precise origin of preeclampsia remains elusive, it is thought to be multifactorial, with the placenta playing a central role. In recent years a clearer picture of the pathophysiology has began to emerge.[3] A 2-stage model has been proposed in which poor placentation, the central initiating event, is believed to occur early. This first stage results from failure of the normal physiologic process in early pregnancy in which endovascular trophoblast invades the maternal vasculature and replaces the smooth muscle normally present in the spiral arterioles with a noncontractile matrix material. The result of this normal but seemingly destructive event is a high-flow, low-resistance vascular conduit that perfuses the intervillous space.[4] This process is reflected by a decrease in the uterine artery resistance with increasing gestation. Failure of the trophoblast invasion leaves a high-resistance vasculature with persistent smooth muscle histology of the maternal blood vessels. This lack of transformation predisposes to hypoperfusion, hypoxia reperfusion injury, oxidative stress, and signs of placental maldevelopment in the second trimester.[5] Recent evidence suggests that a significant part of placental injury is mechanical damage resulting from intermittent perfusion caused by persistence of smooth muscle in the spiral arterioles.[6]

The second stage of preeclampsia pathogenesis is the maternal response to abnormal placentation, which is initially adaptive, but subsequently resulting in widespread systemic injury. Key features of this second phase are systemic endothelial dysfunction[3,7] and an imbalance of circulating vasoactive factors.[8–10] Many of the resulting features can be detected before clinical signs of disease (preeclampsia or IUGR) appear, creating an opportunity for potential predictive tests.

There is emerging evidence that the pathophysiology described earlier is more consistent with preterm preeclampsia with coexisting IUGR than term preeclampsia.[11] For example, placental pathologic studies indicate that preeclampsia or IUGR resulting in preterm delivery before 34 weeks has high rates of thrombotic placental pathologic findings of the villous trees.[12] By contrast, term preeclampsia and/or IUGR was associated with either normal or minimal pathologic findings.[13] Doppler studies also suggest that preterm preeclampsia/IUGR is associated with defective invasion of the spiral arteries, whereas the spiral artery defect plays a smaller role in the cases nearer term.[14] Thus, term preeclampsia and IUGR seem to be associated with normal trophoblast transformation in the first trimester and late atherosclerotic changes in spiral arterioles. Such late changes may be the consequence of increased placental mass as occurs in diabetic and twin pregnancies, senescence of the placenta as in prolonged pregnancy, or placental edema and necrosis as in fetal hydrops.[15]

PRINCIPLES OF SCREENING

Screening tests are commonly used in clinical practice, yet the underlying principles of screening are widely misunderstood.[16] A brief overview is provided of these principles to place the discussion of specific screening tests for preeclampsia and IUGR in perspective.

Screening is the testing of apparently healthy people to find those at increased risk of developing a disease or disorder. Important properties of a screening test are its sensitivity, specificity, negative predictive value, and positive predictive value. Sensitivity is the probability of a screening test being positive when the individual manifests the disease, whereas specificity is the probability that the test is negative when the individual does not develop the disease. In practice, sensitivity and specificity are often inversely related, with increase in sensitivity producing a decrease in specificity and vice versa. For continuous measures, receiver-operator characteristics (ROC) curves are useful in determining the optimum trade-off of sensitivity and specificity. The area under the ROC curve also provides information on the discriminating ability of the screening test, with a value more than 0.75 suggesting a good screening test.

The sensitivity and specificity of a test are intrinsic properties of the test and cannot be used to estimate the probability of the disease in an individual. Positive and negative predictive values designate the probability of developing or not developing a disease given a positive or negative test, respectively. However, they are dependent on the prevalence of the disease in the population and are therefore limited in their ability to be extrapolated from one population to another.

Likelihood ratios are used to circumvent the limitations of predictive values, because they are independent of disease prevalence. They integrate the sensitivity and specificity of screening tests and are dependent only on the ability of a test to distinguish between individuals who will develop the disease and those who will not. Positive and negative likelihood ratios provide information on how many times more or less likely individuals who will develop the disease are to have a positive or negative test result than those who will not develop the disease. Likelihood ratios therefore indicate by how much a given test result increases or decreases the probability of developing a condition. The greater the positive likelihood ratio, the larger the increase in the probability of developing the condition, if the test is positive. On the other hand, the smaller the negative likelihood ratio, the larger the decrease in the probability of the condition, if the test is negative. Thus, the most clinically useful screening tests are characterized by high positive and low negative likelihood ratios. Generally, tests with positive likelihood ratios greater than 10 and negative likelihood ratios less than 0.1 are likely to be clinically useful, whereas those with positive and negative predictive values of less than 5 and greater than 0.2, respectively, have minimal predictive potential.[17] Mathematical conversion permits the use of likelihood ratios and pretest probabilities to estimate the posttest probability that an individual will or will not develop the condition, once the test result is known. An additional advantage is the ability to use likelihood ratios of different screening tests sequentially to produce a final posttest probability. To do this, the posttest probability after one test serves as the pretest probability for the next test.

Although negative and positive likelihood ratios are independent of the prevalence of the disease, the clinical usefulness of screening tests significantly depends on disease prevalence. For preeclampsia, the low overall prevalence (1.3–6.7% in developing countries and 0.4–2.8% in industrialized countries)[18] dictates that any useful predictive test must have a high positive likelihood ratio to significantly increase the probability that individuals with a positive result will develop preeclampsia and low negative likelihood ratio to confidently conclude that individuals with a negative result will not develop preeclampsia. In addition to high positive and low negative likelihood ratios, the ideal test for preeclampsia should be simple, acceptable, rapid, noninvasive, inexpensive, feasible early in pregnancy, and use widely available technology. In addition, results of the test must be valid, reliable, and reproducible.[19]

Because few tests have high enough discriminating characteristics, a common approach is to combine them. Multiple screening tests may be performed sequentially or in tandem (parallel or simultaneously). This approach results in higher sensitivity than would otherwise be possible with any of the tests alone.[20,21]

SPECIFIC SCREENING TESTS

Proposed screening tests for preeclampsia are grouped according to the type as well as the presumed pathophysiologic basis for the test (**Box 1**). We provide a brief discussion of each test or groups of tests and summarize results of studies evaluating their performance in screening for preeclampsia. For brevity, results of recent systematic reviews and meta-analysis are used when available and emphasis is placed on the more recent screening modalities. When tests are uniquely used in either the first or second trimester, the designation is specified.

Clinical Factors

Several prepregnancy- and pregnancy-related factors have been associated with increased risk of preeclampsia and IUGR (**Box 2**). These factors may increase the likelihood of preeclampsia through placental mechanisms or predisposition to maternal cardiovascular disease. The use of clinical risk factors has the advantage of being free of cost, noninvasive, and routinely collected. However, clinical factors have not been found to be an effective screening tool for preeclampsia and IUGR in the general obstetric population because of their poor sensitivity and specificity.[22] The role of risk factor assessment may be in the identification of individuals at higher risk for preeclampsia and IUGR than baseline, in whom other screening tests may be applied.[23] The combination of risk factors with other screening tests may improve their screening efficiency for preeclampsia and IUGR.[24]

Placenta Perfusion Dysfunction–related Factors

Uterine artery Doppler velocimetry
Enhanced uterine artery resistance reflects failure of trophoblastic invasion of the spiral arteries and is associated with the development of preeclampsia and IUGR.[15,25] Increased resistance to vascular flow can be measured noninvasively by Doppler flow studies of the myometrial segments of the arteries supplying the spiral arterioles. Uterine artery Doppler ultrasonography is performed via the transvaginal or transabdominal routes. The uterine artery is identified with the aid of color Doppler, and then pulse-waved Doppler ultrasonography is performed to obtain waveforms from which indices are calculated. The indices include the systolic (S) to diastolic (D) velocity ratio (S/D), pulsatility index (PI)($PI = S - D/V_m$, where V_m is the mean velocity throughout the cardiac cycle), resistive index (RI)($RI = S - D/S$) and early diastolic notching (characteristic waveform indicating decreased early diastolic flow in the uterine artery compared with later diastolic flow). Increased uterine artery resistance as measured by PI or RI greater than a chosen value and/or percentile or the presence of unilateral or bilateral diastolic notches has been investigated for the prediction of preeclampsia and IUGR. The use of different criteria for defining abnormal uterine artery flow is one of the limitations to comparing results across different studies.

Abnormal uterine artery Doppler studies in the the first and second trimesters have been shown to be associated with preeclampsia and IUGR. A recent update of a meta-analysis of studies using uterine artery Doppler indices to predict preeclampsia produced several important conclusions.[19,23] First, irrespective of the Doppler artery

---

Box 1
Candidate screening tests for preeclampsia and IUGR

1. Clinical risk factor screening

2. Placenta perfusion dysfunction–related tests

   Uterine artery Doppler ultrasonography

   Two-dimensional (2D) placenta imaging

   Three-dimensional (3D) placenta imaging

   Placental volume

   Placenta quotient

   Placenta vascular indices

3. Maternal serum analytes

   Down syndrome markers

   α-Fetoprotein (AFP)

   Human chorionic gonadotropin (hCG)

   Estriol

   Inhibin A

   disintegrin and metalloproteases (ADAM)

   Placental protein 13

4. Endothelial dysfunction–related tests

   Circulated angiogenic factors

   Placental growth factor (PlGF)

   Soluble fms-like tyrosine kinase 1

   Vascular endothelial growth factor (VEGF)

   Soluble endoglin (sEng)

   Entholial cell adhesion molecules

   Selectin

5. Markers of insulin resistance

   Tumor necrosis factor

   Sex hormone–binding globulin (SHBG)

   Adiponectin

   Leptin

6. Genomics and proteomics

---

indices used, predictive accuracy in low-risk populations was moderate to minimal, whereas that in high-risk population was minimal. The sensitivities and specificities of uterine artery Doppler indices in low-risk populations varied from 34% to 76% and 83% to 93%, respectively. Second, the best predictor indices were increased PI and the presence of bilateral notching, with positive likelihood ratio of 5. In high-risk populations, all uterine artery Doppler indices had poor predictive ability with positive and negative likelihood ratios of 2.5 to 3.3 and 0.4 to 0.8, respectively. Third, the

Box 2
Risk factors for preeclampsia and IUGR

A. Preeclampsia

  1. Prepregnancy factors

    Chronic hypertension

    Renal disease

    Diabetes mellitus

    Connective tissue disease

    Thrombophilia

    Uncontrolled hyperthyroidism

    Polycystic ovarian syndrome

    Age older than 40 years and younger than 20 years

    Obesity/insulin resistance

    Preeclampsia in a previous pregnancy

    Primipaternity

    Limited sperm exposure

    Pregnancies from artificial reproductive technology

    Partner who fathered preeclamptic pregnancy with another woman

    Smoking (reduced risk)

    Family history of preeclampsia

  2. Pregnancy-related factors

    Multifetal gestation

    Chromosomal abnormality (triploidy, trisomy 13)

B. IUGR

  1. Prepregnancy factors

    Chronic hypertension

    Renal disease

    Diabetes with vasculopathy

    Autoimmune syndromes: antiphospholipid syndrome, lupus

    Thrombophilia

    Maternal hypoxemia (cyanotic heart disease, severe chronic anemia, chronic pulmonary disease)

    Uterine anomalies: large submucous myomas, septate uterus, synechia

    Smoking

    Substance abuse: alcohol, heroin, methadone, cocaine, therapeutic agents

    Malnutrition

    Family history of IUGR

  2. Pregnancy-related factors

    Fetal chromosomal abnormality (trisomy 13, 18, and 21, triploidy, uniparental disomy)

Fetal malformations (gastroschisis, omphalocele, diaphragmatic hernia, congenital heart defect)

Maternal infection: malaria, rubella, cytomegalovirus, herpes, toxoplasmosis

Multiple gestation

predictive accuracy for early onset preeclampsia is moderate to good, irrespective of the index or combination of indices used.

Another recent systematic review and meta-analysis concluded that, for preeclampsia and IUGR, Doppler testing was more accurate in the second than the first trimester. Increased PI with notching in the second trimester emerged as the best predictor of preeclampsia. The investigators strongly recommended their routine use in clinical practice.[26] That review has been strongly criticized and the recommendation labeled premature, as it is based on only 2 studies (one of which included 1757 low-risk women and the other 351 high-risk women) and the tests (increased PI with notching) produced insufficiently high positive likelihood ratios of positive (7.5) and poor negative likelihood ratios for both populations (0.59 and 0.82, respectively).[27] Several methodological concerns were appropriately raised, including absence of formal tests for heterogeneity, publication bias, and the inappropriate pooling of sensitivities and specificities.[27]

Although uterine artery Doppler velocimetry shows promise especially for the prediction of early onset preeclampsia and IUGR, standards are lacking for gestational age of screening and criteria for an abnormal test. Thus, current evidence does not support routine screening with uterine artery Doppler ultrasonography in low- or high-risk populations.

3D placenta imaging

The size of the placenta and the vascular flow patterns within the placental villous tree in early pregnancy may predict adverse pregnancy outcomes, including preeclampsia and IUGR. Small placental volume results from shallow invasive activity of the extravillous trophoblast. This situation may be secondary to a reduction in oxygen tension in the intervillous space and/or the activation of inhibitors of trophoblast differentiation and proliferation.[4] Improvements in sonographic imaging provide a tool for estimating placental volume and villous blood flow using three- and four-dimensional scanning techniques.[28,29] Parameters evaluated for predicting preeclampsia and IUGR include the placental volume itself, placental quotient (PQ), and vascular indices.

PQ

The PQ, defined as the ratio of the placental volume to the fetal crown–rump length, quantifies the size of the placenta in relation to the fetus in the first trimester. Decreased placental volume at 11 to 14 weeks of gestation has been implicated in the subsequent development of preeclampsia and IUGR, with a predictive value similar to and independent of uterine artery Doppler indices.[30,31] Hafner and colleagues[30] reported high negative predictive value of PQ, enabling it to define a subgroup at low risk for perinatal complication. PQ performed better in predicting severe preeclampsia with IUGR requiring delivery before 34 weeks' gestation. However, it was not useful for screening in a low-risk population with sensitivity of 38.5% for preeclampsia and 27.1% for small for gestational age (SGA). Combining the assessment of placental volume with the first trimester uterine artery Doppler screening may improve the detection rate of preeclampsia to values similar to that of late second-trimester screening, with the added advantage of early screening.

Placental Vascular Indices

Vascular indices within the placenta are calculated from three-dimensional data formed by the voxels (the basic information units of volume) for vascularization assessment of organs and structures. These indices represent the total and relative amounts of power Doppler information within the volume of interest. The vascularization index (VI) quantifies the number of color-coded voxels to all voxels within the volume expressed as a percentage, flow index (FI) represents the power Doppler signal intensity from all color-coded voxels and vascularization flow index (VFI) is the mathematical relationship derived from multiplying VI by FI. These indices are believed to reflect the number of blood vessels within the volume (VI), the intensity of flow at the time of the 3D sweep (FI), and blood flow and vascularization (VFI). After acquisition of the 3D image, machine-specific software is used to calculate the placental indices. 3D ultrasound with power Doppler has been shown to be particularly useful and superior to 2D ultrasound in the determination of the distal vascular branches of the fetal placental blood vessels.[32] When the entire image of the placenta cannot be obtained in a single sweep, vascular biopsy or sonobiopsy has been proposed to obtain a representative sample of the placenta.[33] A recent study noted that 2 of the indices obtained from sonobiopsy (VI and VFI) are similar to those from whole placenta evaluation.[34]

Placental flow indices obtained by these techniques have been correlated with gestational age, alterations in fetal growth, amniotic fluid volume, and Doppler biometric parameters of fetoplacental circulation.[35–37] Reduction in these indices may be an early marker of placental dysfunction. A study in normal and growth-restricted pregnancies revealed that FI, which identifies the most severe cases of placental impairment, was the most reliable index.[37] After assessing placental vascularization in 208 normal fetuses between 12 and 40 weeks of gestation and 13 pregnancies with IUGR at 22 to 39 weeks' gestation, Noguchi and colleagues[36] found that VI values in 8 of 13 fetal growth restriction (FGR) pregnancies (61.5%), FI value in one IUGR pregnancy (7.7%) and VFI values of 6 IUGR pregnancies (46.2%) were less than −1.5 standard deviations of the reference ranges for VI, FI, and VFI, respectively.

Although this technology shows promise, no large-scale studies have been performed to validate its use. In addition, technical and methodological issues must be addressed before its general application.[38–41] First- and second-trimester studies using standardized techniques are under way to clarify the usefulness of this tool in predicting adverse pregnancy outcomes including preeclampsia and IUGR.

2D placenta imaging

Examination of the placenta is a normal part of routine obstetric ultrasound examinations. In the standard B-mode, the normal placenta is relatively homogeneous, with areas of differing echogenicity as pregnancy progresses secondary to varying degrees of calcification. Abnormalities in the placenta in 2D imaging, including decreased length and thickness, infarcts, abnormal texture, and presence of echogenic cystic lesions, have been associated with adverse pregnancy outcomes, including preeclampsia and IUGR. A method for systematic 2D placental ultrasound examination has been described and used, often in combination with other parameters for screening.[42] Abnormal placental morphology is defined by shape, texture, or both and determined by measurement of the maximal placental length and thickness with placental thickness greater than 4 cm or greater than 50% of placental length, defining an abnormal shape; categorizing placental texture as normal (homogeneously granular), heterogeneous (echogenic patches alternating with normal texture), or abnormal when the placenta contains either multiple echogenic cystic lesions or assumes a jelly-like appearance with turbulent uteroplacental flow visible because of lack of normal villous development; and defining placental cord insertion as normal (>2 cm from the placental disc margin), lateral (within 2 cm of the margin), marginal (on the margin), or velamentous (inserting into the surrounding membranes).[42]

Using this method of placenta examination Toal and colleagues[25] in a cohort of 60 high-risk women with abnormal uterine artery Doppler indices, found higher odds of IUGR in patients with abnormally shaped placentas when compared with those with normally shaped placentas. The same group used placental morphology from 2D imaging in combination with maternal serum screening and uterine artery Doppler indices to define a placenta function profile, which was then used to screen for placenta-related adverse pregnancy outcomes, including IUGR and preeclampsia in 212 high-risk pregnancies.[43] Although the combined test proved useful in predicting women who would and would not have adverse pregnancy outcomes, no data were reported on the predictive performance of the placental morphology from 2D imaging of the placenta alone.

To date, no large-scale prospective studies have validated the use of 2D placenta imaging in the prediction of preeclampsia or IUGR. This modality has significant limitations including poor resolution, difficulty assessing nonanteriorly located placentas, and wide variability in the morphology of normal placentas. Three- and four-dimensional scanning techniques are significant improvements that are likely to prove more useful than 2D imaging in delineating placental structure.

Maternal Serum Analytes

Maternal serum analytes provide minimally invasive tests of fetal and placental endocrine function as well as endothelial dysfunction. Current understanding of the pathophysiology of preeclampsia and IUGR provides the basis for these screening tests. The failure of trophoblastic invasion may be related to dysregulated secretory activity of the trophoblasts, whereas alteration in the surface layer of the syncytiotrophoblast may contribute to leakage of hCG and AFP into the maternal circulation.[44,45] Reduced placental size or defective syncytiotrophoblast formation may result in reduced production of placenta-derived proteins, such as pregnancy-associated protein A (PAPP-A).[46] Hypoxia-reoxygenation may be responsible for the increased secretion of proinflammatory cytokines, such as tumor necrosis factor α (TNF-α) and interleukin 1β, and antiangiogenic factors, such as the soluble receptor for VEGF (sFlt-1).[47–49] Hypoxia-reoxygenation may also result in increased apoptosis in trophoblasts, leading to the release of free fetal DNA into maternal circulation.[49] Endothelial cell damage, platelet activation dysfunction, and disturbances in coagulation may be responsible for increased P-selectin and markers of insulin resistance.[7,50,51]

Many of the tests of fetal and placental endocrine function are measured in the first and/or second trimester as part of routine prenatal care. The use of these analytes is attractive because results are routinely available. However, they have generally yielded poor predictive characteristics, increasing interest in the development and testing of novel markers.

Fetal and placental endocrine dysfunction–related tests
Down syndrome markers Second-trimester serum screening for Down syndrome is routinely offered to women, either as the triple test (AFP, hCG, and unconjugated

estriol) or with the addition of inhibin A as the quadruple test. More recently, first-trimester screening with fetal nuchal translucency, hCG and PAPP-A is in use. Because of their origin and sites of metabolism these biochemical markers may be useful in the prediction of preeclampsia and IUGR. Several studies have investigated their role as predictive tests for preeclampsia and IUGR.

A recent meta-analysis summarized results of relevant studies to determine the accuracy of the 5 serum analytes used in Down serum screening (hCG, AFP, uncon-jugated estriol, PAPP-A and inhibin A) for prediction of preeclampsia and/or SGA.[52] A total of 44 studies, including 169,637 pregnant women (4376 preeclampsia cases) and 86 studies, including 382,005 women (20,339 FGR cases) met the selection criteria. The results showed low predictive accuracy overall. For preeclampsia, the best predictor was inhibin A level greater than 2.79 multiples of the median (MoM) with positive likelihood ratio of 19.5 (95% confidence interval [CI] 8.3–45.8) and negative likelihood ratio of 0.3 (95% CI 0.1–0.7). For SGA the best predictor was AFP level greater than 2.0MoM with positive likelihood ratio of 28.0 (95% CI 8.0–97.5) and negative likelihood ratio of 0.8 (95% CI 0.6–1.1). The investigators acknowledged methodological and reporting limitations in the included studies as well as heterogeneity, which resulted in wide confidence intervals of the pooled estimates.

Although an attractive screening modality because of its widespread availability, Down serum screening analytes by themselves have low predictive accuracy for preeclampsia and SGA. However, they may be a useful means of risk assessment or used in combination with other screening tests.

ADAM ADAM12 is a placenta-derived multidomain glycoprotein involved in control-ling fetal and placental growth and development. ADAM12-S (the short isoform) is the secreted form and can bind to adhesion receptors and mediate shedding of oxy-tocinase, which may be associated with progressive growth of the placenta.[53,54] Reduced ADAM12 has been shown to be a potential marker of preeclampsia and IUGR in the first trimester.[55–57] Concentration of ADAM12 in normal pregnancies varies with gestational age, African American race, and maternal weight, necessitating adjustment for these variables before comparing results with pathologic pregnancies.[58]

The screening performance of first-trimester ADAM12 alone is poor. For a 5% false-positive rate, it can detect only 26.6% of the preeclampsia pregnancies and 7% to 20% of the SGA pregnancies.[56–58] After adjusting for maternal weight and race in a case-control study, Poon and colleagues[58] noted that maternal serum ADAM12 concentration at 11 to 13 + 6 weeks of gestation in pregnancies developing preeclampsia or gestational hypertension was neither significantly different from normotensive pregnancies nor associated with the severity of preeclampsia. These investigators concluded that the development of preeclampsia associated with low levels of ADAM12 may be a reflection of the association between the development of preeclampsia and increasing maternal weight.

Studies to date suggest that ADAM12 may have a limited or no role as a predictive test for preeclampsia and IUGR. Results of ongoing studies may further clarify these observations.

Placental protein 13 Placental protein 13 (PP13), a member of the galectin family, is produced by syncytiotrophoblast. It binds to proteins on the extracellular matrix between the placenta and the endometrium and is believed to be involved in placental implantation and maternal vascular remodeling.[59,60] A decrease in the PP13 mRNA expression noted in trophoblasts obtained from women at 11 weeks' gestation who subsequently develop preeclampsia suggests that alteration in PP13 expression may be involved in the pathogenesis of preeclampsia.[61]

Several studies have evaluated serum PP13 levels as a predictive test for preeclampsia and IUGR with conflicting results.[62–65] In a prospective nested case-control study, Chafetz and colleagues[60] reported that when serum PP13 at 9 to 12 weeks was expressed as MoM, sensitivities for preeclampsia and IUGR were 79% and 33%, respectively, at a 90% specificity rate. In another study, sensitivity of 100% was obtained for early onset preeclampsia at 80% specificity.[63] In addition, 2 prospective studies suggest a potential role for first-trimester PP13 levels in combination with the slope between the first and second trimester for predicting preeclampsia.[64,65] In contrast, a case-control study by Akolekar and colleagues[66] found that the addition of serum PP13 did not significantly improve the prediction of early preeclampsia provided by a combination of maternal factors, uterine artery PI, and PAPP-A. Other studies also found no association between low levels of PP13 and subsequent development of preeclampsia and IUGR.[62]

PP13 shows promise as a predictor of preeclampsia and IUGR, but results of preliminary studies are conflicting and limited by their case-control design and small sample sizes. It is expected that results of current larger prospective studies will resolve these conflicting results and clarify its potential role in the prediction of preeclampsia and IUGR.

Endothelial dysfunction–related tests

Circulating angiogenic factors Growing evidence suggests that an imbalance between proangiogenic factors (such as VEGF and PIGF) and antiangiogenic factors (such as sFlt-1 and sEng) is related to the development of preeclampsia.[67] Generally, levels of proangiogenic factor levels are lower and antiangiogenic factors are increased in maternal circulation before the onset and during active disease.[67] Angiogenic factors are believed to contribute to normal trophoblastic proliferation and implantation. sFlt-1 blocks the effects of VEGF and PIGF by inhibiting interaction with their receptors.[68] This situation deprives maternal vascular endothelium of these essential proangiogenic factors and causes systemic endothelial dysfunction that may culminate in preeclampsia.[69,70]

Several studies suggest that PIGF concentration in the first trimester is reduced in women who go on to develop preeclampsia/IUGR and the levels inversely correlate with severity of the disease.[69,71–77] Kusanovic and colleagues[78] examined the role of maternal plasma PIGF, sEng, and sFlt-1 concentrations in early pregnancy (6–15 weeks) and midtrimester (20–25 weeks) for predicting preeclampsia. They found that individual proangiogenic and antiangiogenic factors had a poor predictive value for preeclampsia. However, a combination of these analytes (PIGF/sEng ratio, its delta and slope) had great predictive performance with sensitivity of 100%, specificity of 98% to 99%, and positive likelihood ratios of 57.6, 55.6 and 89.6, respectively, for predicting early onset preeclampsia.

Urinary PIGF has also been explored as a possible screening test for preeclampsia, with disappointing results. Savvidou and colleagues[79] reported that first-trimester urinary PIGF levels were not significantly different between pregnancies that developed preeclampsia and normotensive controls. Also, serum VEGF is unlikely to serve as a useful screening marker because it binds sFlt-1 with a higher affinity than PIGF, and free VEGF is extremely low in the sera, less than the detection limit of currently available assays.[71,73]

Circulating sEng levels have been shown to increase earlier and more distinctly in pregnancies with subsequent preeclampsia compared with normal pregnancies.[80]

This effect was particularly pronounced in gestations affected by early onset preeclampsia.[81] Baumann and colleagues[82] reported that increased levels of sEng were paralleled by increased sFlt-1/PlGF ratios and similar to sFlt-1 levels. There are conflicting results among studies on sEng levels in the first trimester and subsequent development of preeclampsia.[80,82]

The current interest in angiogenic factors for the prediction of preeclampsia is promising, but most studies to date are limited by their retrospective design, nonstandardized assays and small sample sizes. Results of an ongoing large international prospective study are expected to define the role for angiogenic factors in the prediction of preeclampsia.

Endothelial cell adhesion molecules P-selectin, a member of the selectin family of cell adhesion molecules expressed in platelets and endothelial cells, is involved in leukocyte-endothelial interactions.[83,84] Because preeclampsia is associated with increase in cytokine levels, endothelial cell damage and platelet activation, increased P-selectin expression is believed to play an important role in the pathophysiology of preeclampsia.[7,50,51]

P-selectin levels are significantly increased at as early as 10 to 14 weeks in women destined to develop preeclampsia.[85] Banzola and colleagues[86] evaluated the performance of P-selectin, total activin A and VEGF receptors at 11 to 15 weeks' gestation in predicting preeclampsia. P-selectin was identified as the marker with the best discriminant ability between controls and preeclampsia. Bosio and colleagues[51] reported an area under the ROC curve of 0.93 at 10 to 14 weeks and a negative predictive value of close to 100% for P-selectin in predicting preeclampsia. These results are yet to be validated by a large study.

Markers of insulin resistance

Insulin resistance has long been implicated in the pathogenesis of preeclampsia. Possible mechanisms are endothelial dysfunction and disturbances in coagulation.[22] Fasting insulin levels have been shown to be increased before the onset of disease.[87] Several investigators have attempted to use markers of insulin resistance (TNF-α, SHBG, adiponectin, and leptin) to predict preeclampsia, with mixed results.[87–93] Overall, none of them proved useful as a predictive test.

Genomics and proteomics Studies in recent years suggest that genetic polymorphisms may play a role in the development of preeclampsia. Maternal susceptibility loci for preeclampsia have been found on the short arm of chromosome 2 and the long arm of chromosome 4.[94,95] There is also evidence suggesting genetic or immunologic discordance between the mother and fetus as etiologic factors in preeclampsia.[22] Using villous sampling, Farina and colleagues[96] reported altered gene expressions relating to angiogenesis and oxidative stress in first-trimester trophoblasts of pregnancies that went on to develop preeclampsia. Founds and colleagues[97] reported 36 differentially expressed genes, providing promising potential biomarkers for preeclampsia and clues to pathogenesis. However, genetic contribution to preeclampsia is likely complex and involves the interaction of multiple genes and environmental factors.[19] Therefore, it is unlikely that any single genetic test reliably predicts preeclampsia.

Cell-free fetal DNA (ffDNA) has been reported as a potential noninvasive marker for placenta-related complications such as preeclampsia and IUGR.[98,99] Several studies have reported increased numbers of fetal cells and ffDNA in pregnancies complicated by preeclampsia.[100,101] Although the exact mechanism for this observation is unclear, the leading hypothesis is the release of DNA fragments by apoptosis, which is known to be widespread in preeclampsia.[102] To date, studies evaluating the use of ffDNA for the prediction of preeclampsia have yielded largely disappointing results, with some studies suggesting no difference in the amount of ffDNA in preeclamptic women compared with normotensive controls.[103,104]

These preliminary findings suggest that genomic studies can improve our understanding of the early pathophysiology of preeclampsia/IUGR at the molecular level and provide potential targets for the development of clinical biomarkers in maternal blood. However, small sample sizes and differences in methodology limit their generalizability. Current use of ffDNA in maternal blood is limited to pregnancies with male fetuses, because only male fragments of DNA can be clearly detected with certainty.[19] Large prospective studies using improved techniques are needed to investigate the role of ffDNA in the prediction of pregnancy complications, including preeclampsia and IUGR.[105]

Combination of tests Because no single screening test is sufficiently predictive of preeclampsia and IUGR to permit routine clinical use, many investigators have attempted to improve the predictive value of tests by combining them.[56,59,82,86,106,107] The use of multiple parameters attempts to increase the specificity and sensitivity by exploring the different possible pathways to preeclampsia and IUGR. Generally, abnormal uterine artery Doppler indices, a reflection of inadequate trophoblastic invasion of the maternal spiral arteries, is combined with abnormal biomarkers, presumably resulting from dysregulated secretory activity of trophoblasts.[77,108] We review representative studies incorporating multiple tests, to illustrate the usefulness and limitations of the combined approached.

In a prospective cohort study including 3348 women, Espinoza and colleagues[109] noted that the combination of abnormal uterine artery Doppler indices and maternal plasma PlGF in the second trimester improved the specificity and positive likelihood ratio for prediction of any preeclampsia, early onset preeclampsia, and severe preeclampsia, but similar negative likelihood ratios as the individual tests. Their results showed that among women with abnormal uterine artery Doppler indices, maternal plasma concentration of PlGF of less than 280 pg/mL identified most patients who would develop early onset and/or severe preeclampsia.

Poon and colleagues[110] showed that uterine artery PI combined with maternal factors, mean arterial pressure (MAP), serum PlGF and PAPP-A improved detection rate of early preeclampsia to about 90% with a false-positive rate of 5%. Recently, the same group reported that combination of the maternal factor-derived a priori risk, uterine artery PI, and MAP, produced detection rates of 89% for early and 57% for late preeclampsia at a 10% false-positive rate.[111]

Plasencia and colleagues[107] reported that uterine artery PI at 11 to 13 + 6 weeks combined with the ratio of the PI at 21 to 24 + 6 weeks to the PI at 11 to 13 + 6 weeks reduced the false-positive rate from 15% to 5% for a 91% detection rate of early preeclampsia. Nicolaides and colleagues[59] showed that for a 10% false-positive rate with early preeclampsia, the detection rates were 80% for PP13 (95% CI, 44%–98%), 40% for uterine artery PI (95% CI, 12%–74%), and 90% for the markers combined (95% CI, 55%–100%). Spencer and colleagues[56] reported that when ADAM12-S was combined with mean uterine artery PI, the area under the ROC curve increased to 0.88, but addition of PAPP-A to ADAM12-S increased detection by only 1%.

Results of these combined screening studies have several features that provide useful insights for future research. First, combination screening is more effective in predicting early than late preeclampsia, reflecting the likely different pathogenesis of late-onset preeclampsia.[28,72,106] Second, some combinations produced no additive benefits, likely secondary to correlation between the markers. Therefore, future research should focus on combining independent biochemical and/or sonographic markers. Third, sequential measurements of markers may improve risk assessment because changes in individual markers from the first to second trimester herald onset in some cases of preeclampsia and IUGR. Fourth, in deriving patient-specific risks for adverse outcomes using multiple markers, it is important to control for confounders. The goal of any combinations should be to obtain cost-effective screening protocols with high sensitivities and acceptable false-positive rates, which are applicable in general practice. To this end, large prospective studies are needed to determine the best parameters and the optimum methods of combination to effectively predict preeclampsia and/or IUGR.

SUMMARY

Accurate prediction of preeclampsia and IUGR is important for identifying those women who require more intensive monitoring, permitting earlier recognition and intervention, allowing targeting of potential preventive measures to those at risk, and timing interventions before the underlying condition is established. The ideal screening test for preeclampsia and IUGR must have high positive and low negative likelihood ratios to overcome their low incidence rates, and be simple, acceptable, rapid, noninvasive, inexpensive, and feasible early in pregnancy with widely available technology. Currently, none of the screening tests meets these criteria. Although different measures of placental dysfunction have been associated with increased risk of adverse pregnancy outcomes, the ability of any single one to accurately predict these outcomes is poor. Attempts to use predictive models combining analytes and measurements of placental structure and blood flow have so far produced mixed results, but provide useful insights for future research. The use of first- and second-trimester biochemical markers in combination with uterine artery Doppler screening may have the greatest potential as a screening tool. Adequately powered prospective studies using standardized methodology are necessary to further evaluate the choice of parameters and strategies of combination to achieve the best predictive models. Improvement in our knowledge of the pathogenesis of preeclampsia and IUGR will facilitate the development of novel modalities for prediction and intervention.

REFERENCES

1. McIntire DD, Bloom SL, Casey BM, et al. Birth weight in relation to morbidity and mortality among newborn infants. N Engl J Med 1999;340(16):1234–8.
2. Kaufmann P, Black S, Huppertz B. Endovascular trophoblast invasion: implications for the pathogenesis of intrauterine growth retardation and preeclampsia. Biol Reprod 2003;69(1):1–7.
3. Roberts JM, Cooper DW. Pathogenesis and genetics of pre-eclampsia. Lancet 2001;357(9249):53–6.
4. Caniggia I, Winter J, Lye SJ, et al. Oxygen and placental development during the first trimester: implications for the pathophysiology of pre-eclampsia. Placenta 2000;21(Suppl A):S25–30.
5. Scifres CM, Nelson DM. Intrauterine growth restriction, human placental development and trophoblast cell death. J Physiol 2009;587(Pt 14):3453–8.
6. Burton GJ, Woods AW, Jauniaux E, et al. Rheological and physiological consequences of conversion of the maternal spiral arteries for uteroplacental blood flow during human pregnancy. Placenta 2009;30(6):473–82.

7. Roberts JM, Taylor RN, Musci TJ, et al. Preeclampsia: an endothelial cell disorder. Am J Obstet Gynecol 1989;161(5):1200–4.
8. Hsu CD, Iriye B, Johnson TR, et al. Elevated circulating thrombomodulin in severe preeclampsia. Am J Obstet Gynecol 1993;169(1):148–9.
9. Mills JL, DerSimonian R, Raymond E, et al. Prostacyclin and thromboxane changes predating clinical onset of preeclampsia: a multicenter prospective study. JAMA 1999;282(4):356–62.
10. Taylor RN, Crombleholme WR, Friedman SA, et al. High plasma cellular fibronectin levels correlate with biochemical and clinical features of preeclampsia but cannot be attributed to hypertension alone. Am J Obstet Gynecol 1991; 165(4 Pt 1):895–901.
11. Vatten LJ, Skjaerven R. Is pre-eclampsia more than one disease? BJOG 2004; 111(4):298–302.
12. Moldenhauer JS, Stanek J, Warshak C, et al. The frequency and severity of placental findings in women with preeclampsia are gestational age dependent. Am J Obstet Gynecol 2003;189(4):1173–7.
13. Egbor M, Ansari T, Morris N, et al. Morphometric placental villous and vascular abnormalities in early- and late-onset pre-eclampsia with and without fetal growth restriction. BJOG 2006;113(5):580–9.
14. Melchiorre K, Wormald B, Leslie K, et al. First-trimester uterine artery Doppler indices in term and preterm pre-eclampsia. Ultrasound Obstet Gynecol 2008;32(2):133–7.
15. von Dadelszen P, Magee LA, Roberts JM. Subclassification of preeclampsia. Hypertens Pregnancy 2003;22(2):143–8.
16. Schulz KF, Grimes DA, editors. The Lancet handbook of essential concepts in clinical research. Philadelphia (PA): Elsevier; 2006. p. 79.
17. Jaeschke R, Guyatt GH, Sackett DL. Users' guides to the medical literature. III. How to use an article about a diagnostic test. B. What are the results and will they help me in caring for my patients? The Evidence-Based Medicine Working Group. JAMA 1994;271(9):703–7.
18. Villar J, Say L, Shennan A, et al. Methodological and technical issues related to the diagnosis, screening, prevention, and treatment of pre-eclampsia and eclampsia. Int J Gynaecol Obstet 2004;85(Suppl 1):S28–41.
19. Lindheimer MD, Roberts JM, Cunningham FG, editors. Chesley's hypertensive disorders in pregnancy. 3rd edition. Oxford (UK): Elsevier; 2009.
20. Lang TA, Secic M. How to report statistics in medicine. Philadelphia: American College of Physicians; 1997.
21. Riegelman RK, Hirsch R, editors. Studying a study and testing a test. 2nd edition. Boston: Little, Brown and Co; 1987.
22. Farag K, Hassan I, Ledger WL. Prediction of preeclampsia: can it be achieved? Obstet Gynecol Surv 2004;59(6):464–82 [quiz: 485].
23. Conde-Agudelo A, Villar J, Lindheimer M. World Health Organization systematic review of screening tests for preeclampsia. Obstet Gynecol 2004;104(6):1367–91.
24. Pilalis A, Souka AP, Antsaklis P, et al. Screening for pre-eclampsia and fetal growth restriction by uterine artery Doppler and PAPP-A at 11–14 weeks' gestation. Ultrasound Obstet Gynecol 2007;29(2):135–40.
25. Toal M, Keating S, Machin G, et al. Determinants of adverse perinatal outcome in high-risk women with abnormal uterine artery Doppler images. Am J Obstet Gynecol 2008;198(3):330, e1–7.
26. Cnossen JS, Morris RK, ter Riet G, et al. Use of uterine artery Doppler ultrasonography to predict pre-eclampsia and intrauterine growth restriction: a systematic review and bivariable meta-analysis. CMAJ 2008;178(6):701–11.

27. Conde-Agudelo A, Lindheimer M. Use of Doppler ultrasonography to predict pre-eclampsia. CMAJ 2008;179(1):53 [author reply: 53–4].
28. Pretorius DH, Nelson TR, Baergen RN, et al. Imaging of placental vasculature using three-dimensional ultrasound and color power Doppler: a preliminary study. Ultrasound Obstet Gynecol 1998;12(1):45–9.
29. Konje JC, Huppertz B, Bell SC, et al. 3-dimensional colour power angiography for staging human placental development. Lancet 2003;362(9391):1199–201.
30. Hafner E, Metzenbauer M, Höfinger D, et al. Comparison between three-dimensional placental volume at 12 weeks and uterine artery impedance/notching at 22 weeks in screening for pregnancy-induced hypertension, pre-eclampsia and fetal growth restriction in a low-risk population. Ultrasound Obstet Gynecol 2006;27(6):652–7.
31. Rizzo G, Capponi A, Pietrolucci ME, et al. Effects of maternal cigarette smoking on placental volume and vascularization measured by 3-dimensional power Doppler ultrasonography at 11 + 0 to 13 + 6 weeks of gestation. Am J Obstet Gynecol 2009;200(4):415, e1–5.
32. Matijevic R, Kurjak A. The assessment of placental blood vessels by three-dimensional power Doppler ultrasound. J Perinat Med 2002;30(1):26–32.
33. Merce LT, Barco MJ, Bau S. Reproducibility of the study of placental vascularization by three-dimensional power Doppler. J Perinat Med 2004;32(3):228–33.
34. Tuuli MG, Houser M, Odibo L, et al. Validation of placental vascular sonobiopsy for obtaining representative placental vascular indices by three-dimensionalpower Doppler ultrasonography. Placenta 2010;31(3):192–6.
35. Merce LT, Barco MJ, Bau S, et al. Assessment of placental vascularization by three-dimensional power Doppler "vascular biopsy" in normal pregnancies. Croat Med J 2005;46(5):765–71.
36. Noguchi J, Hata K, Tanaka H, et al. Placental vascular sonobiopsy using three-dimensional power Doppler ultrasound in normal and growth restricted fetuses. Placenta 2009;30(5):391–7.
37. Guiot C, Gaglioti P, Oberto M, et al. Is three-dimensional power Doppler ultrasound useful in the assessment of placental perfusion in normal and growth-restricted pregnancies? Ultrasound Obstet Gynecol 2008;31(2):171–6.
38. Raine-Fenning NJ, Welsh AW, Jones NW, et al. Methodological considerations for the correct application of quantitative three-dimensional power Doppler angiography. Ultrasound Obstet Gynecol 2008;32(1):115–7 [author reply: 117–8].
39. Raine-Fenning NJ, Nordin NM, Ramnarine KV, et al. Determining the relationship between three-dimensional power Doppler data and true blood flow characteristics: an in-vitro flow phantom experiment. Ultrasound Obstet Gynecol 2008;32(4):540–50.
40. Raine-Fenning NJ, Nordin NM, Ramnarine KV, et al. Evaluation of the effect of machine settings on quantitative three-dimensional power Doppler angiography: an in-vitro flow phantom experiment. Ultrasound Obstet Gynecol 2008;32(4):551–9.
41. Schulten-Wijman MJ, Struijk PC, Brezinka C, et al. Evaluation of volume vascularization index and flow index: a phantom study. Ultrasound Obstet Gynecol 2008;32(4):560–4.
42. Viero S, Chaddha V, Alkazaleh F, et al. Prognostic value of placental ultrasound in pregnancies complicated by absent end-diastolic flow velocity in the umbilical arteries. Placenta 2004;25(8–9):735–41.
43. Toal M, Chan C, Fallah S, et al. Usefulness of a placental profile in high-risk pregnancies. Am J Obstet Gynecol 2007;196(4):363, e1–7.

44. Redman CW. Current topic: pre-eclampsia and the placenta. Placenta 1991; 12(4):301–8.
45. Thomas RL, Blakemore KJ. Evaluation of elevations in maternal serum alpha-fetoprotein: a review. Obstet Gynecol Surv 1990;45(5):269–83.
46. Costa SL, Proctor L, Dodd JM, et al. Screening for placental insufficiency in high-risk pregnancies: is earlier better? Placenta 2008;29(12):1034–40.
47. Cindrova-Davies T, Spasic-Boskovic O, Jauniaux E, et al. Nuclear factor-kappa B, p38, and stress-activated protein kinase mitogen-activated protein kinase signaling pathways regulate proinflammatory cytokines and apoptosis in human placental explants in response to oxidative stress: effects of antioxidant vitamins. Am J Pathol 2007;170(5):1511–20.
48. Hung TH, Charnock-Jones DS, Skepper JN, et al. Secretion of tumor necrosis factor-alpha from human placental tissues induced by hypoxia-reoxygenation causes endothelial cell activation in vitro: a potential mediator of the inflammatory response in preeclampsia. Am J Pathol 2004;164(3):1049–61.
49. Tjoa ML, Cindrova-Davies T, Spasic-Boskovic O, et al. Trophoblastic oxidative stress and the release of cell-free feto-placental DNA. Am J Pathol 2006; 169(2):400–4.
50. Redman CW. Platelets and the beginnings of preeclampsia. N Engl J Med 1990; 323(7):478–80.
51. Bosio PM, Cannon S, McKenna PJ, et al. Plasma P-selectin is elevated in the first trimester in women who subsequently develop pre-eclampsia. BJOG 2001;108(7):709–15.
52. Morris RK, Cnossen JS, Langejans M, et al. Serum screening with Down's syndrome markers to predict pre-eclampsia and small for gestational age: systematic review and meta-analysis. BMC Pregnancy Childbirth 2008;8:33.
53. Ito N, Nomura S, Iwase A, et al. ADAMs, a disintegrin and metalloproteinases, mediate shedding of oxytocinase. Biochem Biophys Res Commun 2004; 314(4):1008–13.
54. Iba K, Albrechtsen R, Gilpin B, et al. The cysteine-rich domain of human ADAM 12 supports cell adhesion through syndecans and triggers signaling events that lead to beta1 integrin-dependent cell spreading. J Cell Biol 2000;149(5): 1143–56.
55. Laigaard J, Sørensen T, Placing S, et al. Reduction of the disintegrin and metalloprotease ADAM12 in preeclampsia. Obstet Gynecol 2005;106(1):144–9.
56. Spencer K, Cowans NJ, Stamatopoulou A. ADAM12s in maternal serum as a potential marker of pre-eclampsia. Prenat Diagn 2008;28(3):212–6.
57. Cowans NJ, Spencer K. First-trimester ADAM12 and PAPP-A as markers for intrauterine fetal growth restriction through their roles in the insulin-like growth factor system. Prenat Diagn 2007;27(3):264–71.
58. Poon LC, Chelemen T, Granvillano O, et al. First-trimester maternal serum a disintegrin and metalloprotease 12 (ADAM12) and adverse pregnancy outcome. Obstet Gynecol 2008;112(5):1082–90.
59. Nicolaides KH, Bindra R, Turan OM, et al. A novel approach to first-trimester screening for early pre-eclampsia combining serum PP-13 and Doppler ultrasound. Ultrasound Obstet Gynecol 2006;27(1):13–7.
60. Chafetz I, Kuhnreich I, Sammar M, et al. First-trimester placental protein 13 screening for preeclampsia and intrauterine growth restriction. Am J Obstet Gynecol 2007;197(1):35, e1–7.
61. Sekizawa A, Sekizawa A, Purwosunu Y, et al. PP13 mRNA expression in trophoblasts from preeclamptic placentas. Reprod Sci 2009;16(4):408–13.

62. Cowans NJ, Spencer K, Meiri H. First-trimester maternal placental protein 13 levels in pregnancies resulting in adverse outcomes. Prenat Diagn 2008; 28(2):121–5.
63. Romero R, Kusanovic JP, Than NG, et al. First-trimester maternal serum PP13 in the risk assessment for preeclampsia. Am J Obstet Gynecol 2008;199(2):122, e1–11.
64. Gonen R, Shahar R, Grimpel YI, et al. Placental protein 13 as an early marker for pre-eclampsia: a prospective longitudinal study. BJOG 2008;115(12): 1465–72.
65. Huppertz B, Sammar M, Chefetz I, et al. Longitudinal determination of serum placental protein 13 during development of preeclampsia. Fetal Diagn Ther 2008;24(3):230–6.
66. Akolekar R, Syngelaki A, Beta J, et al. Maternal serum placental protein 13 at 11–13 weeks of gestation in preeclampsia. Prenat Diagn 2009;29(12):1103–8.
67. Maynard S, Epstein FH, Karumanchi SA. Preeclampsia and angiogenic imbalance. Annu Rev Med 2008;59:61–78.
68. Powers RW, Roberts JM, Cooper KM, et al. Maternal serum soluble fms-like tyrosine kinase 1 concentrations are not increased in early pregnancy and decrease more slowly postpartum in women who develop preeclampsia. Am J Obstet Gynecol 2005;193(1):185–91.
69. Maynard SE, Min JY, Merchan J, et al. Excess placental soluble fms-like tyrosine kinase 1 (sFlt1) may contribute to endothelial dysfunction, hypertension, and proteinuria in preeclampsia. J Clin Invest 2003;111(5):649–58.
70. Sugimoto H, Hamano Y, Charytan D, et al. Neutralization of circulating vascular endothelial growth factor (VEGF) by anti-VEGF antibodies and soluble VEGF receptor 1 (sFlt-1) induces proteinuria. J Biol Chem 2003;278(15):12605–8.
71. Taylor RN, Grimwood J, Taylor RS, et al. Longitudinal serum concentrations of placental growth factor: evidence for abnormal placental angiogenesis in pathologic pregnancies. Am J Obstet Gynecol 2003;188(1):177–82.
72. Crispi F, Llurba E, Domínguez C, et al. Predictive value of angiogenic factors and uterine artery Doppler for early- versus late-onset pre-eclampsia and intrauterine growth restriction. Ultrasound Obstet Gynecol 2008;31(3):303–9.
73. Thadhani R, Mutter WP, Wolf M, et al. First trimester placental growth factor and soluble fms-like tyrosine kinase 1 and risk for preeclampsia. J Clin Endocrinol Metab 2004;89(2):770–5.
74. Teixeira PG, Cabral AC, Andrade SP, et al. Placental growth factor (PIGF) is a surrogate marker in preeclamptic hypertension. Hypertens Pregnancy 2008; 27(1):65–73.
75. Lam C, Lim KH, Karumanchi SA. Circulating angiogenic factors in the pathogenesis and prediction of preeclampsia. Hypertension 2005;46(5):1077–85.
76. Moore Simas TA, Crawford SL, Solitro MJ, et al. Angiogenic factors for the prediction of preeclampsia in high-risk women. Am J Obstet Gynecol 2007; 197(3):244, e1–8.
77. Akolekar R, Zaragoza E, Poon LC, et al. Maternal serum placental growth factor at 11 + 0 to 13 + 6 weeks of gestation in the prediction of pre-eclampsia. Ultrasound Obstet Gynecol 2008;32(6):732–9.
78. Kusanovic JP, Romero R, Chaiworapongsa T, et al. A prospective cohort study of the value of maternal plasma concentrations of angiogenic and anti-angiogenic factors in early pregnancy and midtrimester in the identification of patients destined to develop preeclampsia. J Matern Fetal Neonatal Med 2009;22(11):1021–38.

79. Savvidou MD, Akolekar R, Zaragoza E, et al. First trimester urinary placental growth factor and development of pre-eclampsia. BJOG 2009;116(5):643–7.
80. Rana S, Karumanchi SA, Levine RJ, et al. Sequential changes in antiangiogenic factors in early pregnancy and risk of developing preeclampsia. Hypertension 2007;50(1):137–42.
81. Signore C, Mills JL, Qian C, et al. Circulating soluble endoglin and placental abruption. Prenat Diagn 2008;28(9):852–8.
82. Baumann MU, Bersinger NA, Mohaupt MG, et al. First-trimester serum levels of soluble endoglin and soluble fms-like tyrosine kinase-1 as first-trimester markers for late-onset preeclampsia. Am J Obstet Gynecol 2008;199(3):266, e1–6.
83. Hsu-Lin S, Berman CL, Furie BC, et al. A platelet membrane protein expressed during platelet activation and secretion. Studies using a monoclonal antibody specific for thrombin-activated platelets. J Biol Chem 1984;259(14):9121–6.
84. Larsen E, Celi A, Gilbert GE, et al. PADGEM protein: a receptor that mediates the interaction of activated platelets with neutrophils and monocytes. Cell 1989;59(2):305–12.
85. Halim A, Kanayama N, el Maradny E, et al. Plasma P selectin (GMP-140) and glycocalicin are elevated in preeclampsia and eclampsia: their significances. Am J Obstet Gynecol 1996;174(1 Pt 1):272–7.
86. Banzola I, Farina A, Concu M, et al. Performance of a panel of maternal serum markers in predicting preeclampsia at 11–15 weeks' gestation. Prenat Diagn 2007;27(11):1005–10.
87. Spencer K, Yu CK, Rembouskos G, et al. First trimester sex hormone-binding globulin and subsequent development of preeclampsia or other adverse pregnancy outcomes. Hypertens Pregnancy 2005;24(3):303–11.
88. Williams MA, Farrand A, Mittendorf R, et al. Maternal second trimester serum tumor necrosis factor-alpha-soluble receptor p55 (sTNFp55) and subsequent risk of preeclampsia. Am J Epidemiol 1999;149(4):323–9.
89. Serin IS, Ozçelik B, Basbug M, et al. Predictive value of tumor necrosis factor alpha (TNF-alpha) in preeclampsia. Eur J Obstet Gynecol Reprod Biol 2002; 100(2):143–5.
90. Schipper EJ, Bolte AC, Schalkwijk CG, et al. TNF-receptor levels in preeclampsia–results of a longitudinal study in high-risk women. J Matern Fetal Neonatal Med 2005;18(5):283–7.
91. Leal AM, Poon LC, Frisova V, et al. First-trimester maternal serum tumor necrosis factor receptor-1 and pre-eclampsia. Ultrasound Obstet Gynecol 2009;33(2): 135–41.
92. Wolf M, Sandler L, Muñoz K, et al. First trimester insulin resistance and subsequent preeclampsia: a prospective study. J Clin Endocrinol Metab 2002;87(4): 1563–8.
93. D'Anna R, Baviera G, Corrado F, et al. Adiponectin and insulin resistance in early- and late-onset pre-eclampsia. BJOG 2006;113(11):1264–9.
94. Moses EK, Lade JA, Guo G, et al. A genome scan in families from Australia and New Zealand confirms the presence of a maternal susceptibility locus for preeclampsia, on chromosome 2. Am J Hum Genet 2000;67(6):1581–5.
95. Harrison GA, Humphrey KE, Jones N, et al. A genomewide linkage study of preeclampsia/eclampsia reveals evidence for a candidate region on 4q. Am J Hum Genet 1997;60(5):1158–67.
96. Farina A, Sekizawa A, De Sanctis P, et al. Gene expression in chorionic villous samples at 11 weeks' gestation from women destined to develop preeclampsia. Prenat Diagn 2008;28(10):956–61.

97. Founds SA, Conley YP, Lyons-Weiler JF, et al. Altered global gene expression in first trimester placentas of women destined to develop preeclampsia. Placenta 2009;30(1):15–24.

98. Alberry MS, Maddocks DG, Hadi MA, et al. Quantification of cell free fetal DNA in maternal plasma in normal pregnancies and in pregnancies with placental dysfunction. Am J Obstet Gynecol 2009;200(1):98, e1–6.

99. Caramelli E, Rizzo N, Concu M, et al. Cell-free fetal DNA concentration in plasma of patients with abnormal uterine artery Doppler waveform and intrauterine growth restriction–a pilot study. Prenat Diagn 2003;23(5):367–71.

100. Holzgreve W, Ghezzi F, Di Naro E, et al. Disturbed feto-maternal cell traffic in preeclampsia. Obstet Gynecol 1998;91(5 Pt 1):669–72.

101. Lo YM, Leung TN, Tein MS, et al. Quantitative abnormalities of fetal DNA in maternal serum in preeclampsia. Clin Chem 1999;45(2):184–8.

102. DiFederico E, Genbacev O, Fisher SJ. Preeclampsia is associated with widespread apoptosis of placental cytotrophoblasts within the uterine wall. Am J Pathol 1999;155(1):293–301.

103. Cotter AM, Martin CM, O'leary JJ, et al. Increased fetal DNA in the maternal circulation in early pregnancy is associated with an increased risk of preeclampsia. Am J Obstet Gynecol 2004;191(2):515–20.

104. Crowley A, Martin C, Fitzpatrick P, et al. Free fetal DNA is not increased before 20 weeks in intrauterine growth restriction or pre-eclampsia. Prenat Diagn 2007; 27(2):174–9.

105. NCI-NHGRI Working Group on Replication in Association Studies, Manolio T, Chanock SJ, et al. Replicating genotype-phenotype associations. Nature 2007;447(7145):655–60.

106. Poon LC, Maiz N, Valencia C, et al. First-trimester maternal serum pregnancy-associated plasma protein-A and pre-eclampsia. Ultrasound Obstet Gynecol 2009;33(1):23–33.

107. Plasencia W, Maiz N, Poon L, et al. Uterine artery Doppler at 11 + 0 to 13 + 6 weeks and 21 + 0 to 24 + 6 weeks in the prediction of pre-eclampsia. Ultrasound Obstet Gynecol 2008;32(2):138–46.

108. Sibai B, Dekker G, Kupferminc M. Pre-eclampsia. Lancet 2005;365(9461): 785–99.

109. Espinoza J, Romero R, Nien JK, et al. Identification of patients at risk for early onset and/or severe preeclampsia with the use of uterine artery Doppler velocimetry and placental growth factor. Am J Obstet Gynecol 2007;196(4):326, e1–13.

110. Poon LC, Kametas NA, Maiz N, et al. First-trimester prediction of hypertensive disorders in pregnancy. Hypertension 2009;53(5):812–8.

111. Poon LC, Karagiannis G, Leal A, et al. Hypertensive disorders in pregnancy: screening by uterine artery Doppler imaging and blood pressure at 11–13 weeks. Ultrasound Obstet Gynecol 2009;34(5):497–502.

Prenatal Screening for Thrombophilias: Indications and Controversies

Jeanine F. Carbone, MD[a],*, Roxane Rampersad, MD[b]

KEYWORDS

- Thrombophilia • Inherited thrombophilia
- Acquired thrombophilia • Pregnancy
- Venous • Thromboembolism

Pregnancy is considered to be a hypercoagulable state and encompasses all 3 elements of Virchow's triad. There are numerous physiologic changes in pregnancy to account for this hypercoagulable state. In pregnancy, there is an increase in fibrinogen, von Willebrand factor, and clotting Factors II, VII, VIII, IX, and X.[1,2] There is a decrease in physiologic anticoagulants manifested by a decrease in protein S (PS) and an increase in protein C (PC) resistance. There are decreases in fibrinolytic activity, increased venous stasis, and vascular injury associated with delivery. Pregnancy is associated with increased clotting potential, decreased anticoagulant activity, and decreased fibrinolyis.[3,4]

A thrombophilia is defined as a disorder of hemostasis that predisposes a person to a thrombotic event.[5] Data suggest that at least 50% of cases of venous thromboembolism[6] in pregnant women are associated with an inherited or acquired thrombophilia.[7,8] Inherited and acquired thrombophilias can lead to an increased risk of maternal thromboembolism and adverse pregnancy outcomes such as recurrent pregnancy loss, intrauterine fetal demise (IUFD), preterm preeclampsia, and intrauterine growth restriction (IUGR). Thrombophilias have been associated with an increased risk of maternal and perinatal morbidity and mortality. Sometimes inherited and acquired thrombophilias are used interchangeably, which is a misconception. Inherited and acquired thrombophilias have different indications for testing. It is important as a clinician to identify what patient is at risk, what are the indications for testing, what laboratory testing should be performed, and what patient should receive

[a] Division of Maternal-Fetal Medicine, Department of Obstetrics and Gynecology, Washington University School of Medicine, Campus Box 8064, 660 South Euclid, Saint Louis, MO 63110, USA
[b] Division of Maternal-Fetal Medicine, Department of Obstetrics and Gynecology, Washington University School of Medicine, Campus Box 8064, 4911 Barnes-Jewish Hospital Plaza, Saint Louis, MO 63110, USA
* Corresponding author.
E-mail address: carboneje@wudosis.wustl.edu

Clin Lab Med 30 (2010) 747–760
doi:10.1016/j.cll.2010.05.003   **labmed.theclinics.com**
0272-2712/10/$ – see front matter © 2010 Elsevier Inc. All rights reserved.

treatment. It is best for the clinician to perform a thrombophilia workup preconceptually because thrombophilia manifestations can start in early pregnancy.

INHERITED THROMBOPHILIAS

Inherited thrombophilias result from deficiencies from components of the coagulation system. Inherited thrombophilias have been associated with venous thromboembolism (VTE) and adverse pregnancy outcomes. Included in the category of inherited thrombophilias are factor V Leiden (FVL) mutation, prothrombin (PT) gene (G20210A) mutation, antithrombin (AT) deficiency, PC deficiency, PS deficiency, and hyperhomocysteinemia.

Factor V Leiden

FVL mutation is the most common inherited thrombophilia and is present in about 5% to 9% of the white European population (**Table 1**).[9] FVL mutation is inherited in an autosomal dominant fashion and arises from a point mutation where glutamine is substituted for an arginine at position 506. This amino acid substitution impairs PC and PS activity; therefore, FVL is the leading case of activated PC resistance. Screening can be performed by assessing activated PC (aPC) resistance using a second-generation coagulation assay followed by genotyping for the FVL mutation. Alternatively, patients can simply be genotyped for FVL.[3] FVL can be accurately diagnosed in pregnancy.

Prothrombin Gene (G20210A) Mutation

PT gene mutation is present in 2% to 3% of the white European population (see **Table 1**).[10] PT gene mutation occurs due to a point mutation causing a guanine to adenine substitution at nucleotide position 20210. Polymerase chain reaction (PCR) methods have been used to detect the G20210A PT gene mutation in genomic DNA.[10,11] Prothrombin gene mutation is associated with elevated plasma levels of PT, but it should not be used for screening.[10–12] Prothrombin gene mutation can be tested in the setting of pregnancy.

AT Deficiency

AT deficiency is present in 0.02% to 0.2% of the population, and is the most thrombogenic of the inherited thrombophilias (see **Table 1**).[2,9] AT III has a 70% to 90% lifetime risk of thromboembolism.[13] Deficiencies in AT III result from numerous point mutations, deletions, and insertions, and are usually inherited in an autosomal dominant fashion.[14] Although AT is most often inherited, it can also be acquired due to liver

Table 1
Risk of VTE with inherited thrombophilias

Thrombophilia	Population Frequency in Caucasians	Frequency of VTE in Asymptomatic Pregnancies	Frequency of VTE in Symptomatic Pregnancies
FVL	5%–9%[9]	0.26%[40]	10%–17%[40]
G20210A PT	2%–3%[10]	0.37%[40]	16.9%[11]
AT	0.02–0.2%[9]	7.2%[40]	60%[41]
PC	0.2–0.5%[17,18]	0.18%[40]	2%–17%[40]
PS	0.03–0.13%[22]	0.8%[40]	0%–22%[40]

Symptomatic pregnancy includes personal and/or family history of VTE.

failure, increased consumption secondary to disseminated intravascular coagulation and/or sepsis, or increased renal excretion in severe nephritic syndrome. AT deficiency is diagnosed with an AT-heparin cofactor assay. This assay will detect all currently recognized subtypes of familial AT deficiency and is therefore the best single laboratory screening test for this disorder. AT deficiency should not be screened for in the setting of pregnancy, acute thrombosis, or during anticoagulation.

Hyperhomocycsteinemia

Hyperhomocysteinemia can be seen with deficiencies in vitamins B6, B12, folic acid, and methylenehydrofolate reductase (MTHFR). Normal circulating plasma levels of homocysteine range from 5 to 16 µmol/L. Hyperhomocysteinemia can be diagnosed with fasting homocysteine levels and can further be classified as severe (>100 µmol/L), moderate (25–100 µmol/L), and mild (16–24 µmol/L).[9] MTHFR can be a cause of mild to severe hyperhomocysteinemia. Frosst and colleagues[15] explained the thermolability of MTHFR and how the mechanism was caused by a cytosine to thymine substitution at base pair 677 in the MTHFR gene.[16] Homozygosity for MTHFR is a relatively common cause of mildly elevated plasma homocysteine levels in the general population, often occurring in association with low serum folate levels.

Protein C

PC deficiency is present in 0.2% to 0.5% of the general population (see **Table 1**).[17,18] Heterozygous PC deficiency is inherited in an autosomal dominant pattern. Most affected patients are heterozygous with the plasma PC concentration being approximately 50% of normal in both immunologic and functional assays. PC is a vitamin K–dependent protein synthesized in the liver. The gene for PC is located on chromosome 2 (2q13–14).[19,20] PC circulates as a zymogen and exerts its anticoagulant function after activation to the serine protease, aPC. The primary effect of aPC is to inactivate coagulation factors Va and VIIIa, which are necessary for efficient thrombin generation and factor X activation.[21] The inhibitory effect of aPC is markedly enhanced by PS, another vitamin K–dependent protein. PC is affected by pregnancy therefore should be tested for preconceptually.

Protein S

PS deficiency is present in 0.03% to 0.13% of the general population (see **Table 1**).[22] PS deficiency is inherited predominately in an autosomal dominant pattern. The gene for PS is located on chromosome 3.[23,24] PS is a vitamin K–dependent glycoprotein and is a cofactor to PC. In the presence of PS, aPC inactivates factors Va and VIIIa, resulting in reduced thrombin generation.[25] Type I is the classical type of PS deficiency and is associated with 50% of the normal total S antigen level, marked reductions in free PS antigen, and reduced PS functional activity.[26–28] There are assays available to measure plasma total and free PS antigen and PS function. Measurement of free PS concentration is the preferred screening test.[29] Patients with levels of total or free PS antigen less than 65 IU/dL are considered to be deficient.[30] PS deficiency should be tested for outside of pregnancy.

ACQUIRED THROMBOPHILIAS
Antiphospholipid Antibody Syndrome (APLS)

APLS is considered to be an acquired thrombophilia, and can be primary or secondary. Primary APLS refers to patients with no other underlying autoimmune disorder. Secondary APLS occurs in the setting of an underlying autoimmune disorder such as systemic lupus erythematosus.[31] APLS is an autoimmune disorder defined by the presence of characteristic clinical features and specified levels of circulating anti-phospholipid antibodies. The combination of VTE and/or adverse obstetric outcomes, and antiphospholipid antibodies encompass this syndrome. The international consensus statement for APLS states that a patient must have one clinical criterion and one laboratory criterion to make the diagnosis.[32]

The clinical criteria for APLS testing can be separated into 2 categories: obstetric outcomes and thrombosis. Obstetric criteria are 3 or more consecutive euploid spontaneous abortions before the 10th week of gestation, unexplained fetal deaths in one or more morphologically normal fetus at 10 weeks or later, and preterm delivery at less than or equal to 34 weeks' gestation resulting from severe preeclampsia or placental insufficiency.[29] Encompassed in the category of placental insufficiency is nonreassuring fetal testing suggestive of fetal hypoxemia, abnormal umbilical Doppler flow velocimetry, oligohydramnios (amniotic fluid index $\leq$5 cm), or birth weight less than 10th percentile (IUGR) requiring delivery at 34 weeks' gestation. There is no actual universal definition of placental insufficiency, nor are there any characteristic placental abnormalities seen on pathology. The criterion for thrombosis is one or more clinical episodes of arterial, venous, or small-vessel thrombosis, in any tissue or organ.[32]

Once clinical criteria are met, antiphospholipid antibody testing should be performed to establish laboratory criteria. Patients should be tested for lupus anticoagulant, anticardiolipin antibody, and anti-β_2-glycoprotein-1 antibody. If any of these laboratory criteria are positive, a confirmatory test must be performed in 12 weeks.[32]

Antiphospholipid Antibodies

Lupus anticoagulants are antibodies directed against plasma proteins that bind to anionic or hexagonal phase phospholipids.[33,34] Lupus anticoagulants paradoxically block phospholipid-dependent clotting assays by interfering with the assembly of the PT complex. Because there are other inhibitors and analytical variables that can cause abnormal test results, several different tests are used to confirm the presence of a lupus anticoagulant. Typically these may include partial thromboplastin time, prothrombin time, dilute or modified Russell viper venom screen (dRVVT or MRVVT), and a hexagonal (II) phase phospholipid assay (Staclot-LA test) or kaolin clotting time. Regardless of the assay used, the result will be reported as present or absent. If the lupus anticoagulant is present, testing must be repeated in 12 weeks to establish if lupus anticoagulant is transient or chronic.

Anticardiolipin antibodies react to the complex of negatively charged phospholipids. These antibodies are detected using conventional immunoassays using purified cardiolipin as the phospholipid matrix. Anticardiolipin antibodies IgG or IgM must be present in medium to high titers of greater than 40 GPL/MPL (IgG/IgM phospholipid) units. Antibodies may be transient, so the testing must be repeated again in 12 weeks for confirmation.

Anti-β_2-glycoprotein-1 is a phospholipid-dependent inhibitor of coagulation. These antibodies are measured by standardized enzyme-linked immunosorbent assay. Antibodies IgG and IgM must have titers greater than the 99th percentile to be considered positive. Like lupus anticoagulant and anticardiolipin antibodies, titers must be tested for again 12 weeks from the first sample. Antiphospholipid antibodies can be tested for during pregnancy.

HISTORY OF VTE

Data suggest that approximately 50% of cases of VTE in pregnant women are associated with an inherited or acquired thrombophilia[7,8]; however, the incidence of VTE is low, estimated at 0.76 to 1.72 per 1000 pregnancies.[35,36] Due to the low incidence of VTE in pregnancy, universal screening of pregnant women is not cost effective nor is it indicated. All patients with a personal history of venous thrombosis, regardless of thrombophilia status, are prone to recurrent thromboses for many years after the first incident.

APLS has been associated with VTE, arterial thrombosis, stroke, amaurois fugax, and transient ischemic attacks. VTE accounts for 32% of APLS-associated clinical events,[37,38] and up to 25% of thrombotic events occur during pregnancy or the post-partum period.[39]

FVL gene mutation is seen in 40% of patients presenting with a VTE in pregnancy.[10] The probability of VTE in FVL heterozygotes and homozygotes with a personal or family history of VTE is 10% to 17% (see **Table 1**).[40] Prothrombin gene mutation is associated with 16.9% of VTE in pregnancy (see **Table 1**).[10] The relative risk of VTE in pregnancy with PT gene mutation is 15.2 (95% confidence interval 4.2–52.6).[10] Patients with severe deficiencies of AT, PC, and PS are associated with increased risk of VTE in pregnancy and the postpartum period. Seligsohn and Lubetsky[41] found that venous thrombosis occurred during pregnancy and the puerperium in up to 60% of women with an antithrombin deficiency and in up to 20% of women with a deficiency of either PC or PS.[13,37] A case-control study showed that in 129 asymptomatic female relatives of patients with a deficiency of antithrombin, PC, or PS, those who also had a deficiency of one of these proteins had a risk of venous thrombosis during pregnancy and the puerperium that was 8 times as high as the risk in those without a deficiency.[41] Robertson and colleagues[42] found that all heritable thrombophilias, with the exception of MTHFR, were found to be significantly associated with an increased risk of VTE.

MTHFR is associated with decreased enzyme activity and mild hyperhomocysteinemia, and is the most common cause of hyperhomocysteinemia.[16,43] There have been several published studies that have shown an increased relative risk for venous thrombosis with elevated homocysteine levels. Meta-analysis of prospective and retrospective studies demonstrated an association of homocysteine with venous thrombosis.[44] This finding supports the hypothesis that MTHFR can be associated with VTE. However, there are also negative studies that have shown no increased risk of VTE in women with MTHFR and with elevated homocysteine levels with history of VTE.[16,45,46] The VITRO study, a randomized placebo-controlled trial of supplementation with folic acid, pyridoxine, and vitamin B12 in patients with elevated homocysteine levels, showed that supplementation with B vitamins lowers homocysteine values but does not show a risk reduction in recurrent venous thrombosis.[47] If hyperhomocysteinemia is indeed a risk factor for VTE, then lowering the levels should be associated with a reduced risk. In the VITRO study there was no difference in recurrence risk of VTE between the treated group and the placebo group.

KNOWN THROMBOPHILIA WITH NO HISTORY OF VTE

There is some controversy among practitioners of how patients with an incidental finding of thrombophilia without a personal history of VTE should be treated. Venous thromboembolism is a multifactorial disorder in which acquired and genetic risk factors can interact dynamically.[8,40] There are no prospective data examining the risks and benefits of prophylactic anticoagulation in this patient population who have no history of VTE or adverse pregnancy outcome but who test positive for a thrombophilia. The probability of VTE in patients without a history is 0.26% for FVL heterozygote, 1.5% for FVL homozygote, 0.37% for PT carrier, and 4.7% for compound heterozygosity. The probability of thrombosis with antithrombin deficiency and PC deficiency is 7.2% and 0.8%, respectively.[40] Friederich and colleagues[48] studied 129 asymptomatic female relatives of patients with a deficiency of antithrombin, PC, or PS. Those subjects who also had a deficiency of one of these proteins had a risk of venous thrombosis during pregnancy and the puerperium that was 8 times as high as the risk in those without a deficiency. Patients who are incidentally found to have antiphospholipid antibodies have a risk of thrombosis of less than 1% each year,[37,49] and currently there is no evidence to recommend thromboprophylaxis.

ADVERSE PREGNANCY OUTCOMES

Many agree that patients with a personal history of VTE should be tested for thrombophilias, but controversy arises on what tests should be performed on patients with adverse pregnancy outcomes.

Pregnancy Loss

Pregnancy loss can be separated into 2 categories: recurrent early pregnancy loss (>3 before 10 weeks' gestation) and late fetal loss ($\geq$1 loss after 10 weeks). APLS is associated with both recurrent early pregnancy loss (<10 weeks) and late fetal loss.[48] A greater proportion of pregnancy losses related to antiphospholipid antibodies are second or third trimester fetal deaths.[50] There have been 3 randomized control trials examining the effect of treatment of APLS patients with recurrent pregnancy loss with low-dose aspirin (acetylsalicylic acid; ASA) alone or low-dose ASA plus heparin.[51–53] Two of these studies showed a significantly better pregnancy outcome and higher rate of live births in women with APLS and recurrent pregnancy loss: 71% to 80% with use of heparin and ASA versus 42% to 72% with ASA alone.[51,52] The study by Farquharson and colleagues[53] did not show an improved outcome; however, the patients in this study did not meet laboratory criteria for the diagnosis for APLS.

There is some controversy about whether patients with recurrent or late pregnancy loss should be tested for inherited thrombophilias. Alfirevic and colleagues[54] performed a systematic review and found that unexplained stillbirth, when compared with controls, was more often associated with heterozygous FVL mutation, PS deficiency, and aPC resistance. A meta-analysis by Rey and colleagues[55] showed that FVL, PT gene mutation, and PS deficiency were associated with recurrent early pregnancy loss and late fetal loss. MTHFR, PC, and antithrombin deficiencies were not significantly associated with fetal loss. Kovalevsky and colleagues[56] performed a systematic review on published case-control studies. The combined odds ratios for the association between recurrent pregnancy loss and FVL and PT gene mutation were 2.0 (95% confidence interval 1.5–2.7; P<.001) and 2.0 (95% confidence interval 1.0–4.0; P = .03), respectively. Lissalde-Lavigne and colleagues[57] performed a case-control study nested in a cohort of 32,683 women, and found that patients with FVL and PT gene mutation were more likely to have a pregnancy loss after 10 weeks' gestation. Contrary to other studies, Roque and colleagues[58] examined a cohort of 491 patients with a history of adverse pregnancy outcomes and evaluated the cohort for acquired and inherited thrombophilias. This study showed the presence of one maternal thrombophilia, or more than one thrombophilia were found to be protective of recurrent losses at less than10 weeks (1 thrombophilia: odds ratio 0.55, 95% confidence interval 0.33–0.92; >1 thrombophilia: odds ratio 0.48, 95% confidence interval 0.29–0.78). In contrast, the presence of maternal thrombophilia(s) was modestly associated with an increased risk of losses at greater than 10 weeks (1 thrombophilia: odds ratio 1.76, 95% confidence interval 1.05–2.94; >1 thrombophilia: odds ratio 1.66, 95% confidence interval 1.03–2.68).[58]

There is only one prospective trial that has studied patients with a history of unexplained pregnancy loss and known inherited thrombophilia. Patients were randomized to receive low-dose ASA or low molecular weight heparin (LMWH). There was a significantly higher number of live births in patients treated with LMWH versus low-dose ASA (odds ratio 15.5, 95% confidence interval 7–34; $P<.0001$).[59] Although this study was not blinded and had no placebo arm, it is the only one looking at possible treatment for history of fetal loss. This positive study can support the argument of testing patients with a history of fetal loss at greater than 10 weeks' gestation for inherited as well as acquired thrombophilias.

Severe Preeclampsia

The association of severe preeclampsia and thrombophilias is controversial. Branch and colleagues[60] performed an observational study and showed that 50% women with APLS developed preeclampsia despite treatment while 25% had severe preeclampsia.[31] A meta-analysis by Robertson and colleagues[42] showed the risk of preeclampsia was significantly associated with heterozygous FVL (odds ratio 2.19; 95% confidence interval 1.46–3.27), heterozygous PT (odds ratio 2.54; 95% confidence interval 1.52–4.23), MTHFR homozygosity (odds ratio 1.37; 95% confidence interval 1.07–1.76), anticardiolipin antibodies (odds ratio 2.73; 95% confidence interval 1.65–4.51), and hyperhomocysteinemia (odds ratio 3.49, 95% confidence interval 1.21–10.11). However, when restricting the analysis to severe preeclampsia only, an odds ratio of 2.04 (95% confidence interval 1.23–3.36) was obtained. Meta-analysis by Alfirevic and colleagues[54] showed that women with preeclampsia/eclampsia were more likely to have heterozygous FVL mutation, heterozygous G20210A PT gene mutation, homozygous MTHFR C677 T mutation, PC deficiency, PS deficiency, or aPC resistance than controls. Roque and colleagues[58] showed an increased risk of preeclampsia (odds ratio 3.21, 95% confidence interval 1.20–8.58) among patients with acquired and inherited thrombophilias.

INTRAUTERINE GROWTH RESTRICTION

IUGR is a term used to describe a fetus whose estimated weight appears to be less than the 10th percentile for gestational age. IUGR is associated with an increase in fetal and neonatal mortality and morbidity rates. Although as a specialty we are becoming more proficient in diagnosing IUGR prenatally, we still do not have the ability to prevent IUGR or its recurrence. IUGR has been shown to complicate pregnancies with inherited and acquired thrombophilias.

IUGR occurs in approximately one-third of patients diagnosed with APLS[60,61] despite treatment seen in retrospective studies. This risk may be higher in untreated pregnancies. Data from Yasuda and colleagues[62] showed a significant association with IUGR observed with anticardiolipin antibodies (odds ratio 6.91, 95% confidence interval 2.70–17.68). IUGR is most often seen in the presence of severe preeclampsia, therefore it is difficult to establish causality. Some prospective studies did not see an association. A prospective cohort study of 95 nulliparous women with elevated antiphospholipid (aPL) levels at their initial prenatal visit had an increase in fetal loss but no increase in low birth weight or IUGR.[63] Pattison and colleagues[64] found no increases in IUGR, but noted increases in preeclampsia in a small cohort of 22 women.

The association between inherited thrombophilias and IUGR has not been consistently demonstrated. A recent meta-analysis examining the relationship between

IUGR and FVL, PT gene mutation, and MTHFR was performed. This analysis showed that the only association seen was with FVL and MTHFR in case-control studies. Funnel plot analysis suggested the existence of publication bias, given the small number of negative studies.[65]

There are limited studies examining AT III, PC, and PS and their association with IUGR. Roque and colleagues[58] found PC to be associated with an increased risk of IUGR (odds ratio 12.93, 95% confidence interval 2.72–61.45). Alfirevic and colleagues[54] found that women with IUGR had a higher prevalence of heterozygous G20210A PT gene mutation, homozygous MTHFR C677 T gene mutation, PS deficiency, and aPL than controls.

Placental Abruption

Some studies have shown a possible association between abruption and thrombophilias. Roque and colleagues[58] reported a significant increase in the rate of abruption with thrombophilias (odds ratio 3.60, 95% confidence interval 1.43–9.09). Robertson and colleagues[42] showed thrombophilias to be associated with an increased risk of placental abruption, but significant associations were only observed with heterozygous FVL (odds ratio 4.70, 95% confidence interval 1.13–19.59) and heterozygous PT (odds ratio 7.71, 95% confidence interval 3.01–19.76). Alfirevic and colleagues[54] found that when compared with controls, placental abruption was more often associated with homozygous and heterozygous FVL mutation, heterozygous G20210A PT gene mutation, homocysteinemia, aPC resistance, or anticardiolipin IgG antibodies. Although there appears to be an association with both inherited and acquired thrombophilia, there are no prospective trials looking at this association and how to prevent recurrence.

THROMBOPHILIA TESTING

Patients that should be tested for inherited thrombophilias are those with a personal history of VTE, a first-degree relative with a diagnosed inherited thrombophilia, or a history of IUFD when all other causes have been excluded (**Table 2**). Based on recent literature, hyperhomocysteinemia in connection with MTHFR should not be tested for. The only inherited thrombophilias that should be tested for are FVL, PT gene mutation, AT, PC, and PS. Patients that have had adverse pregnancy outcomes such as early onset preeclampsia and IUGR requiring delivery before 34 weeks, IUFD greater than 10 weeks, and recurrent pregnancy loss (>3 losses at less than 10 weeks) should undergo APLS testing. The only adverse pregnancy outcome for which an

Table 2
Recommendations for thrombophilia testing

Thrombophilia	Indications for Testing
Inherited thrombophilia	Personal history of VTE Family history of a diagnosed inherited thrombophilia[a] IUFD (when all other causes have been excluded, severe IUGR, or severe placental pathology)
Acquired thrombophilia	Personal history of VTE Recurrent pregnancy loss (>3 losses at <10 wk) IUFD (>10 wk) Severe preeclampsia (requiring delivery <34 wk) Placental insufficiency/IUGR (requiring delivery <34 wk)

[a] Need for testing is controversial.

inherited thrombophilia panel should be sent is for a fetal loss at greater than 10 weeks. The American College of Obstetrics and Gynecology (ACOG) recommends testing for inherited thrombophilias after an IUFD in cases of severe placental pathology, severe IUGR, or a family or personal history of VTE.[66] The only inherited thrombophilias that can be adequately tested for in pregnancy are FVL and PT gene mutations. FVL and PT mutations are gene mutations and are not affected by pregnancy. Testing for APLS can also be performed during pregnancy. Thrombophilia screening should be postponed during pregnancy with a new diagnosis of VTE. Thrombophilia testing should be done outside of the current thrombotic event and current anticoagulation. Diagnosis of a thrombophilia will not change management in this setting of a current VTE.

THROMBOPROPHYLAXIS

Despite the increased risk of thrombosis in pregnancy secondary to a hypercoagulable state, not every woman with a thrombophilia needs to be anticoagulated. The clinician must make sure that the benefits of anticoagulation outweigh the risks. Maternal complications with heparin and LMWH can be as high as 2%.[67–69] If the decision is made to treat, anticoagulation with heparin or LMWH should be given throughout pregnancy and up to 6 weeks postpartum. Patients can be converted to warfarin postpartum.

The clinician must first look at whether the patient has a personal history of clot and if the thrombotic event was associated with a temporary risk factor. Temporary risk factors include pregnancy, trauma, and oral contraceptive (OCP) use, surgery, immobility, and chemotherapy. Brill-Edwards and colleagues[70] prospectively studied 125 women with history of a single episode of VTE. Eighty-four of these episodes were associated with a temporary risk factor and no known thrombophilia. Anticoagulation was withheld in the antepartum period, and started for 4 to 6 weeks postpartum. Of the 84 women with an initial episode of VTE associated with a temporary risk factor, there were only 2 recurrences. Because the risk of recurrence is so low in this clinical scenario, many would consider withholding prophylactic anticoagulation until post partum in this patient population. The American College of Chest Physicians (ACCP) recommends clinical antepartum surveillance and prophylactic anticoagulation postpartum in women with a single episode of VTE associated with a temporary risk factor and without a known thrombophilia. If the temporary risk factor is pregnancy, the ACCP recommends prophylactic anticoagulation during pregnancy and post partum.[71]

Treatment of women with APLS without a thrombotic event but with an adverse pregnancy outcome remains controversial. There have only been prospective trials looking at recurrent pregnancy loss and treatment with heparin plus ASA versus ASA alone. These studies show that treatment with ASA and heparin leads to a significantly higher rate of live births in women with recurrent pregnancy loss and APLS.[51,52] Further prospective studies need to be performed looking at treatment in patients with APLS associated with history of IUFD, early-onset preeclampsia, and uteroplacental insufficiency requiring delivery before 34 weeks. Most experts and the ACOG recommend prophylactic anticoagulation and ASA during pregnancy and 6 to 8 weeks postpartum.

Treatment of women with APLS with a history of a thrombosis is much less controversial. Most experts recommend therapeutic anticoagulation plus ASA during pregnancy and 6 to 8 weeks postpartum.

Treatment of women with a known thrombophilia without a thrombotic event is also controversial. At present there is no data to support treating these patients in pregnancy. A patient with a highly thrombogenic thrombophilia such as AT deficiency, PC, or PS may warrant therapeutic anticoagulation during pregnancy and post partum. Also patients who are homozygous for an FVL or PT gene mutation may benefit from prophylactic anticoagulation as well as compound heterozygotes for FVL and PT gene mutation; however, no data exist to support this treatment. Patients with a diagnosed inherited thrombophilia associated with IUFD may benefit from prophylactic anticoagulation.[59]

ACCP and ACOG recommend therapeutic anticoagulation in patients with history of VTE with AT III deficiency, FVL homozygous, PT gene mutation homozygous, and compound heterozygosity for FVL and PT gene mutation.[2,71] It is not clear whether patients with a history of thrombosis with PC or PS deficiency should be treated with prophylactic or therapeutic anticoagulation during pregnancy and post partum.[2]

SUMMARY

Thrombophilias have been associated with an increased risk of thrombosis and adverse pregnancy outcomes. All patients with a history of a thrombotic event should be tested for inherited and acquired thrombophilias. Given the high incidence of thrombophilia in the population and the low incidence of VTE, universal screening is not cost effective. There is some controversy regarding which patients should be screened for thrombophilias in the setting of adverse pregnancy outcomes. Women with thrombophilias appear to be at an increased risk for adverse pregnancy outcomes. With the exception of recurrent pregnancy loss in the setting of APLS, there is no clear evidence supporting that thromboprophylaxis during pregnancy improves outcome. Further randomized control trials are needed to assess the association of adverse pregnancy outcomes and whether thromboprophylaxis improves pregnancy outcome. Until it is shown that thromboprophylaxis prevents recurrent adverse pregnancy, pregnancy outcomes universal screening should not become the standard of care.

REFERENCES

1. Brenner B. Thrombophilia and adverse pregnancy outcome. Obstet Gynecol Clin North Am 2006;33(3):443–56, ix.
2. Barbour LA. ACOG educational bulletin. Thromboembolism in pregnancy. Number 234, March 1997. American College of Obstetricians and Gynecologists. Int J Gynaecol Obstet 1997;57(2):209–18.
3. Creasy RK, Resnik R, Iams JD. Creasy and Resnik's maternal-fetal medicine: principles and practice. 6th edition. Philadelphia: Saunders/Elsevier; 2009.
4. Hellgren M. Hemostasis during normal pregnancy and puerperium. Semin Thromb Hemost 2003;29(2):125–30.
5. Haemostasis and Thrombosis Task Force, British Committee for Standards in Haematology. Investigation and management of heritable thrombophilia. Br J Haematol 2001;114(3):512–28.
6. Marik PE, Plante LA. Venous thromboembolic disease and pregnancy. N Engl J Med 2008;359(19):2025–33.
7. Greer IA. Thrombosis in pregnancy: maternal and fetal issues. Lancet 1999; 353(9160):1258–65.
8. Rosendaal FR. Venous thrombosis: a multicausal disease. Lancet 1999; 353(9159):1167–73.
9. Lockwood CJ. Inherited thrombophilias in pregnant patients: detection and treatment paradigm. Obstet Gynecol 2002;99(2):333–41.

10. Gerhardt A, Scharf RE, Beckmann MW, et al. Prothrombin and factor V mutations in women with a history of thrombosis during pregnancy and the puerperium. N Engl J Med 2000;342(6):374–80.
11. Poort SR, Rosendaal FR, Reitsma PH, et al. A common genetic variation in the 3'-untranslated region of the prothrombin gene is associated with elevated plasma prothrombin levels and an increase in venous thrombosis. Blood 1996; 88(10):3698–703.
12. Kierkegaard A. Incidence and diagnosis of deep vein thrombosis associated with pregnancy. Acta Obstet Gynecol Scand 1983;62(3):239–43.
13. Girling J, de Swiet M. Inherited thrombophilia and pregnancy. Curr Opin Obstet Gynecol 1998;10(2):135–44.
14. Lane DA, Bayston T, Olds RJ, et al. Antithrombin mutation database: 2nd (1997) update. For the Plasma Coagulation Inhibitors Subcommittee of the Scientific and Standardization Committee of the International Society on Thrombosis and Haemostasis. Thromb Haemost 1997;77(1):197–211.
15. Frosst P, Blom HJ, Milos R, et al. A candidate genetic risk factor for vascular disease: a common mutation in methylenetetrahydrofolate reductase. Nat Genet 1995;10(1):111–3.
16. Morelli VM, Lourenco DM, D'Almeida V, et al. Hyperhomocysteinemia increases the risk of venous thrombosis independent of the C677 T mutation of the methyl-enetetrahydrofolate reductase gene in selected Brazilian patients. Blood Coagul Fibrinolysis 2002;13(3):271–5.
17. Miletich J, Sherman L, Broze G Jr. Absence of thrombosis in subjects with hetero-zygous protein C deficiency. N Engl J Med 1987;317(16):991–6.
18. Tait RC, Walker ID, Reitsma PH, et al. Prevalence of protein C deficiency in the healthy population. Thromb Haemost 1995;73(1):87–93.
19. Foster DC, Yoshitake S, Davie EW. The nucleotide sequence of the gene for human protein C. Proc Natl Acad Sci U S A 1985;82(14):4673–7.
20. Plutzky J, Hoskins JA, Long GL, et al. Evolution and organization of the human protein C gene. Proc Natl Acad Sci U S A 1986;83(3):546–50.
21. Clouse LH, Comp PC. The regulation of hemostasis: the protein C system. N Engl J Med 1986;314(20):1298–304.
22. Dykes AC, Walker ID, McMahon AD, et al. A study of protein S antigen levels in 3788 healthy volunteers: influence of age, sex and hormone use, and estimate for prevalence of deficiency state. Br J Haematol 2001;113(3):636–41.
23. Ploos van Amstel JK, van der Zanden AL, Bakker E, et al. Two genes homologous with human protein S cDNA are located on chromosome 3. Thromb Haemost 1987;58(4):982–7.
24. Schmidel DK, Tatro AV, Phelps LG, et al. Organization of the human protein S genes. Biochemistry 1990;29(34):7845–52.
25. Esmon CT. The protein C anticoagulant pathway. Arterioscler Thromb 1992;12(2): 135–45.
26. Schwarz HP, Fischer M, Hopmeier P, et al. Plasma protein S deficiency in familial thrombotic disease. Blood 1984;64(6):1297–300.
27. Broekmans AW, Bertina RM, Reinalda-Poot J, et al. Hereditary protein S defi-ciency and venous thrombo-embolism. A study in three Dutch families. Thromb Haemost 1985;53(2):273–7.
28. Holmes ZR, Bertina RM, Reitsma PH. Characterization of a large chromosomal deletion in the PROS1 gene of a patient with protein S deficiency type I using long PCR. Br J Haematol 1996;92(4):986–91.

29. Zoller B, Berntsdotter A, Garcia de Frutos P, et al. Resistance to activated protein C as an additional genetic risk factor in hereditary deficiency of protein S. Blood 1995;85(12):3518–23.

30. MacCallum PK, Cooper JA, Martin J, et al. Associations of protein C and protein S with serum lipid concentrations. Br J Haematol 1998;102(2):609–15.

31. Esplin SM. ACOG Practice Bulletin #68: antiphospholipid syndrome. Obstet Gynecol 2005;106(5 Pt 1):1113–21.

32. Miyakis S, Lockshin MD, Atsumi T, et al. International consensus statement on an update of the classification criteria for definite antiphospholipid syndrome (APS). J Thromb Haemost 2006;4(2):295–306.

33. Passam F, Krilis S. Laboratory tests for the Antiphospholipid syndrome: current concepts. Pathology 2004;36(2):129–38.

34. Roubey RA. Autoantibodies to phospholipid-binding plasma proteins: a new view of lupus anticoagulants and other "antiphospholipid" autoantibodies. Blood 1994; 84(9):2854–67.

35. Heit JA, Kobbervig CE, James AH, et al. Trends in the incidence of venous thromboembolism during pregnancy or postpartum: a 30-year population-based study. Ann Intern Med 2005;143(10):697–706.

36. James AH, Jamison MG, Brancazio LR, et al. Venous thromboembolism during pregnancy and the postpartum period: incidence, risk factors, and mortality. Am J Obstet Gynecol 2006;194(5):1311–5.

37. Eby C. Antiphospholipid syndrome review. Clin Lab Med 2009;29(2):305–19.

38. Cervera R, Piette JC, Font J, et al. Antiphospholipid syndrome: clinical and immunologic manifestations and patterns of disease expression in a cohort of 1,000 patients. Arthritis Rheum 2002;46(4):1019–27.

39. Silver RM, Draper ML, Scott JR, et al. Clinical consequences of antiphospholipid antibodies: an historic cohort study. Obstet Gynecol 1994;83(3):372–7.

40. Zotz RB, Gerhardt A, Scharf RE. Inherited thrombophilia and gestational venous thromboembolism. Best Pract Res Clin Haematol 2003;16(2):243–59.

41. Seligsohn U, Lubetsky A. Genetic susceptibility to venous thrombosis. N Engl J Med 2001;344(16):1222–31.

42. Robertson L, Wu O, Langhorne P, et al. Thrombophilia in pregnancy: a systematic review. Br J Haematol 2006;132(2):171–96.

43. Kang SS, Zhou J, Wong PW, et al. Intermediate homocysteinemia: a thermolabile variant of methylenetetrahydrofolate reductase. Am J Hum Genet 1988;43(4):414–21.

44. Den Heijer M, Lewington S, Clarke R. Homocysteine, MTHFR and risk of venous thrombosis: a meta-analysis of published epidemiological studies. J Thromb Haemost 2005;3(2):292–9.

45. McColl MD, Ellison J, Reid F, et al. Prothrombin 20210 G–>A, MTHFR C677 T mutations in women with venous thromboembolism associated with pregnancy. BJOG 2000;107(4):565–9.

46. Domagala TB, Adamek L, Nizankowska E, et al. Mutations C677 T and A1298C of the 5,10-methylenetetrahydrofolate reductase gene and fasting plasma homocysteine levels are not associated with the increased risk of venous thromboembolic disease. Blood Coagul Fibrinolysis 2002;13(5):423–31.

47. den Heijer M, Willems HP, Blom HJ, et al. Homocysteine lowering by B vitamins and the secondary prevention of deep vein thrombosis and pulmonary embolism: a randomized, placebo-controlled, double-blind trial. Blood 2007;109(1):139–44.

48. Friederich PW, Sanson BJ, Simioni P, et al. Frequency of pregnancy-related venous thromboembolism in anticoagulant factor-deficient women: implications for prophylaxis. Ann Intern Med 1996;125(12):955–60.

49. Vila P, Hernandez MC, Lopez-Fernandez MF, et al. Prevalence, follow-up and clinical significance of the anticardiolipin antibodies in normal subjects. Thromb Haemost 1994;72(2):209–13.
50. Oshiro BT, Silver RM, Scott JR, et al. Antiphospholipid antibodies and fetal death. Obstet Gynecol 1996;87(4):489–93.
51. Rai R, Cohen H, Dave M, et al. Randomised controlled trial of aspirin and aspirin plus heparin in pregnant women with recurrent miscarriage associated with phospholipid antibodies (or antiphospholipid antibodies). BMJ 1997; 314(7076):253–7.
52. Kutteh WH. Antiphospholipid antibody-associated recurrent pregnancy loss: treatment with heparin and low-dose aspirin is superior to low-dose aspirin alone. Am J Obstet Gynecol 1996;174(5):1584–9.
53. Farquharson RG, Quenby S, Greaves M. Antiphospholipid syndrome in pregnancy: a randomized, controlled trial of treatment. Obstet Gynecol 2002;100(3): 408–13.
54. Alfirevic Z, Roberts D, Martlew V. How strong is the association between maternal thrombophilia and adverse pregnancy outcome? A systematic review. Eur J Obstet Gynecol Reprod Biol 2002;101(1):6–14.
55. Rey E, Kahn SR, David M, et al. Thrombophilic disorders and fetal loss: a meta-analysis. Lancet 2003;361(9361):901–8.
56. Kovalevsky G, Gracia CR, Berlin JA, et al. Evaluation of the association between hereditary thrombophilias and recurrent pregnancy loss: a meta-analysis. Arch Intern Med 2004;164(5):558–63.
57. Lissalde-Lavigne G, Fabbro-Peray P, Cochery-Nouvellon E, et al. Factor V Leiden and prothrombin G20210A polymorphisms as risk factors for miscarriage during a first intended pregnancy: the matched case-control 'NOHA first' study. J Thromb Haemost 2005;3(10):2178–84.
58. Roque H, Paidas MJ, Funai EF, et al. Maternal thrombophilias are not associated with early pregnancy loss. Thromb Haemost 2004;91(2):290–5.
59. Gris JC, Mercier E, Quere I, et al. Low-molecular-weight heparin versus low-dose aspirin in women with one fetal loss and a constitutional thrombophilic disorder. Blood 2004;103(10):3695–9.
60. Branch DW, Silver RM, Blackwell JL, et al. Outcome of treated pregnancies in women with antiphospholipid syndrome: an update of the Utah experience. Obstet Gynecol 1992;80(4):614–20.
61. Lima F, Khamashta MA, Buchanan NM, et al. A study of sixty pregnancies in patients with the antiphospholipid syndrome. Clin Exp Rheumatol 1996;14(2): 131–6.
62. Yasuda M, Takakuwa K, Tokunaga A, et al. Prospective studies of the association between anticardiolipin antibody and outcome of pregnancy. Obstet Gynecol 1995;86(4 Pt 1):555–9.
63. Lynch A, Marlar R, Murphy J, et al. Antiphospholipid antibodies in predicting adverse pregnancy outcome. A prospective study. Ann Intern Med 1994; 120(6):470–5.
64. Pattison NS, Chamley LW, McKay EJ, et al. Antiphospholipid antibodies in pregnancy: prevalence and clinical associations. Br J Obstet Gynaecol 1993;100(10): 909–13.
65. Facco F, You W, Grobman W. Genetic thrombophilias and intrauterine growth restriction: a meta-analysis. Obstet Gynecol 2009;113(6):1206–16.
66. Fretts RC. ACOG Practice Bulletin No. 102: Management of stillbirth. Obstet Gynecol 2009;113(3):748–61.

67. James AH. Prevention and management of venous thromboembolism in pregnancy. Am J Med 2007;120(10 Suppl 2):S26–34.

68. Ginsberg JS, Kowalchuk G, Hirsh J, et al. Heparin therapy during pregnancy. Risks to the fetus and mother. Arch Intern Med 1989;149(10):2233–6.

69. Lepercq J, Conard J, Borel-Derlon A, et al. Venous thromboembolism during pregnancy: a retrospective study of enoxaparin safety in 624 pregnancies. BJOG 2001;108(11):1134–40.

70. Brill-Edwards P, Ginsberg JS, Gent M, et al. Safety of withholding heparin in pregnant women with a history of venous thromboembolism. Recurrence of Clot in This Pregnancy Study Group. N Engl J Med 2000;343(20):1439–44.

71. Bates SM, Greer IA, Pabinger I, et al. Venous thromboembolism, thrombophilia, antithrombotic therapy, and pregnancy: American College of Chest Physicians Evidence-Based Clinical Practice Guidelines (8th edition). Chest 2008;133(6 Suppl):844S–86.

Index

Note: Page numbers of article titles are in **boldface** type.

A

Abortion
    planned, gestational age at, first-trimester screening effects on, 607–608
    spontaneous
        in maternal serum abnormalities, 618
        in nuchal thickening, 614
Abruption, placental, in thrombophilia, 754
Achondrogenesis, in thickened nuchal translucency, 616
ADAM 12 glycoprotein, for preeclampsia screening, 736
Allele drop-out, in preimplantation genetic testing, 524–525
Alpha-fetoprotein
    for Down syndrome screening, 549–552, 566–569, 733
    for neural tube defect screening, **721–725**
American College of Medical Genetics, cystic fibrosis screening guidelines of, 536–538
American College of Obstetricians and Gynecologists screening guidelines
    cystic fibrosis, 536–538
    first-trimester, 605–606
American Society for Reproductive Medicine, preimplantation testing guidelines of, 527
Amniocentesis
    cost-effectiveness analysis of, 634
    counseling for, 644–645
    for cytomegalovirus testing, 715–716
    for multiple pregnancies, 646–648
    for toxoplasmosis, 711
    rate of, first-trimester screening effects on, 606–607
Amnionicity, of twin pregnancies, 574
Analytic framework, in cost-effectiveness analysis, 631–632
Anemia, in parvovirus infections, 713–714
Anencephaly, screening for, 721–725
Aneuploidy. *See also* Down syndrome.
    screening for, in multiple pregnancies, 645–646
Angiogenic factors, for preeclampsia screening, 737–738
Anticardiolipin antibodies, 750
Anticoagulants, for thrombophilias, 755–756
Antiphospholipid antibody syndrome, 749–753
Antithrombin deficiency, thrombosis tendency in, 748–749, 754
Aspirin, for thrombophilias, 755
Avidity test
    for cytomegalovirus, 715
    for toxoplasmosis, 710

Clin Lab Med 30 (2010) 761–773
doi:10.1016/S0272-2712(10)00107-1
0272-2712/10/$ – see front matter © 2010 Elsevier Inc. All rights reserved.

Moving?

Make sure your subscription moves with you!

To notify us of your new address, find your **Clinics Account Number** (located on your mailing label above your name), and contact customer service at:

Email: journalscustomerservice-usa@elsevier.com

800-654-2452 (subscribers in the U.S. & Canada)
314-447-8871 (subscribers outside of the U.S. & Canada)

Fax number: 314-447-8029

Elsevier Health Sciences Division
Subscription Customer Service
3251 Riverport Lane
Maryland Heights, MO 63043

*To ensure uninterrupted delivery of your subscription, please notify us at least 4 weeks in advance of move.

ELSEVIER

Printed and bound by CPI Group (UK) Ltd, Croydon, CR0 4YY

03/10/2024

01040459-0008